RADIATION
THERAPY
PLANNING

RADIATION THERAPY PLANNING

Including Problems And Solutions

GUNILLA C. BENTEL
Duke University Medical Center
Durham, North Carolina

McGRAW-HILL, INC.
Health Professions Division
New York St. Louis San Francisco Auckland Bogotá Caracas Lisbon
London Madrid Mexico Milan Montreal New Delhi Paris San Juan
Singapore Sydney Tokyo Toronto

234567890   VBA VBA   98765432

ISBN 0-07-105382-4

Library of Congress Cataloging-in-Publication Data

Bentel, Gunilla Carleson.
      Radiation therapy planning / Gunilla C. Bentel.
            p.   cm.
      Includes bibliographical references and index.
      ISBN 0-07-105382-4 (softcover)
      1. Cancer–Radiotherapy–Problems, exercises, etc.   2. Radiation–
Dosage–Problems, exercises, etc.
      [DNLM: 1. Neoplasms–radiotherapy.   2. Radiometry.
3. Radiotherapy Dosage.   QZ 269 B475r]
      RC271.R3B45   1991
      616.99′40642–dc20
      DNLM/DLC
      for Library of Congress   91-21034
                                                     CIP
                                                     r91

DEDICATION

Our lives are often touched by many people with whom we work and interact on a regular basis. We often spend more time with our co-workers than we do with our own family members and it is easy to develop a sense of family even at work. When a family member - or a co-worker, is suddenly not there anymore, we feel a tremendous emptiness, a sense of helplessness.

During the development of this text, two of my co-workers were suddenly gone, and so, I would like to dedicate this book to their memory and in recognition of their contributions to radiation oncology:

To Alisa Butler, R.T.T. who worked in our department for almost 12 years. She was devoted to her job as chief technologist, and was very much involved with the continuing education of other technologists in North Carolina. She died in a car accident on a rain-slick highway just before Christmas 1990. Alisa contributed to this manuscript by taking the photograph in Fig. 6.1. Her happy smile and good cooking will long be remembered.

To Lucille P. Harris, L.P.N. who was very devoted to her job as an advanced L.P.N. and who was very active in many professional organizations in North Carolina. She died suddenly of heart failure during the final week of preparation of this manuscript, and only three months after Alisa. Lucille was associated with our department for 14 of the 29 years she worked at Duke University. Her cheerfulness and good humor will be remembered for many years.

We are often affected by the loss of patients, particularly the younger ones, but the loss of these two young long-time associates within only a three-month time-frame has had a profound effect on the sense of family among the remaining staff. We have also quickly learned to put matters into perspective and to value the bad as well as the good times.

TABLE OF CONTENTS

PREFACE

The technology of radiation oncology treatment planning and dose calculation is developing rapidly and is now very complex. The growth has brought with it an increased demand for a text which will better prepare the student for this new technology. The need for a practical guide, written primarily for technologists, dosimetrists, and the radiation physics student, has been met with the publication of my previous book (with Drs. Nelson and Noell) <u>Treatment Planning and Dose Calculation in Radiation Oncology</u>.

The present manuscript has been developed to complement the previous work and gives a more in-depth description of both external beam and brachytherapy dose calculations. The two books are closely related and as a result, the earlier book is frequently referred to in this text. There is of necessity some overlap, for example, in the definition of terms. This overlap eliminates the need to switch from one book to the other while solving the problems.

This new book gives the reader a brief but often forgotten historical perspective of radiation oncology. One chapter describes some of the most commonly used treatment machines and a large section describes methods of calculating dose in a patient at practically any point and under many different circumstances, for example, on and away from the central axis, at the isocenter and at other depths, in an irregular field, under a block, and when using moving-beam treatments. One chapter is dedicated to brachytherapy dose calculations, and, in another very large chapter, the practical application of brachytherapy techniques is described. Two chapters focus on solutions to some of the not-so-common treatment problems in radiation oncology. Each chapter is followed by questions and answers relating to the problems discussed in the text.

There is no textbook available today, including these two books, that will adequately cover <u>all</u> of the knowledge required to solve all treatment planning and dose calculation problems encountered in radiation oncology. The student is therefore encouraged to seek out other text books to gain the understanding of anatomy, physics, and biology which may be needed.

ACKNOWLEDGEMENTS

The development of this book would not have been possible without the advice and many helpful suggestions by colleagues and friends in Radiation Oncology and Physics at Duke University Medical Center. Maturation of this lengthy project has required many hours of my time away from clinical responsibilities and I appreciate everyone's effort in carrying on the clinical work during my absence. I truly value my association with Duke University and the staff from whom I have gained much of the clinical philosophy needed for this work.

I am particularly indebted to Dr. Fearghus O'Foghludha, Professor Emeritus, for his invaluable suggestions and editing skills, and to Dr. Edward Halperin for his helpful suggestions. Special thanks to Ran and Becky Whitehead and their family who helped early on with typing and editing.

As modern technology brings us new tools with which to accomplish our goals, some unfortunate problems sometimes come along which we cannot control. Many of the illustrations in this book were drawn by the author with the help of a computer and while all of the diagrams looked very nice prior to being brought into the text, many now appear as if they were drawn by a nervous hand. Unfortunately, this problem was discovered too late for corrective action, and it is hoped that the reader will be tolerant of this mishap.

DISCLAIMER

Great care has been taken to maintain the accuracy of the information contained in this volume. Treatment plans and dose calculations described in the text are suggested methods only and no responsibility is accepted for their wrongful application. Consideration must be given to a particular patient's contour or target volume, and to the beam data particular to the individual treatment machine.

All radiation doses stated assume fractionation at 180 to 200 cGy per day in a continuous course of 5 fractions per week, unless otherwise indicated.

ABBREVIATIONS

Al...............aluminum
avg.............average
Au..............gold
BSF............Backscatter Factor
Bq..............becquerel
Ca Cl$_2$.........calcium chloride
Ca F$_2$.........calcium fluoride
cGy.............centigray
cGy/min....centigray per minute
cGy/MU.....centigray per Monitor Unit
Ci...............curie
cm..............centimeter
cm^3 ....cubic centimeter
Co ....cobalt
Cs..............cesium
CT.............Computed Tomography
Cu ....copper
D................depth
D$_{max}$..........maximum dose
d$_{max}$...........depth of maximum dose
eq. sq........equivalent square
fs...............field size
f$_{tis}$ ....roentgen to centigray in tissue
g................gram
Gy ....Gray
hr..............hour
HVL...........Half-Value Layer
HVT ....Half-Value Thickness
I ....iodine
ICRU.........International Commission on Radiation Units
ISF.............Inverse Square Factor
keV ....kilo electron volt

kVp............peak kilovoltage
LiF.............lithium fluoride
mCi ....millicurie
mm............millimeter
MeV..........million electron volt
mg hr.........milligram hour
mg Ra eq....milligram radium equivalent
MRI ....Magnetic Resonance Imaging
M.U. ....Monitor Unit
MV............million volt
Na Cl ....sodium chloride
OAR...........Off-Axis Ratio
P ....phosphorus
Pb..............lead
Pt..............platinum
R................roentgen
Ra..............radium
ref..............reference
Rn..............radon
SAD...........Source-Axis Distance
SAR...........Scatter-Air Ratio
sec ....seconds
SMR ....Scatter-Maximum Ratio
Sn..............tin
Sr..............strontium
SSD...........Source-Surface Distance
T$_{avg}$ ....average life
TAR...........Tissue-Air Ratio
TLD ....Thermoluminescent Dosimeters
TMR..........Tissue-Maximum Ratio
TPR...........Tissue-Phantom Ratio
X$_r$...............exposure rate
Yt...............yttrium
%DD..........percentage depth dose

CHAPTER 1

HISTORICAL PERSPECTIVE OF RADIATION THERAPY

THE DISCOVERY OF ROENTGEN RAYS AND RADIOACTIVITY

On Friday, November 8, 1895, while passing an electric current through a Hittorf-Crookes high-vacuum tube, Wilhelm Conrad Röntgen* noticed a light coming from a workbench about a yard away. He identified the shining object as a piece of paper painted with barium platinocyanide. He realized that this light must be caused by a new kind of ray, which he called x-rays and which later became known as roentgen rays. He continued the investigation of these rays and found that when he replaced the fluorescent screen with a photographic plate, he could obtain pictures. The most dramatic picture was one showing the bones in his wife's hand, which was taken on December 22, only 6 weeks following the discovery of the invisible rays. Density variations, depending on the tissues in the path of the rays, were observed, and the value of such radiographic images in the diagnosis of human ailments immediately became evident.

On December 28, 1895, Röntgen delivered a written presentation of his discovery to the Physical-Medical Society of Würzburg. Within a few weeks, this Preliminary Communication entitled *On a new kind of rays* was translated into many languages. On New Year's Day 1896, he mailed copies of his paper along with some radiographs to several European physicists whom he knew. The news of the discovery spread very quickly and was soon known all over the world.

---

* Usually written Roentgen in the English language literature.

1

Only a few weeks after Röntgen's discovery, Henri Becquerel began investigating the possibility of similar rays being produced by known fluorescent or phosphorescent substances. He observed the darkening of photographic plates (Chapter 3) by uranium salts and realized that these rays were emitted spontaneously and continuously from the uranium; thus, radioactivity was discovered.

Marie Curie, who at this time was studying minerals in Paris, became interested in the phenomena of radioactivity and chose this subject for her doctoral thesis. Pierre Curie eventually joined his wife in her research, and in July 1898, they discovered polonium, and in December of the same year, they reported the discovery of radium.

Both Becquerel and Pierre Curie experienced erythema on the skin of the chest from carrying small samples of radium in their vest pockets. Pierre Curie applied radium to his arm and described in detail the various phases of a moist epidermitis and his recovery from it. He also provided radium to physicians, who tested it on patients.

The news of these discoveries spread quickly, and having learned that redness of the skin was observed by the users of these rays, several physicians began investigating their effect on malignant tumors; thus, the use of ionizing radiation in the treatment of cancer began.

THERAPEUTIC USES OF X-RAYS AND RADIOACTIVITY

More than any other innovation, the ability to painlessly visualize the interior of the living human body has governed the practice of medicine during the twentieth century. The radiotherapeutic application of these discoveries also had a profound effect on cancer survival rates. This chapter will focus on the therapeutic uses of x-rays and radioactivity.

The discovery of x-rays and radioactivity was promptly followed by their therapeutic application. The first therapeutic use of x-rays is reported to have taken place on January 29, 1896, when a patient with carcinoma of the breast was treated, and by 1899, the first cancer, a basal cell epithelioma, had been cured by radiation.

The initial dramatic responses observed in the treatment of skin and other superficial tumors generated the hope that a cure for cancer had finally been found. This hope was soon followed by a wave of disillusionment and pessimism when tumor recurrences and injuries to normal tissues began to appear. The treatments often involved single massive exposures aimed at eradication of tumors, and the patients who survived the immediate postirradiation period often developed major complications. Because of these disappointing results, the use of x-rays to treat tumors would soon have been abandoned had it not been for laboratory and clinical work by Claude Regaud and Henri Coutard. They found that by administering fractionated doses of radiation, that is, smaller daily doses rather than a large single dose, they could achieve the same tumor response but without serious injury to the adjacent normal tissues.

From the early experience, it was evident that the unique advantage of radium was in intracavitary and interstitial applications. Here, where the radioactivity was placed directly on or inside the tumor, the radiation did not first have to traverse normal tissue; the short distance and rapid fall-off of dose offered an advantage in this setting. Initially, containers were rather bulky and could be used only for intracavitary gynecologic implants. In 1914, methods were developed for collecting radon (a daughter product of radium) in small glass tubes, which were then placed inside hollow metal seeds, and like radium needles, these could be inserted directly into the tumors. Radium needles and radon seeds were very popular for many years but have more recently been replaced by safer, artificially produced isotopes.

Many of the physical facts of radium were discovered early. The skin burns suffered by Becquerel and Curie served as a warning to other users. The value of filtration and the importance of distance from the source to the treated tissue were soon recognized by the many chemists, physicists, and medical specialists who worked together in the treatment of patients.

Initially, the only countries where radium could be obtained were France and Austria. Later, it was also discovered in Colorado, and in 1911, radium was purified from the Colorado ore. To reduce and purify 1 gram of radium it was necessary to use 500 tons of ore, 10,000 tons of distilled water, 1,000 tons of coal, and 500 tons of chemicals. A gram of radium sold for $120,000.

The first use of radium (imported from Europe) in the United States was around 1908. The radium tubes were primarily used in the treatment of gynecologic malignancies, whereas radium solutions were used to treat arthritis and gout. The latter use was discontinued after a few years.

The clinical pioneers in radiation therapy, mostly surgeons and dermatologists, used the "erythema dose," or radiation dose necessary to cause redness of the skin, to estimate the proper length of the treatments.

It was recognized early that accurate dosimetry was fundamental to success in any type of radiation treatment. In radium therapy this comprised three parts: the accurate measurement of the radium content of the various sources, the determination of the radiation output of each source in terms of an acceptable dose unit, and a knowledge of the distribution of radiation within the tissues under treatment.

Until 1911, there was no satisfactory method to standardize radium. Madame Curie then began to prepare an accurate standard of carefully weighed quantities of pure radium salt. The standard was deposited with the International Bureau of Weights and Measures, at Sèvres near Paris, and continues to serve as the standard for radioactivity.

Madame Curie's standard, developed in 1911, was used for determining the amount of the radioactivity in each source. Output measurements in terms of radiation exposure were very complicated, but following tedious work by many investigators, it was determined that a point source of radium, filtered by 0.5 mm of platinum, delivers what later became known as 8.25 roentgen per hour at 1 cm from the source.

As for the distribution of the sources within the tissues, a dosage system that is still used in many hospitals was begun in 1932 and published in 1939 by Ralston Paterson and Herbert Parker at Christie Hospital in Manchester, England. Their dosage system was developed on the theory that non-uniform spacing of the radioactivity within the the the tissue could result in a relatively uniform dose distribution. In 1941, Edith Quimby, first at Memorial Hospital and later at the College of Physicians and Surgeons in New York, published a dosage system in which the sources were arranged in a uniform pattern and the resulting dose distribution was non-uniform.

Several other systems for radium distribution (Chapter 8) were worked out both in the U.S. and in Europe. The Manchester (Paterson and Parker), Paris, and Stockholm techniques are the most notable and are more or less followed by other institutions.

MEASUREMENTS OF QUALITY AND QUANTITY OF RADIATION BEAMS

During the early years of radiology, the methods of measuring the *quality* (or penetrating power) and the *quantity* of x-ray beams were unsatisfactory. Direct measurements of radiation quality were made by means of a "penetrometer" which was introduced by Benoist in 1901. This instrument consisted of a thin silver disk surrounded by a ring of aluminum wedges arranged like a stair with 12 steps of increasing thicknesses. The aluminum step that matched the silver disk in absorption was fluoroscopically or photographically determined and was used to represent the radiation quality in designated units (Glasser 1956).

Also at the beginning of the century, Holzknecht described a "chromoradiometer," an instrument to measure quantity of dose. It consisted of small disks of a fused mixture of potassium chloride and sodium carbonate. These compounds became discolored when irradiated with x-rays. Holzknecht called the dose producing a minimal degree of discoloration "$_1$H." Doses high enough to produce a skin erythema would be of the order of "$_3$H" (Glasser 1956).

Another device, a "radiometer," was developed in 1904 to measure quantity of dose. This device was used for many years, primarily by dermatologists. A method of measuring dose in calories was also used at the beginning of the century. These methods were unsatisfactory, and during the subsequent 50 years, many efforts were made to develop accurate and reliable methods to determine the amount of dose. From 1914 to 1925, a number of physicists worked on the determination of a unit of dose and built various types of instruments, most notably a primary standard ionization chamber for the determination of the dose unit and a secondary instrument to measure dose on the patient (Glasser 1956).

In 1928, H. Geiger and W. Mueller constructed an improved detector tube based on a counter built as early as 1906. In various modified forms, both of these instruments were used well into the 1960s (Glasser 1956).

Antoine Béclère in Paris, Gösta Forssell in Stockholm, J. J. Thomson in Liverpool, and George Pfahler in Boston were some of the pioneers who laid the groundwork of radiation therapy. They, and many other dedicated scientists, soon recognized the need for an internationally accepted unit of dose and a method by which to define the quality of the rays. In 1913, the term "half-value layer" or HVL (a term now replaced, as in this text, by half-value thickness, or HVT) was suggested as a measure of quality. It was not until 1928 that the roentgen as a unit of measurement for x-rays and gamma rays was internationally accepted, and in 1953, the International Commission on Radiological Units recommended the rad as the unit of absorbed dose. The rad has more recently been replaced by the centigray (cGy).

TECHNICAL DEVELOPMENTS

TECHNICAL DEVELOPMENTS: 1920 - 1940

The equipment used in the treatment of malignant disease during the first years of radiation therapy was primitive, temperamental, and had very low penetrating power. The use of x-rays was limited by the low kilovoltage available, but as the applicability of roentgen rays expanded, the demand for better equipment increased. During the 1920s, Coolidge invented a vacuum x-ray tube capable of operating at peak kilovoltages (kVp) of 200 to 250. With such machines, more deep-seated tumors could be treated without excessive injury to the overlying skin.

Figure 1.1, copied from Albert Bachem's textbook *Principles of X-ray and Radium Dosage*, depicts the use of water bags as compensators, indicating an understanding of isodose distributions and the composition of tissue-equivalent materials prior to 1920 (Bachem 1923). Improved treatment techniques where multiple beams were aimed at the tumor from different directions (Fig. 1.2), the so-called "crossfire" techniques, were also used. Other advances during this era were improved design and reliability of treatment machines.

Much had been learned about the need for filtration of the radiation produced by these machines. The concept of the inverse square law, scattering, and the effect of treatment distance on the percentage depth dose (%DD) were also understood. The treatment times for external beam treatment were expressed in erythema time factors, whereas the standard

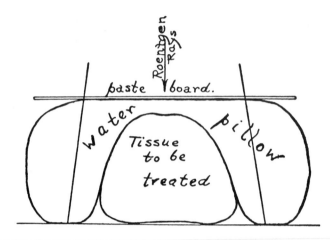

Fig. 1.1. The use of water bags as tissue-equivalent material in this illustration, first published in 1923, indicates an early understanding of isodose distributions and the need for compensators.

Fig. 1.2. A multiple-beam arrangement in the treatment of breast cancer was used early in the history of radiation therapy as depicted in this illustration from Albert Bachem's textbook published in 1923.

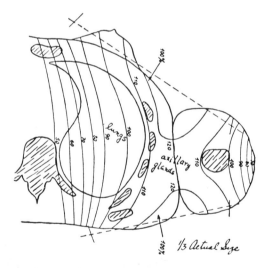

measure of erythema dose in radium treatment consisted of 100 milligram hours or mg hr (Bachem 1923). The erythema dose as a measure of how much dose to deliver was replaced during this era by the first physical unit, the roentgen.

The discovery of artificial radioactivity in 1934 had a profound impact on the future of brachytherapy, however the use of radium continued for many years. It was not until World War II that neutron reactors, which are capable of producing artificial radionuclides in large quantities, were developed; isotopes for medical use were thereafter produced on a large scale.

The combination of external beam treatment with intracavitary radium was used during this time period and elaborate systems for calculating the combined dose were devised.

TECHNICAL DEVELOPMENTS: 1940 - 1960

As cure rates improved and the complication rate declined, radiation therapists were encouraged and looked for even higher energy machines producing better dose distributions. The first use of "supervoltage" radiation therapy equipment, then considered to be anything operating at greater than 1 million volts (MV), was in 1937 at St. Bartholomew's Hospital in London. The clinical experience with this machine clearly showed the advantages of high energy beams. Several investigators (Ising 1924, Wideröe 1928, van de Graaff 1933) described different methods of accelerating particles, and following this initial work, betatrons and linear accelerators for medical use emerged. Machines using reactor-produced cobalt-60 sources became available at about the same time (Chapter 2).

In addition to the improved percentage depth dose with higher energy beams, a skin-sparing effect was gained because the high energy beams deposit the maximum dose at some depth under the skin surface. This skin-sparing effect allowed delivery of high doses even to deep-seated tumors without causing significant skin erythema. Another advantage of the high energy beams was the more forward direction of radiation scattering and the sharper edges (penumbra) of the radiation beam. As physical improvements of the beam were made, along with advances in design and versatility of the treatment machines, and as simulators became available, the doors opened on a new era in radiation therapy.

Instruments capable of mapping the isodose distribution in phantoms were developed. A better understanding of the need to concentrate the radiation dose in the tumor while minimizing the dose to the adjacent normal tissues followed. The need for wedges to produce the desired dose distribution was recognized and a renewed interest in tissue compensators emerged. Treatment planning computers began to appear on the horizon, and the developments that followed have been overwhelming in terms of treatment techniques and equipment.

During this era, radium continued to be the primary source for temporary intracavitary and interstitial therapy. Radon, encapsulated in gold seeds, was used for permanent interstitial implants. Radon seeds were primarily inserted during surgery in deep-seated pelvic or abdominal tumors where subsequent removal of the radioactivity was impractical. Gynecologic intracavitary implants continued to be the primary use of radium.

TECHNICAL DEVELOPMENTS: 1960 - PRESENT

Modern developments in electronics and computers have led to an unbelievable bonanza of equipment to diagnose and treat patients with cancer, to visualize the relationship of the tumor to normal organs, to align and position the patient, and to measure and calculate dose.

Significant improvements have been made in the design and versatility of treatment machines, simulators, treatment-planning computers, and dose measuring and mapping instruments. The development and use of computed tomography (CT) and magnetic resonance imaging (MRI) to define the target volume and to map the patient's external contour, as well as internal organs and target volumes, have had an unprecedented impact on radiation therapy. The use of CT images as an aid in calculating the effect of tissue inhomogeneities has improved the accuracy by which the dose can be calculated. The precision with which radiation therapy can be delivered has been greatly improved and may have an impact on cancer cure rates. As a result of the ability to better localize and treat the target and thus reduce the radiation dose to adjacent normal tissue, the need for improved positioning and immobilization techniques became evident (*Treatment Planning and Dose Calculation in Radiation Oncology*, Bentel 1989*).

The collimators of radiation therapy machines have traditionally been built to produce only square or rectangular field shapes, and other field shapes have had to be formed by the tedious and not very precise addition of lead blocks placed on a tray in the path of the beam. Through the development of customized shielding blocks, the reproducibility of the treatment field design and the sparing of adjacent normal tissue has been greatly improved.

Some modern treatment machines are equipped with multileaf collimators. These multileaf collimators, described on page 38, consist of a large number of individually controlled leaves which can be moved into the beam to the desired extent, thus forming the needed field shape.

In the treatment of cylinder-shaped targets, a rotation or arc technique is well suited. However, in the treatment of irregularly shaped targets, where the shape of the target in the "beam's-eye view" constantly changes as the machine moves around the patient, the need for "conformal" therapy was

---

*   Previously published companion book frequently referred to throughout this text.

recognized. The development of the multileaf collimator, where the shape of the field can be changed to match the shape of the target, has led to very elaborate treatment techniques. Computers can be programmed to drive the leaves of the collimator so that the radiation field always matches the shape of the target as the gantry moves around the patient (Fig. 1.3). This type of conformal therapy, where the field shape and the beam angle change simultaneously, requires very powerful computer systems.

Another less frequently used treatment technique was developed in the early 1960s and consisted of gravity-oriented shielding blocks. The gravity-oriented shield hangs from the collimator within the beam such that it always shadows the desired organ (spinal cord, eye, etc.). The shield is formed to the shape of the organ to be shadowed. As the gantry moves, the gravity-oriented shield will always retain the same position and shape with respect to the organ it is shadowing; thus, the organ is shielded regardless of beam direction. See Chapter 7 of *Treatment Planning and Dose Calculation in Radiation Oncology*.

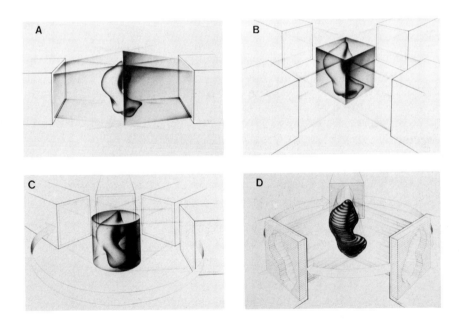

Fig. 1.3. Parallel opposed fields used to treat an irregularly shaped target also deliver high dose to a large volume of normal tissue (A). The volume of normal tissue within the high-dose area can be reduced by the use of a four-field technique (B). A rotational technique will further decrease the volume of normal tissue within the high-dose area (C). By using a conformal therapy technique, the high-dose area can be confined almost exclusively to the target (D). (Courtesy Dr. Alan Lichter, University of Michigan.)

Powerful treatment planning computers, capable of three-dimensional dose calculations, represent a major contribution to radiation therapy. Traditionally, isodose lines were represented by solid lines indicating a particular dose level. In the modern graphical representation, each isodose level is represented by a color for easier visualization. Internal organs can also be color coded for easier recognition when viewed in different planes.

Three-dimensional renditions of CT or MRI images give an improved appreciation of the region at hand. Outlining normal organs and the tumor volume permit a beam's eye view of the intended fields with respect to the tumor and the normal anatomy (Fig. 1.4). Field size and beam angle can be changed in real time until the desired placement is obtained.

Along with the improved techniques by which radiation therapy can be delivered came the need for radiographic imaging of treatment fields. Comparison of radiographs taken on the simulation unit and with the treatment beam to verify reproducibility before and at intervals during the course of treatment is common practice. Systems are currently being used by which the treatment field can be viewed in real time on a video monitor at the treatment console. Misalignments can be discovered and corrected when only a fraction of a particular treatment has been delivered.

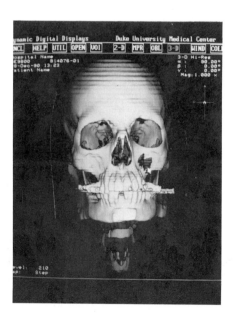 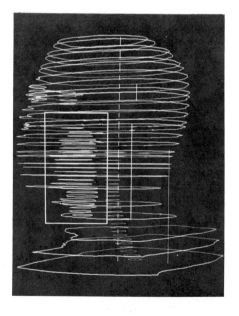

Fig. 1.4. (Left) Three-dimensional rendition of a patient's head showing bone destruction by a left maxillary sinus tumor. (Right) External contours, spinal cord, eyes, and a tumor outlined on several CT images of another patient; a rectangular field, angled to include the tumor without including the spinal cord is shown.

Machines required to generate fast neutrons, pi-mesons, and heavy ions for use in radiation therapy are very complex and expensive. Their use is therefore limited to only a few institutions around the world.

Along with the tremendous popularity of using artificially developed isotopes came the development of afterloading techniques in brachytherapy. Radium fell out of favor and was largely replaced when other less hazardous radioactive materials became available. Cobalt-60 and cesium-137 replaced radium in intracavitary gynecologic applications because they have characteristics somewhat similar to radium, and ribbons carrying radioactive seeds replaced radium needles. The most popular isotope for this use is iridium-192. These ribbons, in addition to being safer than radium, also have the advantage that they can be afterloaded through plastic tubes inserted interstitially.

The development of afterloading techniques was a major step in reducing the exposure to a large number of staff. The benefit of inserting empty intracavitary and interstitial source carriers in the operating room was not limited to the reduced exposure of staff; by freeing staff from the pressure of working quickly in order to reduce exposure, it also led to better placement. Radiographic verification of the placement and, often of the dose calculation prior to inserting the radioactive sources yielded better dose distributions.

More recently, *remote* afterloading equipment for brachytherapy has been developed (page 317, Chapter 9). These devices allow afterloading and removal of radioactive sources from the patient via remote control; thus, the exposure to staff is practically eliminated. The sources are removed and deposited in a shielded safe while, for example, nursing care is provided to the patient. After the staff leaves the room, the sources are again loaded into the patient via a pneumatic tube, and treatment is resumed.

Prior to the introduction of treatment planning computers in radiation therapy, dose calculations were very tedious and time-consuming. Generally, the dose was calculated only at certain points in the vicinity of the implant using standard dose tables developed by early investigators, most notably Paterson and Parker during the 1930s and Quimby during the 1940s. With the use of computers, isodose distributions can quickly be calculated and evaluated, often prior to the insertion of the radioactive sources. Source strengths can thus be selected to yield an acceptable dose distribution.

The diminished use of radium created a need for safe disposal of these highly radioactive sources with a half-life of about 1600 years. Sources that were bought at great expense many years ago are now without value and, because they are still extremely hazardous, can only be disposed of at great expense, if at all.

The benefits of combining external beam treatment with brachytherapy have been known for many years; however, research is still being conducted to improve dose-delivery sequencing. Hyperthermia is a promising new modality which has been added to both external beam and brachytherapy treatments. Quite promising results have been obtained, and research over the next several years is likely to lead to a better understanding of this new treatment modality.

RADIOBIOLOGY

A historical survey of radiation therapy is not complete without some mention of the evolution of radiobiology, although no attempt is made in this text to present a complete history.

The following paragraphs from *Principles of X-ray and Radium Dosage* by Albert Bachem, published in 1923, serve as an example of the understanding of radiobiology held 70 years ago.

"Since tissue congested with blood is more sensitive to radiation, the suggestion has been made to treat the region to be rayed beforehand by diathermy. The congestion produced in this way is supposed to make the tissues more sensitive."

"The cells of the body are most radio-sensitive at the instant of their division. Hence one method which promises to be successful is to distribute the raying over such a period that all the cells go through a division during this time. Of course, the correct exposure time would be different for various tumors depending on their rapidity of growth."

"....Roentgen sickness may be due to three causes; 1) poisonous gases in the treatment room, 2) electrostatic charges influencing the cells of the body, and 3) direct poisoning of some organ due to excessive dosage, particularly in the treatment of the stomach, liver, pancreas and suprarenals.

To avoid roentgen sickness the following must be observed: 1) the production of ozone must be reduced to a minimum; this is best accomplished by installing the rectifier, the spark gap, and the tube in a separate room (couch, cylinder). The treatment room must be well ventilated. A large lead covered tube box with a blower to draw off the air is ideal. 2) Holfelder advises grounding of the patient. If precautions are taken to avoid accidental electric shock, the grounding of the patient is not dangerous and may be beneficial. In the case of the couch, the window and the tube box methods of treatment, it is not necessary. 3) The region rayed should not be too large; a well planned treatment avoids unnecessary exposure. The symptoms may also be mitigated by administering calcium chloride or by injecting it into the veins previous to the treatment. Voltz found a decrease in the chloride contents of the blood after intensive radiation. Pape accordingly increased the chlorine content of the blood by means of 200 cc of physiological NaCl (sodium chloride) and $CaCl_2$ (calcium chloride) solution and avoided roentgen sickness in many cases."

During the first three decades of this century, radiobiologists and radiotherapists worked closely together in an effort to understand the intricate phenomena of the biological effects caused by ionizing radiation.

During the 1920s and 1930s, protracted fractionation methods were formulated and the relative radiosensitivity of different tissues was studied primarily by Claude Regaud and Henri Coutard in France. With the beginning of fractionated radiation therapy, many new biological questions were raised and as improved cancer cure rates were experienced, radiobiologists explored the significance of repair, recovery, reoxygenation, redistribution, and repopulation (Hall 1988).

Adverse effects on normal tissue and radiation sickness necessitated fractionation of the dose, and it was found that higher doses could then be delivered. Careful evaluation of the results of such treatment, along with better understanding of the characteristics of the rays, led to the development of different time-dose fractionation schemes. Much of the current clinical application of radiation therapy has evolved from similar experiments and further refinements in fractionation schedules continue today.

Recognition of the typical patterns of spread of malignancies occurring in various types of tissues and in various sites and the adaptation of treatment strategies for each disease have required many years of dedicated work by many radiation therapists. Collecting data and sharing it with colleagues has led to the development of a foundation on which modern clinical radiation oncology is built. Similarly, careful recording and evaluation of complications and results have yielded a large base on which radiation tolerance and dose requirements for tumor eradication are built.

RADIATION PROTECTION

As early as March of 1896, an x-ray pioneer, Thomas Edison, reported eye irritation and cautioned against the use of x-rays. His laboratory assistant, Clarence M. Dally, developed acute x-ray dermatitis and died later as a result of overexposure. Henri Becquerel and Pierre Curie sustained acute dermatitis on the skin of the chest after carrying small amounts of radium in their vest pockets. The small grains of radium looked totally harmless, and it was only through these events that the injurious effects were first observed. The invisible x-rays were also thought of as being harmless (it was the practice, during the early days, to test the "hardness," or the penetrating power, of the rays by placing the hand of the operator between the tube and the fluorescent screen) until the injuries begun to appear.

Protracted exposure to x-rays was found to cause pain, swelling, redness, and often also blistering. By the end of 1896, numerous reports had been published about x-ray dermatitis and burns. The delayed effect of x-rays caused much of the injuries to occur before the dangers were evident; thus, many of the pioneers sustained radiation injuries. Several cases of radiation-induced cancer were reported during the first 10 years following the discovery of x-rays and radioactivity. There is strong evidence that Madame Curie's long exposure to radium contributed to her illness and death. The early investigators often handled radium directly with their hands, and as a result, many of these workers experienced damage to their fingers, including degeneration in some cases.

The need for protective measures was eventually acknowledged, and the use of x-rays was thereafter limited to physicians' offices. During the ensuing years, much effort was put into improving the equipment and techniques to reduce the radiation exposure.

The recognition, as early as 1900, of increased distance, short exposure time, and the use of shielding as measures to help reduce the incidence of radiation injuries led to the development of shielded storage safes and long-handled tools for handling radium. It is interesting to note that the initial development of radiation protection was aimed at protecting the radium itself, a valuable and expensive commodity, rather than protecting human beings from the radium.

Early on, the practice of what was later to be known as radiology was carried out by electricians, photographers, as well as by physicians. In 1899, a newspaper reporter recommended state licensing for radiographers following a lawsuit in which the courts awarded a $10,000 damage judgement on the behalf of a plaintiff who allegedly suffered an injury from improper application of diagnostic x-rays.

During the 1920s, methods of measuring dose were developed and quantitative measurements of radiation exposure were introduced. The use of film badges was recommended during the 1920s, and during the 1930s, portable survey meters and ionization chambers became standard equipment in most hospitals.

The difference in biological effectiveness of different radiations was recognized and stated in tolerance doses. Tolerance doses gave way to the concept of maximum permissible dose. The whole body maximum permissible exposure, which was set at 30 roentgen (R) per year in 1936, has been reduced a number of times since then and is now 5 rem per year (the unit rem is the sum of the products of the absorbed dose in rad and the quality factor for each radiation producing the exposure). The quality factor was introduced because the biological effectiveness of one radiation may be different from that of another. The rem is the quantity of any radiation which will produce the same biological effect as 1 cGy of cobalt-60 gamma rays, for which the quality factor is 1.0. The change in units to include the quality factor was made necessary by the more complex radiological environment present after the development of nuclear weapons in the 1940s.

The radiation protection practiced prior to World War II was aimed at protecting the operator of the radiation producing equipment, while following the war, radiation protection measures also considered the patient. The importance of radiation protection was generally not recognized until the early 1950s, when the long-term biological effects of exposure to small, fractionated doses of radiation over long periods was appreciated. A large proportion of the world's population was exposed to low levels of radiation when the testing of nuclear weapons began and thus, the biological damage became a matter of concern.

Medical radiation protection has become very complex with the use of sophisticated diagnostic and therapeutic equipment but the basic principles understood at an early stage still apply. The modern era has also brought further increases in regulatory control such as mandatory licensing of radionuclides and radiation sources, educational requirements for the operator of radiation machines, and the institution of radiation protection programs based on ALARA (As Low As Reasonably Achievable). ALARA is based on the concept that the radiation exposure should *always* be minimal and all reasonable precautions should be exercised even when the exposure is well below the permissible levels.

THE LIFE OF OUR PIONEERS

The following short descriptions of some of the pioneers in radiation therapy are extracted from a series of articles entitled "Our History and Heritage," written by Dr. Juan A. del Regato, himself a pioneer of radiation therapy in the United States.

WILHELM CONRAD RÖNTGEN

Wilhelm Conrad Röntgen was born on March 27, 1845 in Lennep, Germany. His family later moved to Holland, and Röntgen attended primary school there. At age 17, he registered at a private technical school in Utrecht from which he eventually was expelled because he refused to reveal the name of the artist who drew a disrespectful caricature of one of the teachers on the blackboard and was therefore considered an accomplice (del Regato 1975).

Röntgen learned that the Zürich Polytechnikum accepted students without the traditional credentials. He was admitted and eventually received a Ph.D. from the University of Würzburg, the university where he discovered the invisible rays 25 years later. He left the University of Würzburg in 1872, but he returned in 1888 as Chairman of Physics and as Director of the Physikalische Institut.

Röntgen was very interested in experimental research and, because of his increased academic responsibilities, he worked at night in his laboratory. He focussed his attention on cathode rays which had been shown to produce fluorescence, and this led him to discover x-rays.

Many honors were bestowed upon Röntgen during the ensuing years, the highest being the first Nobel Prize for Physics. He refused all suggestions that he profit by his discovery. For example, he turned over the Nobel cash prize to the University of Würzburg. Röntgen died on February 10, 1923, from cancer. His ashes are buried in Alte Friedhof in Giessen, Germany.

MARIE SKLODOWSKA CURIE

Marie Sklodowska was born on November 7, 1867, in Warsaw. She finished school at age 16. Under Tzarist domination, women were denied higher education, so she tried to obtain education through clandestine organizations. In 1885, one of her sisters decided to study medicine in Paris. Marie took various jobs to help and support her sister, thinking that later on she might need help herself. After a couple of disappointing jobs, she decided to move to Paris (del Regato 1976).

After two years of hard work, she finished first in her class at the Sorbonne, and then went back to Poland to visit her father. When she returned to Paris, she began to study the magnetic properties of various minerals. During this time, she met Professor Pierre Curie, the Chief of the Laboratories at the Industrial School of Physics and Chemistry. She obtained a master's degree in mathematical sciences and returned to Poland again to visit her father. She returned to Paris and married Pierre in 1895. In December, 1898, they discovered radium.

In 1903, Madame Curie presented her thesis at the Sorbonne and obtained her doctor's degree. Shortly thereafter, she prematurely delivered a baby girl, who died shortly afterwards. Later the same year, the Swedish Academy of Science announced that the Nobel Prize for Physics had been awarded to Henri Becquerel and to Marie and Pierre Curie. Marie was later (1911) to receive the Nobel Prize in Chemistry also. Twenty-four years later, the Curies' daughter, Irene, and her husband, Frederic Joliot, received the Nobel Prize in Chemistry for the discovery of artificial radioactivity, an unparalleled accomplishment by this scientific family.

Pierre Curie died on April 19, 1906, when he was run over by a horse-drawn wagon as he tried to cross a street in Paris. Marie was promoted to the chair left vacant by her husband. She had dreamed of a special research institution devoted to the study of radioactivity and its medical applications. In 1911, her dream became a reality with the establishment of the Institut de Radium under the auspices of the Pasteur Institute and the University of Paris. It was at the Radium Institute that the pioneers of radiobiology, Henri Coutard, Antoine Lacassagne, Octave Monod, and others, through years of dedicated work, established the foundations of modern clinical radiotherapy.

Marie Curie died in Paris on July 6, 1934, of complications resulting from long exposure to radiation.

ANTOINE BÉCLÈRE

Antoine Béclère was born on March 17, 1856, in Paris. A physician with a keen interest in experimental medicine, he became intrigued with Röntgen's discovery and he eventually became one of the world's leading personalities in the unfolding of the medical applications of radium (del Regato 1978).

His first experiments were in the use of roentgen rays for diagnostic purposes, but he soon became interested in the therapeutic potential of these invisible rays as well. He obtained the necessary equipment for his office and began the practice of "Radiology," a word which he coined. His first roentgen tube relied on a hand-cranked electrical generator, but he later used a battery-operated tube.

As was the custom then, the radiologists would check the performance of the roentgen ray tube by testing the ability to see the bones of their own hand (del Regato 1978). Béclère soon recognized the adverse effects on the skin of his own hands and many of his colleagues suffered similar injuries. He therefore advocated measures to protect physicians and patients. He also insisted that the roentgen rays be kept under the control of physicians and not be entrusted to photographers and other laymen.

Béclère developed an increasing interest in radiation therapy and obtained some radium soon after its discovery. He treated some patients using radium and though the radiations had somewhat different depth doses, etc., he observed effects similar to those of roentgen rays.

During the 1920s, Béclère became interested in using roentgen rays in the treatment of deep-seated tumors. For this, he insisted on careful dosimetry and urged the appointment of a Commission on Measurements and Units to establish a common dose unit in radiation therapy to be adopted around the world.

Béclère also foresaw the need for dose fractionation and the necessity of combining external roentgen therapy and intracavitary "Curie therapy" in the treatment of gynecologic malignancies.

Having laid much of the groundwork in radiology, Antoine Béclère died unexpectedly of a heart attack on February 24, 1939.

SOME IMPORTANT MILESTONES IN THE HISTORY OF RADIATION THERAPY

The following is extracted from *Physical Foundations of Radiology* (4th ed.) by Goodwin, Quimby, and Morgan and represents an abbreviated list of achievements by many scientists who have laid the basis of radiation therapy (Goodwin 1970).

1895 -   (November 8) - Wilhelm Conrad Röntgen discovered the invisible rays, which he subsequently called x-rays.

1896 -   (January) - The first x-ray treatment of a cancer patient was delivered.

         Antoine Henri Becquerel discovered radioactivity.

1897 -   Joseph John Thomson announced the finding of negatively charged particles which he called electrons.

         Ernest Rutherford found two types of radiations from uranium which he called alpha and beta rays.

1898 -   (December) - Marie and Pierre Curie discovered radium.

         P. von Villard discovered gamma rays and found them to be similar to x-rays.

1901 -   Röntgen was awarded the first Nobel Prize in Physics for his discovery of x-rays.

1902 -   Guido Holzknecht presented his chromoradiometer, a device built to measure the quantity of radiation administered.

1903 -   Becquerel was awarded a Nobel Prize in Physics for the discovery of radioactivity.

         Marie and Pierre Curie were awarded a Nobel Prize in Physics for their work on radioactivity.

1906 -   H. Geiger and Ernest Rutherford developed an instrument to count alpha particles. With the assistance of W. Mueller, this device was later improved to detect and count other types of radiation.

1908 -   P. von Villard proposed a unit of dose based on ionization of air by x-rays.

1913 -   The half-value layer was suggested as a term for the expression of the quality of roentgen rays.

1922 -   Arthur Holly Compton discovered the change in wavelength of scattered x-rays, the "Compton effect."

1925 -   H. Fricke and Otto Glasser developed the thimble ionization chamber.

1928 -   The Commission on Measures and Units proposed the roentgen as an international unit of dose.

Geiger and Mueller developed an improved Geiger-counter tube on the basis of the Geiger-Rutherford point counter built in 1906.

Glasser, Portmann and Seitz built the condenser dosimeter for the measurement of x-rays and radiations from radioactive substances. This type of dosimeter has subsequently become known as the Victoreen condenser R-meter.

1932 - E. O. Lawrence invented the cyclotron.

Lauriston S. Taylor developed a standard air-ionization chamber to determine the value of the roentgen.

1933 - R. J. van de Graaff built electrostatic generators capable of producing up to 12 million volts.

1934 - Frederic Joliot and his wife, Irene Joliot-Curie (Marie and Pierre Curie's daughter), produced artificial radioactivity by bombarding aluminum with alpha particles.

1937 - The Fifth International Congress of Radiology (Chicago) accepted the roentgen as an international dosage unit for x-rays and gamma radiation.

1939 - The treatment of cancer patients with a neutron beam from a cyclotron was begun.

1940 - Kerst constructed the betatron with which electrons were accelerated to energies of 20 million electron-volts and later to 300 million electron-volts.

1951 - The first cobalt-60 teletherapy units were used in radiation therapy (Saskatoon, Saskatchewan, and London, Ontario, Canada).

1952 - The first electron linear accelerator designed for radiotherapy was installed (Hammersmith Hospital, London, England).

1953 - The Seventh International Congress of Radiology (Copenhagen, Denmark) adopted the rad as a unit of absorbed dose of any ionizing radiation.

1960s - Treatment planning computers were developed.

1971 - Geoffrey N. Hounsfield invented computerized tomography.

REFERENCES

Bachem, A., Principles of x-ray and radium dosage, Albert Bachem, Chicago, IL, 1923.

Bentel, G.C., Nelson, C.E., Noell, K.T., Treatment Planning and Dose Calculation in Radiation Oncology, Pergamon Press, Inc. Elmsford, NY, 1989.

Del Regato, J.A., Our history and heritage. Wilhelm Conrad Röntgen, Int. J. Radiat. Oncol. Biol. Phys. 1, 133 (1975).

Del Regato, J.A., Our history and heritage. Marie Sklodowska Curie, Int. J. Radiat. Oncol. Biol. Phys. 1, 345 (1976).

Del Regato, J.A., Our history and heritage. Antoine Béclère, Int. J. Radiat. Oncol. Biol. Phys. 4, 1069 (1978).

Glasser, O., Technical development of Radiology. Am. J. Roentgenol. Radium Ther. Nucl. Med. 75, 7 (1956).

Goodwin, P.N., Quimby, E.H., Morgan, R.H., Physical Foundations of Radiology (4th ed.), Harper & Row, New York, NY, 1970.

Hall, E. J., Radiobiology for the Radiologist (3rd ed), J.B. Lippincott Company, Philadelphia, PA, 1988.

Ising, G., Principle of method for production of canal rays at high voltages. Arch. för Matematik, Astronomi och Fysik 18, 1 (1924).

Van de Graaff, R.J., Compton, K.T., Van Atta, C.L., Electrostatic production of high voltages for nuclear investigators, Phys. Rev. 43, 149 (1933).

Wideröe, R., Über ein neues Prinzip zur Herstellung hoher Spannungen, Arch. Elektrotech. 21, 387 (1928).

PROBLEMS

1. X-rays were discovered by

    a) Henri Coutard
    b) Wilhelm Conrad Röntgen
    c) Henri Becquerel
    d) Marie Curie

2. Radioactivity was discovered by

    a) Wilhem Conrad Röntgen
    b) Henri Coutard
    c) Pierre Curie
    d) Henri Becquerel

3. Radium was discovered by

    a) Wilhelm Conrad Röntgen and Henri Becquerel
    b) Pierre and Marie Curie
    c) Henri Coutard and Claude Regaud

4. The erythema dose

    a) was the dose which was found to cure all cancer
    b) was the only measure of dose by which the early pioneer could estimate the necessary length of the treatments
    c) was the highest dose which could be given without causing complications

5. That one could achieve the same tumor response with less injury to normal tissue by fractionating the dose was discovered by

    a) Henri Coutard and Claude Regaud
    b) Pierre and Marie Curie
    c) Wilhelm Conrad Röntgen and Henri Becquerel

6. The Manchester system of radium distribution was developed by

    a) Edith Quimby
    b) Wilhelm Conrad Röntgen and Henri Becquerel
    c) Ralston Paterson and Herbert Parker

7. The "penetrometer" to measure quality of x-rays was introduced by

    a) Benoist
    b) Holzknecht
    c) J.J. Thomson

8. The roentgen was internationally accepted as a unit of measurement for x-rays and gamma rays in

    a) 1953
    b) 1936
    c) 1928

9. The rad as a unit of absorbed dose was recommended by ICRU in

    a) 1936
    b) 1953
    c) 1928

10. Artificial radioacitivity was discovered in

    a) 1936
    b) 1953
    c) 1934
    d) 1928

11. Artificial radioactivity was discovered by

    a) Irene Curie and Frederic Joliot
    b) Pierre and Marie Curie
    c) Ralston Paterson and Herbert Parker

12. Which of the following statements is *not* true:

    a) Becquerel was awarded a Nobel Prize in Physics for the discovery of radioactivity;
    b) Röntgen was awarded the first Nobel Prize in Physics;
    c) Marie and Pierre Curie were awarded a Nobel Prize in Physics for their work on radioactivity;
    d) Holzknecht was awarded the Nobel Prize for his work on a "radiometer."

SOLUTIONS

1. b

2. d

3. b

4. b

5. a

6. c

7. a

8. c

9. b

10. c

11. a

12. d

CHAPTER 2

EXTERNAL-BEAM RADIATION THERAPY EQUIPMENT

Prior to 1950, nearly all external beam radiation therapy was carried out using x-rays generated at voltages up to approximately 300 kVp. Following the development of cobalt-60 (Co) machines in the early 1950s, this type of treatment machine remained the most popular source of radiation for radiotherapy for many years. High energy betatrons were introduced at approximately the same time as Co-60 machines, but their popularity has diminished in recent years and both are now largely replaced by high energy linear accelerators. Other machines, which are impractical and economically not feasible for installation in the average radiation therapy department, are cyclotrons and gigantic linear accelerators producing intense beams of neutrons, protons, mesons, and other particles useful in the treatment of malignant tumors (Catterall 1975, 1976, Chen 1979, von Essen 1985, Saunders 1985). This text is intended as a brief overview of the most commonly used equipment only.

SUPERFICIAL MACHINES

Radiation therapy units operating in the approximate range of 50 to 120 kVp, are referred to as superficial machines. The penetrating ability of x-rays produced at this low kVp is very poor. Addition of filters, typically aluminum (Al), of variable thickness, removes the very soft non-penetrating x-rays and thus hardens the beam. The degree of hardening, or beam quality, depends on the energy at which the beam is generated and on the filter thickness and is expressed as the half-value thickness (HVT). The HVT, which is also discussed in Chapter 3 (page 55), is defined as the thickness of a specified material which, when introduced into the path of the beam, reduces the intensity of the beam to half of its original value. Typical HVTs in the superficial range are 1.0 to 8.0 mm Al.

The custom of expressing the *quality* of a beam in terms of HVT of tin (Sn), Copper (Cu), and aluminum (Al) is not to be confused with the filters just described and consisting of the same materials.

Superficial beams, as one can deduce from the name, are used in the treatment of superficial lesions. Treatment fields are often defined by a cone which is attached to the head of the machine near the focal point and with the distal end placed directly on the skin surface. Alternatively, lead shielding can be placed directly on the patient's skin to shield areas surrounding the lesion. Treatment distances are usually in the range of 15 to 20 cm to decrease depth dose. The dose rate is fairly high in superficial treatments due to the short treatment distance. The backscatter (page 66, Chapter 3) is relatively high at these low energies and increases rapidly with increased field size. The maximum dose is on the surface and falls off very rapidly with depth, due to the low energy and short source-surface distance (SSD).

ORTHOVOLTAGE MACHINES

X-ray machines operating in the range of 150 to 500 kVp are referred to as orthovoltage units. Filters used to harden the beam in these units consist of Cu and sometimes Sn in addition to Al. The Al is placed distal to the Cu in the path of the beam to remove soft secondary radiation produced when the beam strikes the Cu. Copper, on the other hand, is added distal to the Sn filter in the path of the beam to remove soft secondary radiation produced when the beam interacts with the Sn filter. Various combinations of filters have been designed to achieve HVTs of up to 4 mm Cu in the orthovoltage energy range.

Orthovoltage equipment usually operates at SSDs of 50 to 70 cm and can be used with or without a cone. Movable lead shields in the head of some of these machines can be used to define the size of square and rectangular radiation fields but, as with superficial beams, additional beam-defining lead shields can be placed directly on the patient. Quite small thicknesses of lead are needed to reduce the dose by 95% in this energy range; the actual thickness depends on the voltage.

The penetrating capability of orthovoltage beams is better than that of superficial beams; thus, the fall-off of dose with depth is less rapid. In a typical orthovoltage beam, the maximum dose occurs at, or very close to, the skin surface, falling to about 90% at approximately 2 cm of depth. A single field would thus not adequately treat a lesion at a greater depth without delivering prohibitive dose to the overlying skin.

The backscatter is quite large in the orthovoltage range and, as with superficial beams, increases with increased field size. Dose rates from orthovoltage units are relatively low due to the fairly long SSD and also due to the heavy filtration of the beam.

BETATRONS

The betatron, developed by Kerst in 1941, is a machine in which electrons are accelerated in a circular orbit via a changing magnetic field (Kerst 1941, 1943). The electrons can be extracted from this orbit to produce an electron beam used for radiation therapy or can be directed to hit a target inside the machine to produce an x-ray beam.

Betatrons were first used for radiation therapy during the 1950s but are now largely replaced by linear accelerators. Low dose rates and very limited field sizes have primarily led to the decline of new betatron installations. Most betatrons are physically very large and require tremendously large treatment rooms. Due to their size, they also have very limited motions, compromising beam direction and flexibility of patient setup.

LINEAR ACCELERATORS

The first linear accelerator was developed by Wideröe in 1928 to accelerate heavy ions (Wideröe 1928). Electron linear accelerators were first developed during the late 1940s and early 1950s by Fry (Fry 1947, 1948), Ginzton (Ginzton 1948), and by Chodorow (Chodorow 1955). Various types of modern linear accelerator designs are available. Linear accelerators use high-frequency electromagnetic waves to accelerate charged particles, such as electrons, to high energies through a linear tube. These electrons, as in the betatron, can be extracted from the unit and used for treatment of shallow lesions or can be directed to strike a target to produce high-energy x-rays used for treatment of deep-seated tumors.

Figure 2.1 shows a typical medical linear accelerator and treatment couch and Fig. 2.2 shows a diagram of the major accelerator components. A power supply provides power to the modulator. High-voltage pulses from the modulator are delivered to the magnetron or the klystron and simultaneously to the electron gun. A wave-guide system injects pulsed microwaves from the magnetron or the klystron into the accelerator tube. At precisely the right instant, electrons produced by the electron gun are injected into the accelerator structure. The accelerator structure consists of a copper tube divided by multiple discs of varying diameter and spacing, which is evacuated to a high vacuum. The electrons, injected at an energy of about 50 kilo electron volt (keV), interact with the electromagnetic field of the microwaves and gain energy from the electric field by an acceleration process analogous to that of a surf rider. The spacing between the discs in the wave guide is narrower near the site where the electrons are injected and gradually increases down the guide; this causes the electromagnetic radiation (and the electrons carried along by it) to speed up as it travels along the guide.

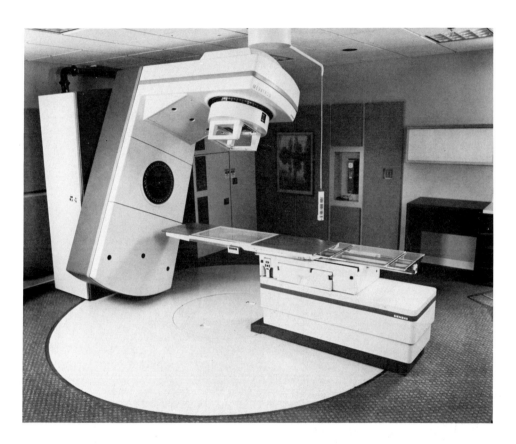

Fig. 2.1. Isocentrically mounted medical linear accelerator and treatment couch. See also Fig. 2.6. (Courtesy Siemens Medical Systems, Inc.)

In lower energy machines, as the high-energy electrons emerge from the accelerator structure window, they are allowed to proceed straight on and strike a target, thus producing x-rays. In higher energy machines, where the accelerator structure is too long and therefore may have to be placed at an angle, the electrons are bent at an appropriate angle (typically 90° or 270°) before striking the target. This is accomplished via a beam transport system consisting of bending magnets, focusing coils, and other components. When the linear accelerator is in the electron mode, the target and the flattening filter are moved aside and the electrons emerge without striking either, but striking instead a scattering foil. The very narrow electron beam (about 3 mm in diameter) is spread by the scattering foil, which also causes a fairly uniform electron distribution across the beam.

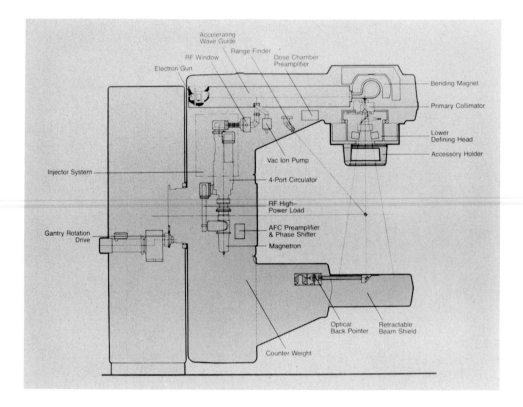

Fig. 2.2. Cutaway view of a medical linear accelerator. See also Fig. 2.6. (Courtesy Siemens Medical Systems, Inc.)

Since electrons scatter readily in air, the beam collimation must extend as close as possible to the skin surface of the patient. Electron cones of variable sizes attached to the collimator and extending to the patient's skin surface are therefore used to collimate electron beams (Fig. 2.3). Secondary beam shaping can be accomplished by adding lead cutouts at the end of a cone. Due to electron scattering, the dose distribution in electron fields depends strongly on the collimation system and must be determined for each individual setup. The x-ray beam, both in high- and in low-energy machines, is defined by a primary collimating system and is intercepted by a flattening filter and multiple ion chambers before exiting the head of the machine through a secondary collimator consisting of movable leaves (Fig. 2.4).

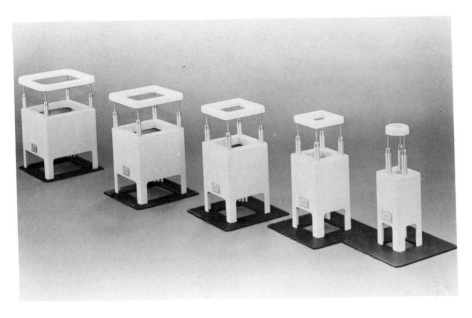

Fig. 2.3. Typical electron cones. (Courtesy Siemens Medical Systems, Inc.)

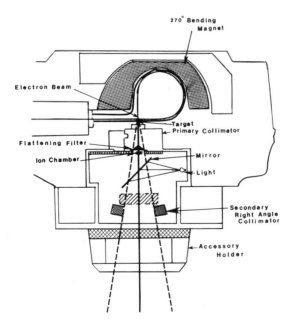

Fig. 2.4. Cutaway view of the head of a typical medical linear accelerator.

The flattening filter is placed in the x-ray beam to reduce the intensity of the forward peaked dose in the center of the field. Flattening filters, usually made of lead, are shaped to produce dose uniformity across the radiation field at a specified depth. Flattening filters made of other materials such as tungsten and uranium are also used. A typical flattening filter is shown in Fig. 2.1 in *Treatment Planning and Dose Calculation in Radiation Oncology* (Bentel 1989).

A dose monitoring system, consisting of several ion chambers or alternatively a single chamber with multiple plates, is built into the path of the beam. This system monitors the dose rate, integrated dose, and the beam symmetry.

A light, projected via mirrors in the head of the machine, is arranged to be congruent with the radiation field and is used in the alignment of the radiation beam and the treatment field marked on the patient's skin surface. Frequent checks of the congruency of the light field and the radiation beam are necessary to ensure continuous treatment field alignment.

Another light, projected from some point outside the collimator, casts a scale indicating the treatment distance. The scale is mounted such that the distance from the target is indicated when the scale intersects the central axis of the beam (Fig. 2.5).

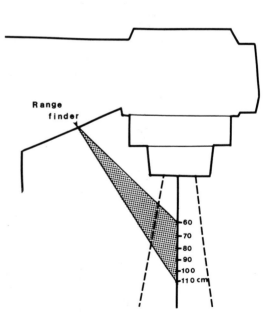

Fig. 2.5. A distance scale, projected by a range finder, indicates the treatment distance at the central axis of the beam.

A typical linear accelerator installation is shown in Fig. 2.6. For further details on linear accelerators the reader is directed to a review article by Karzmark (Karzmark 1973) and to other literature (Sable 1970, Johns 1983, Khan 1984).

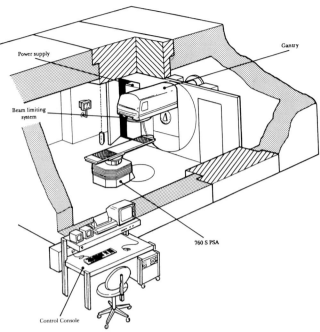

Fig. 2.6. A typical linear accelerator installation. (Courtesy General Electric Company.)

MACHINES USING ISOTOPES

Prior to 1951, machines for external beam irradiation (teletherapy[*]) using an isotope were made for use with radium. The prohibitive cost, the "self-filtration" caused by the front layer of the source filtering out radiation from the back portion of the large radium source, and the low dose rates are some of the reasons teleradium units never gained much popularity.

The development of very strong sources of cobalt-60 in Canada in 1951 led to the introduction of cobalt-60 units for teletherapy (Johns 1952). Figure 2.7 shows a diagram of a typical cobalt-60 machine and treatment couch. The cobalt-60 source usually consists of a double-encapsulated cylinder filled with discs or pellets of the isotope (Fig. 2.8). The double steel capsule, which is sealed by welding, is necessary to prevent escape of radioactive material. The Co-60 source typically has the shape of a cylinder with a diameter of from 1 to 1.5 cm. The circular end of the cylinder faces the collimator opening from which the radiation escapes when the machine is in the "on" position.

---

[*] Teletherapy refers to treatments in which the source of radiation is at some distance from the patient. In brachytherapy, on the other hand, the source is very close to the treated tissue (in molds) or may even be embedded in it (nterstitial).

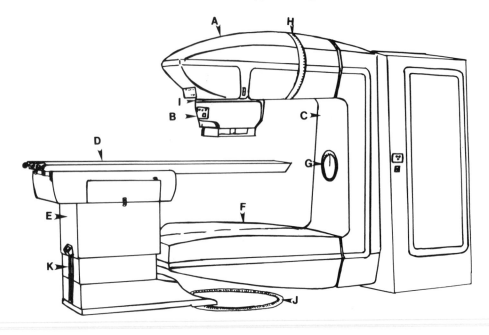

Fig. 2.7. Diagram of a typical cobalt-60 machine and treatment couch.

A = Source head   G = Gantry scale
B = Collimator   H = Head swivel scale
C = Gantry   I = Collimator scale
D = Couch top (stretcher)   J = Couch rotation scale
E = Treatment couch   K = Vertical couch scale
F = Beam stopper (optional)

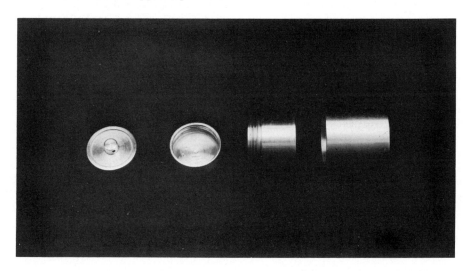

Fig. 2.8. Cobalt-60 source capsule. The circular end of the double encapsulated cylinder, which faces the opening, is typically 1 to 1.5 cm in diameter.

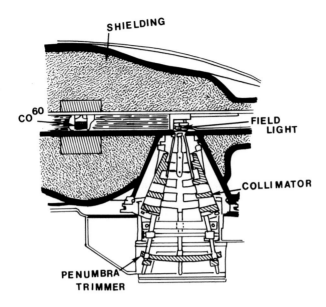

Fig. 2.9. Diagram of the head of a typical cobalt-60 machine.

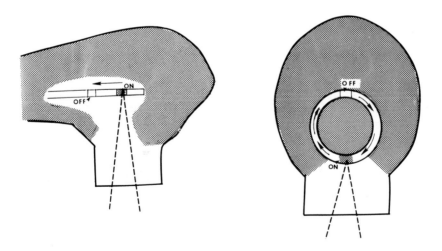

Fig. 2.10. Diagram showing two typical arrangements for "on" and "off" positions for a cobalt-60 source; a sliding drawer mechanism to move the source (left), and a wheel to carry the source from the shielded "off" position to its "on" position at the collimator port (right).

Unlike linear accelerators or other electrically operated machines, the cobalt-60 source emits radiation constantly; thus, the source must be shielded when the machine is in the "off" position to protect personnel.

Isotope machines consist of a lead-filled container in which the radioactive source is placed near the center (Fig. 2.9). An opening is provided for the radiation beam to exit when the machine is in the "on" position. Various types of mechanisms exist for bringing the source into a position opposite this opening. In one arrangement, the source is mounted on a wheel, itself a good radiation shield, which can be rotated 180° to carry the source between the "on" and "off" positions (Fig. 2.10). In another arrangement, the source is mounted in a drawer and the source slides horizontally between the "on" and "off" positions. Should the power fail while the source is in the "on" position, the source will automatically move to the "off" position via a fail-safe system.

All isotope machines must be equipped with this fail-safe mechanism because, unlike accelerators, these machines are very quiet in their operation and the operator has no audible warning that the source is in the "on" position.

COBALT-60 MACHINES

Cobalt-60, which is further discussed in Chapter 8 (page 224), emits two photons per disintegration (1.17 and 1.33 MeV), which are useful in radiation therapy. It decays with time and has a half-life of 5.26 years. The half-life is the time required for an isotope to decay to half of its original strength (page 223, Chapter 8). The dose rate is therefore constantly decreasing and an adjustment of treatment times must be made periodically. In the case of cobalt-60, this is typically once a month.

Due to the large size of a cobalt source, the penumbra, or unsharp edge of the beam, is larger than in the beam from a linear accelerator which has a very small focal point. The penumbra, which is further discussed in Chapter 3 and in *Treatment Planning and Dose Calculation in Radiation Oncology*, can be reduced by allowing the beam collimating tunnel to extend further along the path of the beam. This, however, reduces the clearance between the collimator and the patient, a serious disadvantage in isocentrically mounted units. Penumbra can of course be reduced by use of a small source, but when the source is small, the activity, and hence the dose rate, are reduced. Using very high specific activity cobalt, that is, high activity per cm^3, will help overcome this problem.

CESIUM-137 MACHINES

Another teletherapy isotope machine, first described in 1956, is the cesium-137 unit (Brucer 1956). Very few cesium machines are still in use. The source head and the mechanism for moving the source to "on" and "off" positions are similar to that of the cobalt machine. The radiation intensity from a cesium source compared with a cobalt source of equal physical size is relatively low, and sources of sufficient activity to produce a reasonable beam intensity at a long treatment distance are fairly large and cause very large penumbra. This penumbra can be reduced by using a physically smaller source, but then the activity is low. Consequently, most cesium units have been used at fairly short treatment distances, typically on the order of 20 to 30 cm; this seriously reduces the percentage depth dose that would otherwise be available at the 0.662 million electron volts (MeV) photon energy of cesium.

MACHINE CONSTRUCTION

Most modern radiation therapy machines are built to meet the needs of the continually increasing sophistication of treatment techniques in radiation therapy.

Linear accelerators and cobalt machines are compact devices, compared with a betatron; they can be rotated 360° around a patient, thus allowing the beam to be directed from any angle toward the tumor site. In some treatments, delivering radiation while the machine continuously rotates around the patient, may be superior to multiple stationary fields. The point around which the source of the beam rotates is referred to as the isocenter.

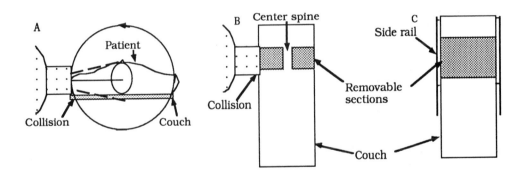

Fig. 2.11. A) The distance between the end of the collimator and the isocenter must be sufficiently long to allow 360° rotation of the treatment unit.

B) Some treatment couches have removable sections to facilitate clearance when the machine is rotated 360°. The removable sections must, however, be longer than the largest dimension of the collimator.

C) A large removable section of the treatment couch, replaced by a mylar sheet or a tennis-racket-type insert, permits treatment of a posterior field without interference by the couch. However, the side rails may interfere with posterior oblique fields.

Adequate distance must be provided between the beam-defining structures and the patient to allow a 360° rotation to take place without colliding with the patient or the treatment couch (Fig. 2.11A). Provision must also be made on the couch to allow a beam of maximum area to enter the patient without interference by attenuating bars or rails on the couch. Most modern treatment couches have removable sections which are replaced by a thin mylar sheet or tennis-racket-type insert to support the patient.   The removable sections, often interchangeable across the couch top, are typically of two different designs. A removable section on each side, with a center spine providing a continuous surface, allows posterior oblique fields to be treated without interference by side rails (Fig. 2.11B).   A large removable section across the width of the couch (Fig. 2.11C) allows a large posterior field to be treated. Side rails offer the link necessary to connect the two segments of the couch separated by the opening.

Figure 2.12 shows a typical modern treatment couch with a large removable section to the right and a removable section on each side of the couch to the left. The couch can be rotated around a pivot point which coincides with the central axis of the beam.

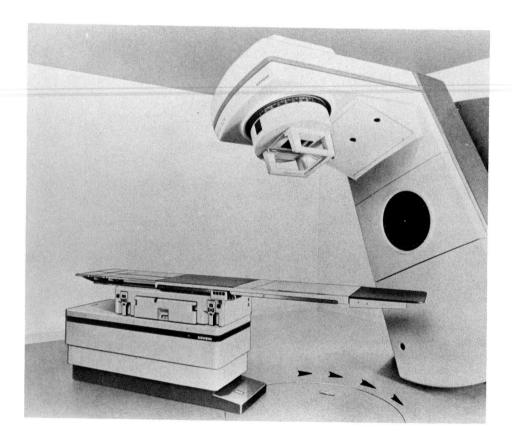

Fig. 2.12. A linear accelerator and a modern treatment table. A large section in one end of the table top can be removed (right) and two sections, one on each side of a center spine, can be removed in the other end (left). The table top can be rotated 180° around the pedestal, so that either end of the table top can be positioned in the beam. The pedestal of the treatment table can be rotated around the central axis of a vertical beam (arrows). (Courtesy Siemens Medical Systems, Inc.)

Some older radiation therapy machines are not capable of rotating around the patient but can be moved up and down to adjust the treatment distance. These non-rotating units are usually swivel mounted, meaning that the head of the machine can be angled around its own horizontal axis with the beam sweeping across the room (Fig. 2.13).

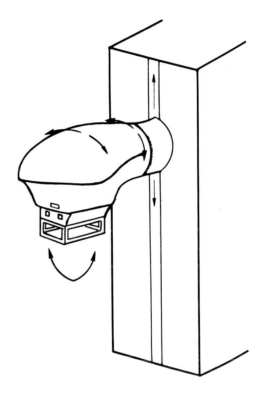

Fig. 2.13. Non-rotating machines are often mounted to allow rotation of the head around its own horizontal axis with the beam sweeping across the room.

The head of a treatment machine using isotopes consists of high-density shielding material such as lead or tungsten, inside which the source is housed. Inside the head, there is also a light localization system, a collimator through which the radiation beam exits, and in the case of a linear accelerator, also the x-ray target, scattering foil, a beam flattening filter, and ion chambers.

The design of the collimating system varies, but basically consists of a primary fixed collimator located immediately beyond the target in the direction of the beam and secondary movable collimators which shape the beam to square or rectangular fields. The secondary collimators are largely responsible for the sharpness of the edge of the beam and are therefore placed as far down toward the patient as can safely be done without causing secondary electron contamination of the patient's skin or colliding with the patient in the case of rotating equipment. The secondary collimators consist of two pairs of leaves which can be moved in and out from the central axis of the beam to decrease or increase the size of the radiation field. This opening can be totally closed by moving the leaves together or opened to its widest position to provide the maximum radiation field. In most linear accelerators or cobalt-60 machines, the largest field is 30 x 30 cm to 40 x 40 cm at standard treatment distances such as 80 or 100 cm.

Many collimators are constructed so that these leaves move only in pairs. They can therefore define only square and rectangular fields, symmetrically centered about the central axis of the beam; however, secondary beam-shaping blocks can be inserted in the path of the beam to produce irregularly shaped fields. (See Chapter 4 in *Treatment Planning and Dose Calculation in Radiation Oncology*.) More modern treatment machines have been built in which each of the four collimator leaves moves independently. This offers the capability of using the collimator leaves to define treatment fields that are asymmetric about the central axis.

Currently being introduced for use in linear accelerators are multileaf collimators which are attached to the head of the machine in the path of the beam. Multileaf collimators (Fig. 2.14) consist of a large number (20 to 30) of pairs of narrow rods with motors that drive the rods in or out of the treatment field, thus creating the desired field shape. The width of these rods varies between manufacturers, but are usually made to cast a shadow of 0.5 to 1.0 cm at the isocenter (100 cm). The resulting treatment fields thus have jagged edges rather than the smooth, sharp edges achieved with customized beam-shaping blocks described in Chapter 4 of *Treatment Planning and Dose Calculation in Radiation Oncology*.

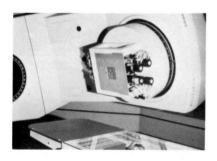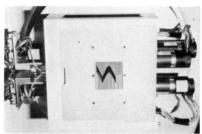

Fig. 2.14. A multileaf collimator system with individually driven rods forming an S-shaped treatment field. (Courtesy Siemens Medical Systems, Inc.)

The capability to change the shape of the field by modifying the distance to which each rod is moved into the beam is particularly useful in moving-beam therapy. The computer-driven rods can be programmed to change the shape of the beam to match the shape of the target as the machine moves around the target, a technique referred to as "dynamic beam-shaping."

Dynamic beam-shaping techniques are very complex, but are superior to fixed-beam therapy and conventional moving-beam techniques in terms of normal tissue sparing. Figure 1.3D demonstrates the concept of dynamic beam-shaping.

The maximum field size which can be treated using multileaf collimator is usually limited by the weight of this accessory; adding it below the fixed collimator system also reduces the clearance between the head of the treatment machine and the patient, thus increasing the risk of collisions.

Selection of radiation therapy units must be made with clinical needs in mind. A wide range of beam energies is needed to adequately treat tumors at various depths without compromising normal tissue tolerance. Treatment of skin lesions requires a beam which produces the highest dose on the skin surface and then falls off very rapidly within a few millimeters of depth, thus sparing deeper normal tissue. Thick surface lesions require treatment with a beam which produces the maximum dose on the surface and maintains a high dose within the first few centimeters and then falls off very rapidly to spare underlying normal tissue. Deep-seated lesions require treatment with a beam which has great penetrating power and provides some sparing of overlying normal tissues. From this, it is obvious that a variety of beam energies is necessary in each modern radiation therapy department.

Other considerations in the selection of equipment are related to the physical capabilities of the machine and the couch, and to the dosimetry of the beam.

A.   Machine considerations

1)   field size range
2)   maximum wedged field (width and length)
3)   rotational capabilities
4)   clearance of the collimator around the couch and the patient
5)   accessories (trays, wedges, electron cones, etc.) and the ease
        with which they can be inserted, weight, etc.
6)   outer dimensions of the collimator
7)   accuracy of motions (isocenter, angles, field size, distance)

B.   Couch considerations

1)   maximum vertical motion
2)   maximum lateral motion
3)   couch rotation capabilities
4)   stability of the couch (no sagging or shaking)
5)   weight tolerance
6)   accuracy of motions and read-out of angles

C.   Dosimetric considerations

1)   dose rates

2)   depth of maximum dose
3)   energy (single or dual photon energy and range of electron
        energies)
4)   penumbra
5)   beam flatness
6)   surface dose

Other considerations are, of course, cost, reliability, service, and maintenance.

SIMULATORS

A treatment simulator is a machine which is capable of duplicating the geometry and mechanical movements of radiation therapy machines but uses a diagnostic x-ray tube. A simulator is primarily used to localize the target volume and normal tissue with respect to skin marks and to visualize the planned treatment fields with respect to tumor and normal tissue. Following confirmation of correct field location and direction, the fields are marked on the skin surface and shielding blocks (discussed in Chapter 4 of *Treatment Planning and Dose Calculation in Radiation Oncology*) are produced to optimize normal tissue sparing.

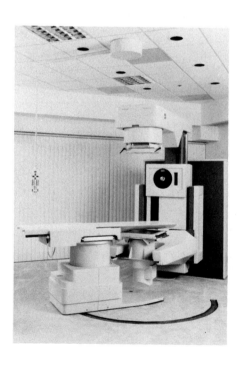

Fig. 2.15. A simulator is an x-ray machine which is designed to simulate the geometry of therapy machines. (Courtesy Siemens Medical Systems, Inc.)

The use of simulators has improved the precision of radiation therapy because it provides a diagnostic x-ray quality radiograph of the treatment field taken with the precise geometric relationship of the treatment beam (Dritschilo 1979).

The range of distances and field sizes of most therapy machines can be reproduced by moving the x-ray tube along an arm which is capable of 360° rotation (Fig. 2.15). The distance from the target to the isocenter can therefore easily be changed. Many simulators have fluoroscopic capabilities, providing real-time visualization (before radiographs are taken) of internal organs, of contrast placed in body cavities, and of lead markers on the skin surface. Field-defining wires, built into the path of the beam, can be moved to simulate the planned treatment field. A small circle or a cross hair indicates the central axis of the beam. Some simulators also can provide a grid which projects a centimeter scale at the isocenter (Fig. 2.16). This facilitates easy measurements of real size on the magnified radiograph. Periodic testing of the accuracy of simulators is necessary for continued precision in radiation therapy (McCullough 1979).

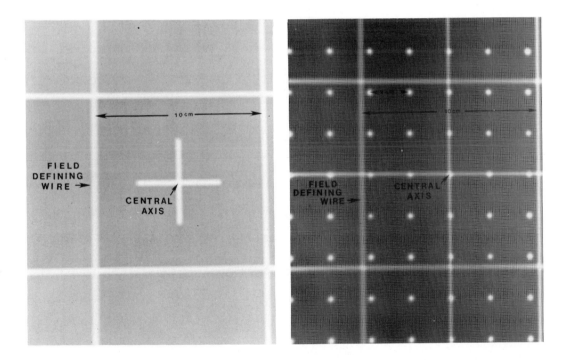

Fig. 2.16. Radiographs of two different simulator units. Radiopaque wires built into the path of the beam indicate the field size, and the central axis (L). A grid is useful in calculating the true dimensions of the images (R).

REFERENCES

Bentel, G.C., Nelson, C.E., Noell, K.T., Treatment Planning and Dose Calculation in Radiation Oncology, Pergamon Press, Inc. Elmsford, NY, 1989.

Brucer, M., An automatic controlled pattern cesium-137 teletherapy machine, Am. J. Radiol. 75, 49 (1956).

Catterall, M., Sutherland, I., Bewley, D.K., First results of a randomized clinical trial of fast neutrons compared with x or gamma rays in treatment of advanced tumours of the head and neck. Report to the Medical Research Council, British Medical Journal 2, 653 (1975).

Catterall, M., Radiology now. Fast neutrons - Clinical requirements, Brit. J. Radiol. 49, 203 (1976).

Chen, G.T.Y., Singh, R.P., Castro, J.R., Lyman, J.T., Quivey, J.M., Treatment planning for heavy ion radiotherapy, Int. J. Radiat. Oncol. Biol. Phys. 5, 1809 (1979).

Chodorow, M., Ginzton, E.L., Hansen, W.W., Kyhl, R.L., Neal, R.B., Panofsky, W.K.H., Stanford high-energy linear accelerator (Mark III), Rev. Sci. Instrum. 26, 134 (1955).

Dritschilo, A., Sherman, D., Emami, B., Piro, A.J., The cost effectiveness of a radiation therapy simulator: A model for the determination of need, Int. J. Radiat. Oncol. Biol. Phys. 5, 243 (1979).

Fry, D.W., Harvie, R.B., Mullett, L.B., Walkinshaw, W., Travelling wave linear accelerator for electrons, Nature 160, 351 (1947).

Fry, D.W., Harvie, R.B., Mullett, L.B., Walkinshaw, W., A travelling wave linear accelerator for 4 MeV electrons, Nature 162, 859 (1948).

Ginzton, E.L., Hansen, W.W., Kennedy, W.R., A linear electron accelerator, Rev. Sci. Instrum. 19, 89 (1948).

Johns, H.E., Bates, L.M., Watson, T.A., 1,000 curie cobalt units for radiation therapy, 1, The Saskatchewan cobalt-60 unit, Brit. J. Radiol. 25, 296 (1952).

Johns, H.E., Cunningham, J.R., The Physics of Radiology, (4th ed.), Charles C. Thomas, Springfield, IL, 1983.

Karzmark, C., Pering, N., Electron linear accelerators for radiation therapy: History, principles and contemporary developments, Phys. Med. Biol. 18, 321 (1973).

Kerst, D.W., Acceleration of electrons by magnetic induction, Phys. Rev. 60, 47 (1941).

Kerst, D.W., The betatron, <u>Radiology</u> 40, 115 (1943).

Khan, F.M., <u>The Physics of Radiation Therapy</u>, Williams & Wilkins, Baltimore, MD, 1984.

McCullough, E.C., Earle, J.D., The selection, acceptance testing, and quality control of radiotherapy treatment simulators, <u>Radiology</u> 131, 221 (1979).

Sable, M., Gunn, W.G., Penning, D., Gardner, A., Performance of a new 4 MeV standing wave linear accelerator, <u>Radiology</u> 97, 169 (1970).

Saunders, W.M., Chen, G.T.Y., Austin-Seymour, M., Castro, J.R., Collier, J.M., Gauger, G., Gutin, P., Phillips, T.L., Pitluck, S., Walton, R.E., Zink, S.R., Precision high dose radiotherapy. II Helium ion treatment of tumors adjacent to critical central nervous system structures, <u>Int. J. Radiat. Oncol. Biol. Phys.</u> 11, 1339 (1985).

Von Essen, C.F., Blattman, H., Bodendoerfer, G., Mizoe, J.E., Pedroni, E., Walder, E., Zimmermann, A., The Piotron: II Methods and initial results of dynamic pion therapy in phase II studies, <u>Int. J. Radiat. Oncol. Biol. Phys.</u> 11, 217 (1985).

Wideröe, R., Über ein neues Prinzip zur Herstellung hoher Spannungen, <u>Arch. Elektrotech.</u> 21, 387 (1928).

PROBLEMS

1. The use of betatrons in radiation therapy became unpopular primarily because they

   a) were difficult to get
   b) were too expensive
   c) were too large
   d) produced low dose rates and limited field sizes

2. Radiation therapy units operating at approximately 50 to 120 kVp are referred to as

   a) linear accelerators
   b) orthovoltage units
   c) superficial units
   d) betatrons

3. The half-value thickness (HVT) is

   a) the thickness of a given material which causes the beam to be more penetrating
   b) the thickness of a given material which, when introduced into the path of the beam, reduces the intensity of the beam to one half its original value
   c) the thickness of a filter which hardens the beam and causes it to be reduced to half of its original value
   d) the thickness of a filter which determines the quantity of the beam

4. Insertion of Al, Cu, and Sn filters into the x-ray beam causes

   a) low-energy x-rays to be absorbed
   b) the kVp to increase
   c) unnecessary dose on the skin surface
   d) the dose to increase

5. Orthovoltage x-ray units usually operate at

   a) 15 to 20 cm source-surface distance (SSD)

    b) 20 to 40 cm source-surface distance (SSD)
    c) 50 to 70 cm source-surface distance (SSD)
    d) 80 to 100 cm source-surface distance (SSD)

6. Orthovoltage x-ray units usually operate in the range of

    a) 20 to 150 kVp
    b) 150 to 500 kVp
    c) 200 to 1200 kVp
    d) any kVp below 200 kVp

7. Orthovoltage x-ray beams are generally

    a) more penetrating than those of linear accelerators
    b) more penetrating than superficial beams
    c) equal to superficial beams in penetration

8. Linear accelerators were first developed

    a) following World War II
    b) during the Depression
    c) following World War I

9. Linear accelerators produce high-energy beams

    a) by accelerating charged particles in a linear tube
    b) by accelerating photons in a circular orbit
    c) by accelerating charged particles in a circular orbit

10. Because electrons scatter readily in air

    a) they are removed before they strike the target
    b) cones extending close to the patient's skin are used
    c) they are bent at 90° to 270° to reduce scattering

11. A collimator

    a) flattens the beam at a specified depth in tissue
    b) defines the beam
    c) determines the dose rate

12. The photon beam from a linear accelerator is intercepted by

   a) a Cu filter which hardens the beam
   b) ionization chambers and a flattening filter
   c) a scattering foil and an ionization chamber

13. A flattening filter

   a) removes all of the electrons from the beam
   b) causes the dose rate to be increased
   c) reduces the dose rate in the center of the unfiltered beam
   d) all of the above

14. The first cobalt-60 machine was introduced during

   a) the 1960s
   b) the 1950s
   c) World War II
   d) the 1940s

15. The half-life of a cobalt-60 source is

   a) 30.3 years
   b) 1600 years
   c) 5.26 years
   d) 74 days

16. The average energy of a cobalt-60 beam is

   a) 0.6 MeV
   b) 1.2 MeV
   c) 2.0 MeV
   d) 4.0 MeV

17. The penumbra of a linear accelerator beam is

   a) smaller than that of a cobalt-60 machine
   b) larger than that of a cobalt-60 machine
   c) the same as that of a cobalt-60 machine

18. The isocenter is

    a) an imaginary point in the beam where the dose is normalized
    b) the point on the central axis where the maximum dose occurs
    c) the point around which the source of the beam rotates

19. The secondary collimator of a linear accelerator is largely responsible for

    a) largely responsible for the sharpness of the beam edges
    b) largely responsible for the flatness of the beam
    c) largely responsible for determining the dose rates

20. Simulators are primarily used to

    a) localize the target
    b) duplicate the geometry of therapy machines
    c) duplicate the mechanical movements of the therapy machine
    d) all of the above

SOLUTIONS

1.	d		11.	b
2.	c		12.	b
3.	b		13.	c
4.	a		14.	b
5.	c		15.	c
6.	b		16.	b
7.	b		17.	a
8.	a		18.	c
9.	a		19.	a
10.	b		20.	d

CHAPTER 3

DOSE DETERMINATION FOR EXTERNAL BEAMS

DOSE MEASUREMENTS

When a radiation beam impinges on a patient, the dose delivered to a point within the patient depends on the depth of the calculation point below the surface (depth), the penetrating power of the beam (energy), the type of tissue, that is, muscle, bone, or fat, that the beam must penetrate (density), the distance from the radiation source to the skin surface (SSD), the size of the field on the skin surface (field size), and, to some extent, the collimator design. The purpose of this section is to give a very brief summary of how these variables are taken into consideration in calculating the dose within the patient.

An essential step in treatment planning is to establish measured data tables for each treatment machine that will be used. Such tables are usually prepared as a result of measurements in dummy patients (phantoms) made of tissue-equivalent material. The phantom material used is often water, which is like soft tissue as far as radiation absorption is concerned. Sheets of various tissue-equivalent plastics are also commonly employed because they are more convenient. The devices called dosimeters, used to measure dose distributions within such phantoms are described briefly below.

Calculation of the dose by the methods in this text with the help of established tables is not enough to insure that the correct dose is being delivered. First, one must be sure that the machine behavior (radiation output, beam energy, beam flatness, etc.) is the same when the patient is treated as when the data tables were prepared, the constancy of the machine must have been routinely checked; otherwise irreversible harm may be

49

caused either by overdosing, which may lead to tissue damage, or by underdosing, which can result in failure to cure, even though all the treatment planning calculations are quite correct. Routine constancy checking is one of the main responsibilities of the radiation physicist. Second, it is advisable, where possible, to measure the dose actually delivered to the patient by means of dosimeters placed in body cavities or in catheters or needles inserted in the tissues. In this way, errors in the dose calculation itself can be corrected.

PRECISION OF DOSE CALCULATIONS

In this text, many dose calculations are carried to four significant figures, that is, they are expressed in a form such as 223.7 cGy. This may give the false impression that the dose is known with certainty to be 223.7 cGy rather than 223.6 or 223.8 cGy. Similarly, tissue-air ratios (TAR), backscatter factors (BSF), SSDs, etc., are frequently given to the same apparent accuracy.

In practice, quantities used in treatment planning and dose calculation are not known to this degree of accuracy; for example, we very rarely know that the %DD is exactly 55.43% rather than 55.42% or 55.44%; indeed, unusually careful measurements, under very favorable experimental conditions, are necessary even to establish the first decimal place value as 55.4%. Similarly, the SSD can not usually be measured to better than, perhaps, 1 mm.

The result of a calculation involving several such uncertainties can not itself be as accurate as results written with several decimal places might suggest. It is convenient, with pocket calculators, to carry a large number of decimal places in the calculations, but the treatment planner must cultivate a habit of rounding off the calculated numbers. Hard and fast rules for rounding out numbers are not available; instead, one must use judgement, which comes with experience. For example, when calculating the number of monitor units required to deliver a prescribed dose, whole numbers are given in the calculation because it is not possible to set fractions of a monitor unit on the machine.

DOSE

Before describing the devices that are used to (1) prepare the data tables, (2) check machine behavior, and (3) measure dose within the patient, it is necessary to have a clear idea of what we mean by dose. The dose (sometimes called the absorbed dose) at a point in an absorber such as tissue is the energy deposited in a small fixed weight of the material surrounding the point in question.

The unit in which the dose is measured is traditionally the rad, which is defined as a dose or energy-deposition of 100 erg* per gram (g).

$$1 \text{ rad} = 100 \text{ erg/g}$$

The rad is rapidly being replaced by the gray (Gy), which is 100 times larger, that is,

$$1 \text{ Gy} = 100 \text{ rad}$$

One rad is therefore the same as one hundredth (prefix centi-) of a gray, or 1 centigray, usually written cGy:

$$1 \text{ rad} = 1/100 \text{ Gy} = 1 \text{ cGy}$$

We shall use the gray or centigray as a dose unit throughout this text just as it was used in *Treatment Planning and Dose Calculation in Radiation Oncology* (Bentel 1989).

Another unit (the roentgen), once widely used in radiation therapy, will not be employed in this text except in connection with brachytherapy, where for mainly historic reasons, it is sometimes retained as a step in the calculations (Chapter 8).

METHODS OF DOSE DETERMINATION

The three devices most commonly used for dose determination in radiation therapy are:

  1. ionization chambers
  2. thermoluminescent dosimeters (TLDs)
  3. photographic film

Though TLDs and photographic films are usually more convenient to use than ionization chambers, it is usually necessary to check their performance by comparing their readings with those of ionization chambers, which must be regarded as the most reliable method of determining dose.

Ionization Chambers
An ionization chamber determines the dose at a point in a rather indirect way. The chamber usually consists of a cylinder (Fig. 3.1) along the center of which runs a rod that is insulated electrically from the cylinder. The chambers used in radiation therapy are usually about as big as a finger-thimble but they can be made small enough to slide along a catheter or to be inserted in a body cavity.

---

* The erg is a very small amount of energy, considerably less than one millionth of a calorie.

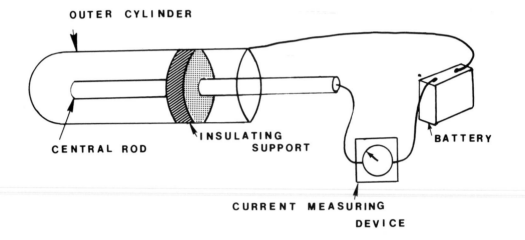

Fig. 3.1. Diagram of an ionization chamber.

No electric current will normally flow around the circuit when the terminals of a battery are connected to the outer wall and central rod of the chamber because the air that fills the chamber does not conduct. If the chamber is exposed to x-rays, the air becomes electrified through the break-up, into charged particles, of atoms that are struck by the x-ray photons. These charged particles (which are called ions, whence the name ionization chamber) drift through the chamber, that is, an electric current flows. The size of the current, measured by means of a sensitive current-measuring device (Fig. 3.1), tells us how much ionization is produced in the air that fills the chamber. If the chamber is embedded in an absorbing material at the time it is irradiated, knowledge of the amount of ionization produced in the air, together with some other data on the absorbing properties of air and of the surrounding medium, allows us to calculate the energy that would be transferred to the medium, that is, the absorbed dose, if the chamber had not been present.

To find the dose in this way from measurements in an air-filled chamber inserted in the absorber, it is first necessary to have the ionization chamber calibrated by the National Institute of Standards and Technology (NIST) or by one of its accredited laboratories. Multiplication of the instrument readings with the calibration factor supplied by one of these laboratories and with certain other tabulated numbers gives the absorber dose at the point where the chamber was placed.

There are requirements both of law and prudence regarding how often a therapeutically used ionization chamber must be calibrated. The qualifications of the expert staff, usually physicists, who make and interpret the measurements are also subject to regulation.

Thermoluminescent Dosimeters

Some crystalline materials retain and store, for very long periods, the energy they absorb when they are exposed to x-rays. The stored energy is released later as visible light, that is, the crystals *luminesce*, if the crystal is heated. Because the luminescence is brought about by thermal (heat) influence, the substances are said to be thermoluminescent. The emitted light can be measured and through previous calibration, it can be expressed in terms of the radiation dose; a thermoluminescent material used in this way is called a thermoluminescent dosimeter (TLD). The most commonly used TLD materials are lithium fluoride (LiF) and calcium fluoride (CaF_2). Commercial TLD materials are available in many forms and sizes (rods, chips, powder, discs, etc.) that are practical for measuring dose in most clinical situations.

The response of each TLD to radiation is unique so each one must be calibrated before it can be used for measuring unknown dose. The dose response is established by exposing a given TLD to a known dose of radiation and determining the amount of light produced on later heating. Once the light produced by the known dose of the same kind of radiation has been found, it is a simple matter to measure an unknown dose by measuring the amount of light that the unknown dose produces.

Photographic Film

Radiographic film consists of a transparent base coated with an emulsion containing silver bromide crystals. When the film is exposed to light or radiation, the exposed crystals form an image. When the film is developed, the unaffected granules are removed, leaving only the clear base, while the affected crystals are reduced to silver, which darkens the film. The darkening of the film is directly related to the absorbed radiation.

The variations in darkness of the film can be measured using a densitometer. A densitometer consists of a light source and a light detector that measures the light transmitted through the film. The relative quantity of dose is obtained by subtracting the reading for a sample which is unexposed but developed under the same circumstances as the film being used for dosimetry; the net density (difference between the exposed and unexposed) is a measure of the dose.

Film dosimetry is not practical for absolute dose determination because of its sensitivity to changes in developing conditions, artifacts on the film, and differences in the emulsion on the film. Dose response of film is very energy-dependent and is therefore not useful in dose determination of orthovoltage radiation. However, it is useful for deducing relative dose distribution, beam-light coincidence, beam flatness, beam symmetry, etc.

DEFINITIONS

The process of determining radiation dose is quite complex and many of the terms used can be difficult to understand. The dose delivery involves two major parts. The first is to determine the output of a machine, that is, the dose delivered at a specified point in the beam, at a specified distance from the target, and in a specified medium. This requires tedious measurements under very specific conditions. The second part is the absorbed dose in the irradiated medium. This requires, for example, knowledge of the composition of the irradiated material, the geometric relationship with the beam, and the size of the irradiated field.

This section will provide definition of some terms used in external-beam dose calculations which are used in this text. Definition of terms used in photon and electron beams will be described separately.

MAXIMUM ELECTRONIC BUILD-UP

Whenever high-energy photon beams strike a medium, secondary electrons are set in motion. These secondary electrons will penetrate the medium to a depth that depends on the photon energy and the composition of the medium. Maximum dose is obtained at the depth where electron equilibrium is reached. This maximum depth is referred to as D_{max}.*

The region between the surface and this depth is referred to as the build-up region. The dose in the build-up region rises rapidly as the secondary electrons contribute to the total dose. Therefore, the surface layer receives a smaller dose than layers between the surface and D_{max}. The skin is thus "spared". The skin-sparing effect observed with high-energy beams is reduced or lost when material such as clothing, treatment couches, positioning devices, etc., are allowed to intercept the beam within a few centimeters of the patient's skin surface. The observed skin-sparing effect is improved with higher energies, and the depth of D_{max} increases with higher energy. The dose at greater depths falls off gradually as the effect of attenuation and increased distance reduce the supply of photons that set the electrons in motion. The %DD falls less rapidly with higher energy as demonstrated in Fig. 3.2.

---

* D_{max} means either the depth (usually written d_{max}) or the dose (usually written D_{max}). The two annotations are often used interchangably, and from the context in which they are used, it should be clear whether depth or dose is intended.

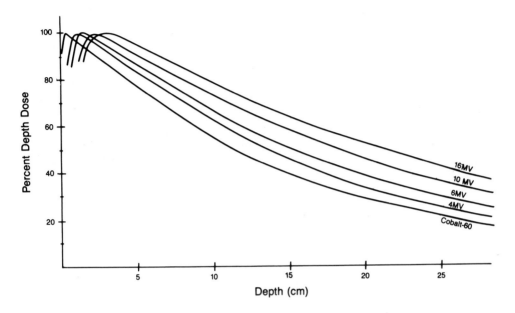

Fig. 3.2. Percentage depth dose for 10 x 10 cm beams of different beam energies, plotted as a function of depth in water.

Measurement of the exact dose at the surface is technically very difficult because the dose gradient is very steep and, therefore, the dose within the instrument used in the dose determination will vary considerably (Gerbi 1990).

HALF-VALUE THICKNESS

A practical way to express the penetration or "quality," or "hardness" of a beam is the half-value thickness (HVT) in a given material. The HVT is the thickness of the material that reduces the intensity of the beam to half its original value. All photon beams can be described in terms of their HVT, however, the quality of high-energy beams is usually described in terms of the accelerating voltage (MV).

The quality of lower energy beams, such as those produced by superficial and orthovoltage equipment, depends not only on the peak accelerating voltage (kVp), but also on the filtration used to filter out the non-penetrating soft x-rays. It is customary to describe the quality of beams in this energy range in terms of their HVT in Al, Cu, or Sn. For example, when we say that the HVT for a given beam is 3 mm Cu, we mean that inserting 3 mm of copper in the path of the beam will reduce its intensity to half of its original value. The practice of expressing beam-penetrating power in the same materials as those used to filter out soft, undesirable x-rays, stems from the early days of radiation therapy when these materials were used to determine the penetration of a given kVp and filter combination and must not be confused with the filters actually used in the beam.

DOSE RATES

Dose rates and dose distributions from radiation therapy machines are ordinarily measured in the absence of a scattering phantom, sometimes referred to as "in air," and in tissue-equivalent material. These measurements, or calibrations, are obtained using very carefully measured variables such as the SSD, field size, depth in tissue-equivalent material, etc. Instruments calibrated against a national standard are used in obtaining these measurements.

It would be impractical to measure the dose at every point within a field at every distance from the source. Measured dose rates plotted at standard distances for multiple field sizes and corresponding isodose curves for multiple field sizes allow one to calculate the dose to practically any point. Since the dose distribution in tissue from cobalt-60 machines are quite predictable, published tables may be used. Dose distributions from linear accelerators with the same nominal energy may vary due to differences in flattening filter and collimator design. The percentage depth dose along the central axis may be reproducible from one linear accelerator to another of the same design using the same energy, and published central axis data may therefore be used.

Dose Rates without a Phantom

Dose rates determined without a scattering phantom are measured with a build-up cap of a thickness equal to the depth of D_{max}. These in air measurements are made on the central axis of the field at the source-axis distance (SAD) for a range of field sizes because the dose rates vary somewhat with the collimator opening.

Dose Rates in Tissue

Dose rates in tissue are ordinarily measured on the central axis at a standard source-surface distance (SSD) at the depth of D_{max} in a phantom, and at other depths and positions if required. Dose rates in a phantom include both the primary dose and the dose due to scatter in the irradiated volume.

Dependence on Field Size

Dose rates increase with increased field size due to scatter within the irradiated volume from the collimator and other beam-shaping devices (Meli 1986). Dose rates increase more rapidly in smaller fields, and as the field size becomes larger (approximately 20 x 20 cm), the increase in dose rates stabilizes and they remain practically unchanged (Fig. 3.3). Since the scatter is greatly dependent on the field size, dose rates must be measured for a large number of field sizes.

It is customary to express dose rates for a cobalt-60 machine in cGy/min for a 10 x 10 cm field (dose rate$_{ref}$) at some fixed distance. An area factor is multiplied into the dose calculation for other field sizes to give the correct dose rate for each particular field size.

Linear accelerators can be altered to change the dose rate per time unit so the dose rates are expressed in cGy/monitor unit (M.U.). A monitor, built into the collimator, indicates a unit on the control console for each measured unit of dose at D_{max}. The monitor unit is often adjusted to be the same as 1 cGy at D_{max} for a given field size (cGy/M.U.$_{ref}$), usually a 10 x 10 cm field, but since the monitor unit is independent of field size, a cGy/M.U. factor for a range of field sizes must be measured and tabulated.

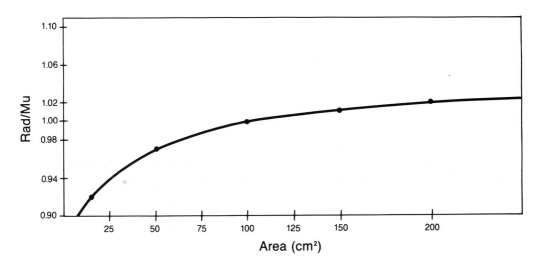

Fig. 3.3. CGy/M.U. measured without a phantom and plotted as a function of field size.

Dependence on Distance

The dose rate for a given energy and field size in principle varies inversely with the square of the distance from the source. However, the inverse square law dependence of dose rates assumes primary radiation only. The collimator or other scattering devices that add to the scattered radiation in the beam may cause deviation from the inverse square law.

Figure 3.4 demonstrates how the area increases as the distance from the target increases. The same number of interactions takes place in this larger area (a$_1$ x b$_1$) as in the smaller area (a x b) at the shorter distance.

An example of calculating the dose rate as a result of increased distance, using the inverse square law, is given below. The dose rate for a 10 x 10 cm cobalt-60 beam at 80.5 cm (SSD + depth of D_{max}) is 117 cGy/min. To find the dose rate at 100.5 cm (SSD + depth of D_{max}) for the same field, but treated at 100 cm SSD, we must find the inverse square factor (ISF).

The inverse square factor is found from

$$ISF = \left(\frac{SSD_1}{SSD_2}\right)^2 \qquad (3.1)$$

so $\left(\frac{80.5}{100.5}\right)^2 = 0.6416$

$117 \times 0.6416 = 75$ cGy/min

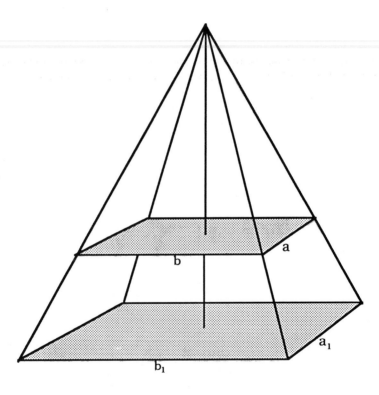

Fig. 3.4. The irradiated area becomes larger as the distance from the target increases. The same number of interactions takes place in the larger area (a_1 x b_1) as in the smaller area (a x b).

One necessary, but often omitted, step in calculation of a treatment prescription which includes an inverse square factor is to do the same calculation without the inverse square factor to find the necessary treatment time, or M.U., if the treatment was delivered at the "normal" SSD. This is a simple way of verifying that the required treatment time or number of M.U. is in fact increased when the SSD is longer, or vice versa when the treatment distance is shortened, and that the inverse square equation was not accidentally inverted. Serious accidents can be prevented by careful checks of these calculations.

PERCENTAGE DEPTH DOSE

Percentage depth dose is the absorbed dose at a given depth expressed as a percentage of the absorbed dose at a reference depth on the central axis of the field. The reference depth is usually taken to be D_{max}, and in this case, the %DD at point A (Fig. 3.5) is 75%.

$$\%DD = \frac{\text{absorbed dose at A}}{\text{absorbed dose at } D_{max}} \times 100\% \qquad (3.2)$$

Percentage depth dose is affected by energy, field size, SSD, and by the composition of the irradiated medium. Of course the %DD also changes with depth.

Percentage depth dose data are usually tabulated for square or rectangular fields (*Brit. J. Radiol.* Supplements No. 11, 1972, and No. 17, 1983, Johns 1983). The majority of treatments encountered in clinical practice require other shapes; therefore, a system of equating clinically used fields to fields with tabulated data is required. This is discussed in greater detail in the irregular field section in Chapter 5.

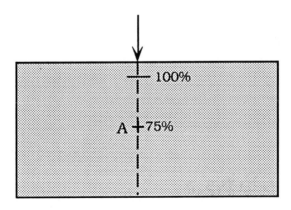

Fig. 3.5. Percentage depth dose is the absorbed dose at a given depth expressed as a percentage of the absorbed dose at a reference depth; in this illustration, the reference depth is at D_{max}.

Dependence on Field Size and Shape

For a 0 x 0 cm field, the dose at a point in a phantom is effectively due to primary radiation only. This method of considering the primary radiation is feasible in theory only, however, it is a reasonable manner in which to consider the primary dose alone. If the collimator were closed entirely, no radiation would be delivered but if the field were *very* small (which we may for convenience show as a 0 x 0 cm field) the dose would effectively be due to primary radiation only. The scattered component of the dose is almost entirely dependent on the size of the radiation field. As the field size is increased, the absorbed dose in a medium is greater due to the increased scatter.

The shape of the field strongly influences the amount of scatter at a given point. A 10 x 10 cm field (100 cm^2) symmetrically placed around the calculation point will produce more scatter at this point than a field which is 2 x 50 cm, also 100 cm^2. This is because the extremes of this field are 25 cm from the calculation point. Large sections of this field are too far from the calculation point to deliver significant amount of scatter there. This is discussed in more detail in Chapter 5.

Furthermore, higher energy photons are scattered in a more forward direction than lower energy photons, thus resulting in less dependence on field size.

Dependence on Energy and Depth

Higher energy beams have greater penetrating power and thus the percentage depth dose at a given depth and SSD is increased. Figure 3.6 illustrates the percentage depth dose along the central axis for a variety of beam energies.

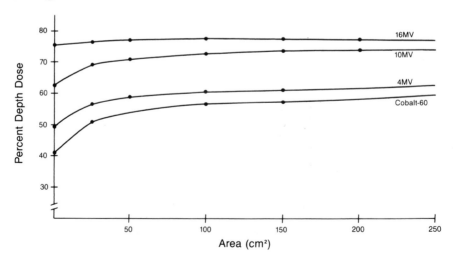

Fig. 3.6. Percentage depth dose plotted as a function of field size for various beam energies. The SSD for the cobalt-60 and the 4 MV photon beam is 80 cm and for the 10 and 16 MV photon beams, the SSD is 100 cm.

Dependence on Distance

Although the absolute dose rate decreases with increased distance from the source, the percentage depth dose, which is a relative dose with respect to a reference point, *increases* with increased SSD. This is illustrated in Fig. 3.7 where it is shown that for a given field size, the volume within which the same number of interactions take place, is smaller when the distance is increased. Grossly simplified, one can say that the interactions are more concentrated when the distance is increased.

The increase of percentage depth dose with increased distance can be determined using the Mayneord F-factor (Mayneord 1941 and *Brit. J. Radiol.* Supplement No. 10, 1961) defined as:

$$F\text{-factor} = \left(\frac{SSD_2 + D_{max}}{SSD_2 + d}\right)^2 \bigg/ \left(\frac{SSD_1 + D_{max}}{SSD_1 + d}\right)^2 \qquad (3.3)$$

so that $\%DD_{SSD_2} = F \times \%DD_{SSD_1}$

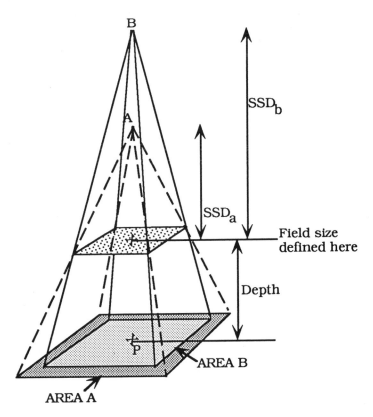

Fig. 3.7. The irradiated volume for a given field size is decreased when the source-surface distance is increased.

The Mayneord F-factor is a reasonably accurate method of calculating the change in percentage depth dose for small fields where the scatter component is small. Significant errors occur when this method is applied under extreme conditions such as low energy, large field, large depth, or large change in SSD.

An example of using the Mayneord F-factor in calculating the change in %DD is given below. The percentage depth dose for a 10 x 10 cm field at 10 cm depth and 80 cm SSD (D_{max} at 1.0 cm) using a 4 MV photon beam is 62.2%. Find the percentage depth dose for the same field size and depth but for 100 cm SSD.

$$\text{F-factor} = \left(\frac{100+1}{100+10}\right)^2 / \left(\frac{80+1}{80+10}\right)^2$$

$$= \left(\frac{101}{110}\right)^2 / \left(\frac{81}{90}\right)^2$$

$$= \frac{0.8431}{0.81} = 1.041$$

Thus the percentage depth dose is the original 62.2 multiplied by the F-factor 1.041:

$$62.2 \times 1.041 = 64.8$$

When making this calculation, caution should be used to prevent any chance of accidentally inverting the equation. One must always remember that as the SSD increase the %DD will also increase.

Dependence on Composition of the Irradiated Medium

In a patient, the beam may traverse tissues of different density such as lung, bone, fat, muscle, and air. These inhomogeneities affect both the penetration of the beam and the scattering characteristics. The effect of these inhomogeneities on the dose depends on the size of the volume, on the density (g/cm^3) of the inhomogeneity, and also on the energy of the beam.

For example, lung tissue, which is largely filled with air, has a much lower density than muscle and thus attenuates the primary photon beam less than an equal thickness of soft tissue. The effect of bone, where the density is higher than in soft tissue, is in the opposite direction.

The density of lung can vary from 0.25 to 1.0 g/cm^3 depending on the amount of air in the lung. A value of 0.25 to 0.33 g/cm^3 is often used. The density of bone is often quoted as 1.8 g/cm^3 but this probably overestimates the attenuation of primary photons. The density of compact bone, for example, is higher than for soft or spongy bone.

The effects of inhomogeneities are in the absorption of the primary beam and in the scatter. For points which lie beyond an inhomogeneity, the dose is primarily affected by the attenuation of the primary beam, while the dose distribution in and near the inhomogeneity is affected more by the scatter. Calculation of dose changes in and beyond an inhomogeneity is very complicated because of variations in density within an inhomogeneity and uncertainties in the three-dimensional shape of the inhomogeneity. Many authors have proposed different methods of calculating the change in dose caused by inhomogeneities (Batho 1964, Greene 1965, Jette and Bielajew 1989, Jette et al. 1989, Sundblom 1965, Young 1970, McDonald 1976, Sontag 1978).

The effect on the dose near the interface between layers of different density is quite complex. For example, there may be loss of electronic equilibrium immediately beyond an air cavity or a layer of low-density material when high-energy beams are used (Epp 1958, 1977, Nilsson 1976, Gillin 1981).

For low-energy x-rays, the absorbed dose within or near the bone may be several times higher than calculated from soft tissue tables. This increased dose is caused by an interaction called photoelectric absorption, which is of major importance only at low energies and in materials of higher atomic number.

In the past the difficulties in calculating dose in a beam that traverses an inhomogeneous volume has been related in part to the difficulties of outlining the boundaries of the inhomogeneity and of determining the density within this volume. The use of computed tomography (CT), in which both detailed outlines of inhomogeneities and some information of the physical composition of that volume can be obtained, has greatly enhanced dose-calculation methods when inhomogeneities are present. Since the CT numbers and the attenuation coefficients have a linear relationship, it is possible to incorporate a density correction in dose calculations.

Though a gradual change to universal introduction of lung inhomogeneity corrections has been proposed (Orton and Herskovic 1984, Orton et al. 1984), generally, there is some reluctance to incorporate inhomogeneity corrections in dose calculations because practically all clinical experience has been gained with dose calculations assuming homogeneity. The validity of using CT information related to the density of an organ is controversial and has been evaluated by several authors (Geise 1977, Sontag 1977, Fullerton 1978, Parker 1979, Van Dyk 1980, 1982, 1983, Cassell 1981, Hogstrom 1981, Mohan 1981, Mira 1982, Badcock 1982, Wong 1983).

TISSUE-AIR RATIO

The concept of tissue-air ratio (TAR) was first introduced for calculation of dose in rotation therapy where the radiation source moves in a circle around the axis of the gantry rotation (isocenter). The axis is usually placed at or close to the center of the tumor. The SAD and the field size at that distance remain unchanged while the SSD, the field area on the patient's surface, and the thickness of overlying tissue may vary depending on the patient's surface contour. The TAR concept is very practical and is now almost universally used; it can be employed not only in rotation treatments, but for calculation of dose using stationary fields, in both SAD and SSD techniques, and for treatments delivered at extended distances using large fields.

Tissue-air ratio is the ratio of the dose at a given point in a medium to the dose at the same point in free space (Fig. 3.8).

$$TAR = \frac{\text{dose in tissue}}{\text{dose in air}} \qquad (3.4)$$

For a given energy, the TAR depends on depth and field size at that depth, but is independent of distance.

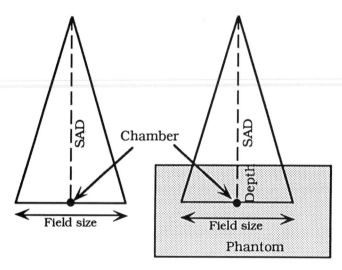

Fig. 3.8. Arrangement for determination of tissue-air ratio. Note that the distance to the chamber and the field size is unchanged.

Tissue-air ratio for a *very* small field represented by a 0 x 0 cm field, which is only an abstraction, represents primary dose only since no scattering material is irradiated. It increases with increasing field size as the scatter from the irradiated volume is added to the primary (0 x 0 cm field).

TISSUE-PHANTOM RATIO

The tissue-phantom ratio (TPR), first introduced by Karzmark in an effort to overcome the limitations of the TAR, is sometimes used instead of TAR in dosimetry of high energy beams (Karzmark 1965, Holt 1970). It retains the properties of the TAR but eliminates difficult and unreliable in air measurements because the determination of dose in free space would require the use of a build-up cap too large to be fully irradiated when small fields are used.

The tissue-phantom ratio is defined as the ratio of dose at a specified point in tissue or in a phantom to the dose at the same distance in the beam at a reference depth, usually 5 cm (Fig. 3.9).

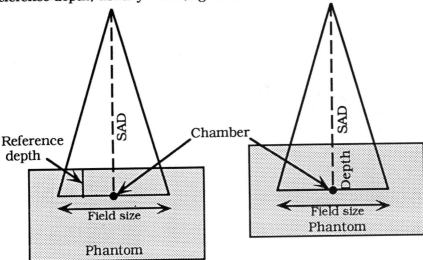

Fig. 3.9. Arrangement for determination of tissue-phantom ratio. Note that the distance to the chamber and the field size is unchanged.

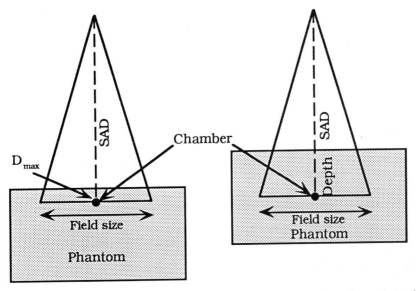

Fig. 3.10 Arrangement for determination of tissue-maximum ratio. Note that the distance to the chamber and the field size are unchanged.

$$TPR = \frac{\text{dose in tissue}}{\text{dose in phantom (ref. depth)}} \qquad (3.5)$$

As with TARs, the dose measurements should be made at the same distance from the source for both determinations, and the field size at the distance of the measuring instrument should also be the same in both cases.

TISSUE-MAXIMUM RATIO

Tissue-maximum ratio (TMR) is a special case of TPR where the reference depth is chosen to be at D_{max}. Tissue-maximum ratio is defined as the ratio of the dose at a specified point in tissue or in a phantom to the dose at the same point when it is at the depth of maximum dose (Fig. 3.10).

$$TMR = \frac{\text{dose in tissue}}{\text{dose in phantom } (D_{max})} \qquad (3.6)$$

SCATTER-AIR RATIO

Scatter-air ratio (SAR) is the ratio of the scattered dose at a given point in a medium to the dose in air at the same point. The SAR, like the TAR, is independent of the treatment distance but depends on the energy, field size, and depth.

Since the scattered dose at a given point in the medium is equal to the total dose minus the primary dose at the same point, scatter-air ratios can be calculated by finding the difference between the TAR for the given field size (primary and scatter are present) and the TAR for a 0 x 0 cm field (primary only). Tissue-air ratio for a 0 x 0 cm field represents the primary component only since no scattering medium is present.

$$SAR (D, fs) = TAR (D, fs) - TAR (D, 0) \qquad (3.7)$$

where D is depth and fs is field size.

Scatter-air ratios are primarily used for the purpose of calculating scattered dose in a medium. Considering the primary and the scattered doses separately is particularly useful in dose calculation for irregularly shaped fields discussed in Chapter 5.

SCATTER-MAXIMUM RATIO

Scatter-maximum ratio (SMR), is really just a variation of SAR and, like scatter-air ratio, is mainly used in calculation of scattered dose in a phantom or tissue. It is defined as the ratio of the scattered dose at a designated point in a phantom to the effective primary dose at the same point at the reference depth of maximum dose. It differs from SAR in that the reference point is different, just as TAR and TMR have different reference points.

BACKSCATTER FACTOR

The backscatter factor (BSF) is defined as the ratio of dose on the central axis at D_{max} to the dose at the same point in air (or free space). The BSF is independent of SSD but depends on the energy and the field size. Backscatter factors and tissue-air ratios at D_{max} are the same.

The BSF is very high for beam energies having a HVT of 0.6 to 0.8 mm Cu and can be as high as 1.5 for large fields at these HVTs (*Brit. J. Radiol.* Supplements No. 11, 1972 and No. 17, 1983, Johns 1983). For megavoltage beams, where the scatter travels in a more forward direction, the BSF is much lower and in beams generated above 8 to 10 MV, the scatter at D_{max} is very small (less than 5% in a 10 x 10 cm field).

COLLIMATOR SCATTER FACTOR

Output measured without a scattering phantom, sometimes referred to as in air, increases as the field size does. The increase is due to increased photon scattering from the collimator, because the surface area of the beam-defining tunnel exposed to the radiation increases as the collimator size is increased.

FIXED SOURCE-AXIS DISTANCE VERSUS FIXED SOURCE-SURFACE DISTANCE TECHNIQUE

A fixed source-axis distance technique is also known as an isocentric, or SAD, technique. In this technique, the axis of machine rotation (the isocenter) is placed in the target volume. The gantry of the machine can then be rotated to any angle while the target remains within the field boundaries. One can either make the machine rotate around the tumor in a complete circle (rotation therapy) or, a partial circle (arc therapy), or treat multiple stationary fields directed at the target from any angle. The tissue surrounding the target volume, outside of the field boundaries, lies in the beam only during a small fraction of the moving beam treatment, while in a stationary technique some tissue between the fields is almost totally spared. The precise dose distribution depends on several factors such as the rotation pattern (arc, full rotation, or stationary), the energy of the beam, the field size, the number of fields, the depth of the isocenter, and the weighting of the beam.

The dose in this technique is normalized at the isocenter. Either TARs and dose rates in air or TPRs and TMRs are used in calculating the dose. Since TARs and TPRs are practically independent of distance (see previous definitions), the precision in measuring the distance to the skin surface is not as important as in an SSD technique where the %DD, the dose rates in air, and the TMR will vary with the distance. In an isocentric technique, small errors in the dose due to small errors in the treatment distance are reduced if an opposing field is used, because there the distance error will be in the opposite direction, thus practically eliminating an error in the dose.

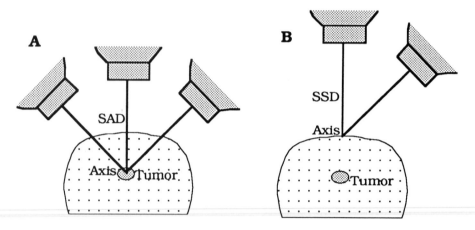

Fig. 3.11. In an isocentric technique (A), the beam is constantly aimed at the tumor (axis), while in a fixed SSD technique (B), the axis of rotation is placed on the patient's skin surface away from the tumor. To prevent missing the tumor, the patient must be moved laterally and, to adjust the SSD, up or down as well.

In a fixed SSD technique, small errors in SSD are not balanced out in an opposing field, as they are in the SAD method, because the patient is moved to adjust the SSD in this technique. The error in dose could in fact be doubled if the distance error is in the same direction in both fields. The only references available in setting up this treatment technique are skin marks. These unreliable references can cause considerable error in field placement. Small errors in angle can also cause geometric misses of the target since the axis of rotation is now placed at considerable distance from the target (Fig. 3.11). In principle, this can be corrected by shifting the patient laterally and, on a curved surface, also higher or lower, but in practice, the correct shift is often difficult to achieve. Another source of error is the difficulty in precisely setting the SSD when the field central axis is on a very steep-sloping surface or on the posterior surface of a supine patient.

The isocentric, or SAD, technique is obviously superior to an SSD technique. However, some therapy units do not have a rotating gantry, thus precluding isocentric techniques (Fig. 2.13 in Chapter 2).

ISODOSE DISTRIBUTION

It is not sufficient to have information about the dose at various depths along the central axis only. In addition, the dose distribution must be known for a large number of field sizes and for different treatment conditions. Dose distributions are usually measured in a phantom for a large number of field sizes and are plotted in terms of *isodose curves*. An isodose curve is one passing through points of equal dose and representing percentage of dose at a reference point.

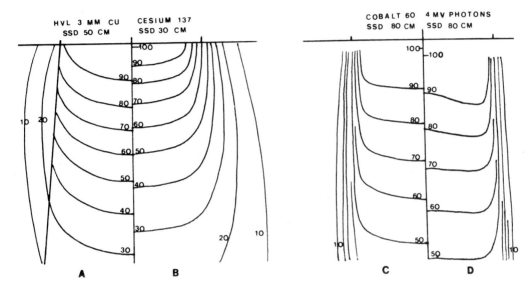

Fig. 3.12. Comparison of isodose charts from various beams all of them normalized to 100% at D_{max}. Only one half of each isodose chart is shown for each beam energy.

ISODOSE CHARTS

Isodose charts consist of a number of isodose curves usually depicted in 10% increments. Dose at other points can be found by interpolating between the lines. Figure 3.12 shows isodose distributions produced of different energy beams. Not only are the %DD along the central axis different for the various beam energies, but the shape of the isodose curves are also quite different.

Field Size

The geometric field size is usually defined by the intersection of the 50% isodose line and the surface (Fig. 3.13). The light source, which coincides with the beam, is aligned to match the 50% isodose line in the majority of treatment units (Figs. 3.15, 3.16, and 3.20). Knowledge of the field size is of particular importance in finding the field separation that will result in optimal dose uniformity across adjoining fields.

Penumbra

Penumbra is the region near the edge of the field margin where the dose falls rapidly. The width of the penumbra depends on the size of the radiation source, the distance from the source to the distal part of the collimator, and the source-to-surface distance (Fig. 3.13). The penumbra of a cobalt-60 beam is relatively wide compared with that of a linear accelerator. This is primarily due to the larger radiation source in the cobalt-60 machine, but also to the target-collimator distance, the SSD, and the scattered dose.

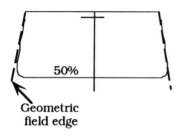

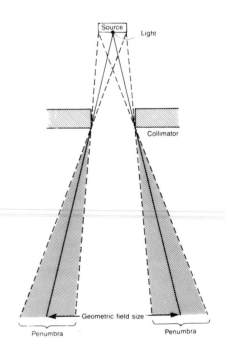

Fig. 3.13. Above: The geometric field size is usually defined by the intersection of the 50% isodose line and the surface. Right: Light field defined by the solid lines compared with the penumbra (hatched lines).

Beam Flatness

Isodose charts reveal information regarding the dose away from the central axis. In Fig. 3.12, it is evident that in the isodose chart for a cobalt-60 machine, the dose decreases away from the central axis, while the isodose distribution for the 4 MV beam shows that the dose away from the central axis is increased. This is particularly evident near the surface and is a result of overflattening of the beam at shallow depths, which is necessary in order to flatten the isodose curves at greater depths (Chapter 2). Without a beam-flattening filter, the dose from a linear accelerator on the central axis would be much higher than away from the central axis. The flattening filter reduces the dose along the central axis and produces a flat beam at a specified depth, usually 10 cm. Figure 3.4 in *Treatment Planning and Dose Calculation in Radiation Oncology* shows the effect of the flattening filter.

Dose Normalization

In isodose charts for a fixed SSD treatment technique, the reference point customarily is at D_{max}. The dose at this point is usually fixed at 100% (normalized to 100%). In an isodose chart for an isocentric technique (fixed SAD), the reference point is at the isocenter.

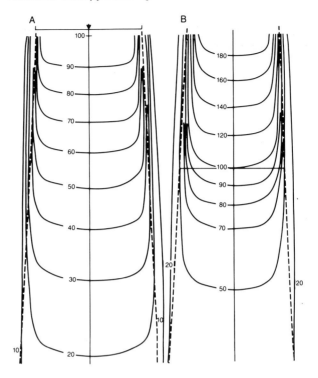

Fig. 3.14. An isodose distribution with fixed SSD (left) is normalized to 100% at D_{max}. In a fixed SAD (right), the dose is normalized to 100% at the isocenter.

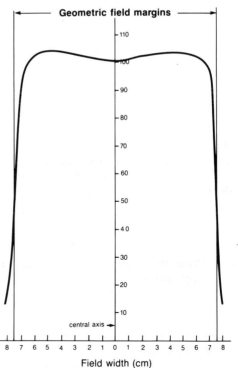

Fig. 3.15. A dose profile plotted across a 15 cm field at D_{max} in Fig. 3.20A. The dose is normalized to 100% on the central axis.

Two methods of normalizing the dose are shown in Fig. 3.14. It is quite easy to determine the dose at any given point in tissue if the dose at the normalization point is known. For example, if 100 cGy is delivered at D_{max} in field A in Fig. 3.14, it is clear that 50 cGy is delivered at any given point along the 50% isodose line.

DOSE PROFILES

Dose variation across a field at a given depth can be ascertained from the corresponding isodose curves and is best represented by a dose profile (Fig. 3.15). The dose profile displays relative doses across a field or across a treatment plan consisting of multiple beams.

BEAM'S-EYE VIEW

Another method of depicting dose variations within a field at a given depth is in the "beam's-eye view" shown in Fig. 3.16. These isodose curves are shown in a plane perpendicular to the central axis of the beam. Although unconventional, this representation of the dose distribution is sometimes useful, particularly in three-dimensional treatment planning.

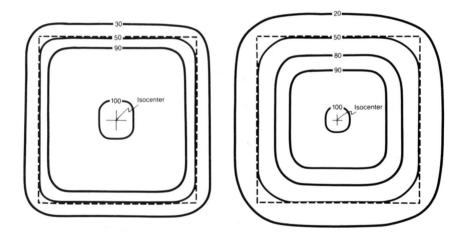

Fig. 3.16. Beam's-eye view of the isodose distribution of a 4 MV photon beam (left) and a cobalt-60 beam (right). The hatched lines indicate the geometric field margins. Note the wider penumbra in the cobalt-60 beam.

WEDGES

Frequently, beam-modifying absorbers (sometimes called filters) are inserted in the path of a beam. The most commonly used beam-modifying filter is a wedge-shaped piece of dense material, usually lead, which attenuates the beam progressively across the field (Fig. 3.17). The thinner side of the wedge attenuates the beam less than the thicker side, resulting in tilted isodose curves as shown in Fig. 3.18. The degree of the resulting tilt depends on the shape and the composition of the wedge.

The wedge angle refers to the angle through which an isodose curve is tilted at the central axis of the beam at a specified depth. The specification of a depth is critical because the degree of tilt changes with depth. The tilt decreases at greater depth because of the increased effect of scattered radiation. While there is no general agreement as to the reference depth, some chose to define the wedge angle at the intersection of the central axis of the beam and the 50% isodose curve. This becomes quite impractical when high-energy beams are used and also because different methods of dose normalization is practiced.

It should be noted that the wedge angle refers to the tilt of the isodose curve, *not* the angle of the actual wedge filter. A wedge that will produce a 45° tilt (wedge angle), for example, is often spoken of as a "45° wedge," though as just explained, the wedge material itself may have quite a different slope.

Wedge filters producing 15°, 30°, 45°, and 60° isodose curves are usually available from the manufacturer of radiation therapy machines. Other angles of isodose tilt can be attained by combining open (unwedged) beams with wedged beams (Tatcher 1970, Zwicker 1985).

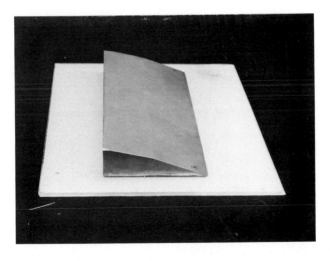

Fig. 3.17. A typical 45° wedge.

The wedge progressively attenuates the beam across the entire field, thus also decreasing the dose rate at the central axis. A wedge transmission factor must therefore be included in the dose calculation. The wedge transmission factor expresses the ratio of the dose rates on the central axis with and without the wedge. Some commercial isodose charts are normalized with the wedge transmission factor included (Fig. 3.18). In such an isodose chart, the isodose line at D_{max} along the central axis represents the wedge transmission factor and the other isodose lines also reflect the attenuation caused by the wedge. No transmission factor should be included in the dose calculation when such prenormalized isodose charts are used.

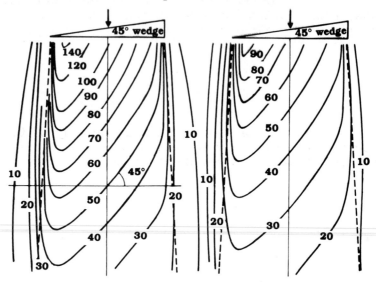

Fig. 3.18. The effect of a 45° wedge inserted in a cobalt-60 beam. On the left, the dose is normalized to 100% at D_{max} on the central axis, meaning that the dose calculation must include the wedge transmission factor. On the right, the isodose distribution includes the effect of the wedge transmission, that is, the dose at D_{max} on the central axis is roughly 70%, meaning the wedge transmission factor is 0.70.

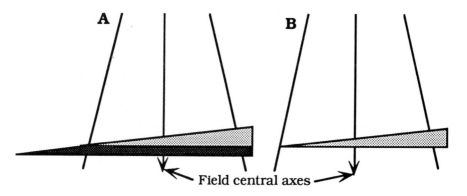

Fig. 3.19. A universal wedge, (A) with the center of the wedge always fixed in the center of the beam and the field can be opened to practically any width. An unused segment of the wedge (darker shading) only reduces the dose rate. In (B) an individualized wedge is used where the thin edge of the wedge is always aligned with the field margin.

A universal wedge is a wedge of a given angle which is fixed in the beam and serves all beam widths up to a designated limit. As illustrated in Fig. 3.19, when a small field is used, only a small thickness of the wedge is needed in producing the isodose tilt. The remainder of the wedge thickness attenuates the beam the same amount across the field, thus unnecessarily reducing the dose rate. For cobalt-60 units, where dose rates are already relatively low, a universal wedge system would be quite impractical as it would further reduce the dose rate. An individualized wedge system is therefore preferred. The individualized system consists of multiple wedges for each isodose tilt. Each wedge is designed for a particular field width and is mounted so that the thin edge of the wedge coincides with the edge of the light field. The beam will, therefore, pass through minimal thickness of wedge material and thus minimally reduce the dose rate.

Wedges inserted in the beam will only reshape already existing isodose curves. Isodose curves from linear accelerators usually show higher dose away from the central axis, especially at shallow depths. A wedge inserted in such a beam will only decrease the already higher dose under the thick section of the wedge. Under the thin section of the wedge, the dose is further increased, resulting in isodose curves shaped as in Fig. 3.20.

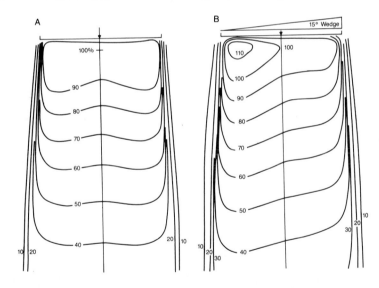

Fig. 3.20. A typical isodose distribution from a 4 MV photon beam in (A). In (B) a 15° wedge is used in the same beam. The isodose curves under the thick part of the wedge is now fairly flat, while under the thin segment the dose with respect to the central-axis dose is increased.

Dynamic Wedging

With modern treatment machines, equipped with independently moving collimator leaves (Chapter 2), a wedge effect can be produced by driving one of the collimator leaves across the field, thus gradually increasing the field size. The side of the field where the starting position of the moving leaf is located will thus receive a higher dose than the side where its final position is located. The speed with which the collimator leaf moves will determine the angle of the sloping isodose curve. This technique is referred to as dynamic wedging and is best explained by Fig. 3.21.

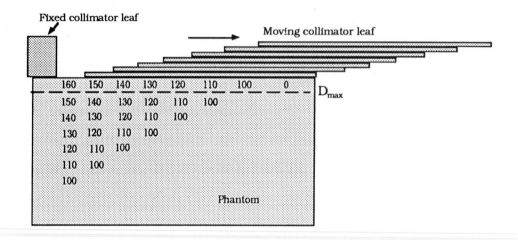

Fig. 3.21. Dynamic wedging is accomplished by having an independently moving collimator leaf move across the field during the treatment. The hatched line represent the depth of D_{max}. The dose at D_{max} on the right in the phantom is 0 because this point is fully shielded during this treatment. At the next step, 100 cGy is delivered at D_{max} because this point is only shielded during part of the treatment. The dose at D_{max} progressively increases towards the left where shielding was provided during progressively shorter time. As the D_{max} dose increases so does the dose at depth and if the points receiving 100 cGy in this case are connected, a sloping isodose curve result.

ELECTRON BEAMS

DOSE RATES

Dose rates and isodose distributions from electron beams are quite different from those of photon beams and are therefore discussed separately. Electron dose rates can vary considerably with field size and energy and from one linear accelerator to another, even when it is the same model. Extensive calibration must therefore be made for every electron energy and with each electron cone and field size. It is customary to fix the cGy/M.U. to 1.0 for a 10 x 10 cm cone at D_{max} and the cGy/M.U. for other cones, and field sizes are expressed as an output factor. Shaping of electron beams with secondary blocks also changes the dose rates and distributions requiring careful measurements of each field (Loevinger 1961, Hettinger 1967, Dutreix 1969, Khan 1976, 1984, 1991, Orton 1978, McGinley 1979, Niroomand-Rad 1986, Khan 1991). Frequent constancy checks of electron dose rates are essential.

PERCENTAGE DEPTH DOSE

The dose distribution from electron beams is characterized by relative uniformity within the first few centimeters in tissue followed by a very rapid fall-off of dose. The depth at which the rapid fall-off of dose sets in depends on the electron energy. As a guideline for selecting the appropriate electron energy for a given tumor, one can say that the electron energy in MeV should be three times the maximum depth of the tumor, that is, for a 3 cm treatment depth, a 9 MeV electron beam should be used. The isodose distribution varies with beam collimation, field size, cone design, etc. Typical depth dose curves for clinically useful electron energies are shown in Figs. 3.5 and 3.6 in *Treatment Planning and Dose Calculation in Radiation Oncology.*

Some skin sparing is afforded with electron beams especially with lower energies. The peak dose (D_{max}) is relatively broad, particularly with the higher energy electron beams.

ISODOSE CHARTS

Isodose curves for electron beams can vary from machine to machine due to differences in the design of the machine, collimating system, and cones. A library of isodose curves for each energy and cone or field size should therefore be obtained for each machine. The converging of the 90% and 80% isodose lines and the bulging out of the 50% and 20% isodose curves near the field edges is of considerable importance in treatment planning. Matching isodose curves of adjacent fields is practically impossible without causing "hot" or "cold" spots (see Chapter 6 in *Treatment Planning and Dose Calculation in Radiation Oncology*). Field margins must also be selected so that the target volume lies within the converging 90% line (Fig. 3.22).

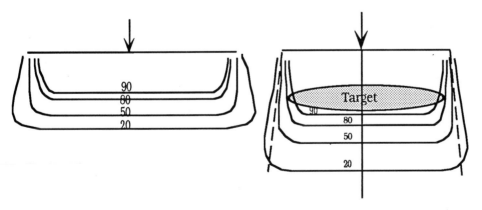

Fig. 3.22. Typical electron isodose curve (left). Field margins must be selected so that the tumor volume lies within the converging 90% isodose line (right).

Radiation Therapy Planning

REFERENCES

Badcock, P.C., Has CT scanning a role to play in radiotherapy planning? Computer dose calculations, Brit. J. Radiol. 55, 434 (1982).

Batho, H.F., Lung corrections in cobalt-60 beam therapy., J. Can. Assoc. Radiol. 15, 79 (1964).

Bentel, G.C., Nelson, C.E., Noell, K.T., Treatment Planning and Dose Calculation in Radiation Oncology, Pergamon Press, Inc. Elmsford, NY, 1989.

Cassell, K.J., Hobday, P.A., Parker, R.P., The implementation of a generalized Batho inhomogeneity correction for radiotherapy planning with direct use of CT numbers, Phys. Med. Biol. 26, 825 (1981).

Central Axis Depth Dose Data for use in Radiotherapy, Brit. J. Radiol. Supplement No. 11, The British Institute of Radiology, London, UK, 1972.

Central Axis Depth Dose Data for use in Radiotherapy, Brit. J. Radiol. Supplement No. 17, The British Institute of Radiology, London, UK, 1983.

Depth Dose Tables for Use in Radiotherapy, Brit. J. Radiol. Supplement No. 10, The British Institute of Radiology, London, UK, 1961.

Dutreix, J., Dutreix, A., Film dosimetry of high energy electrons, Ann. N.Y. Acad. Sci. 161, 33 (1969).

Epp, E.R., Lougheed, M.N., McKay, J.W., Ionization build-up in upper respiratory air passages during teletherapy units with cobalt-60 radiation, Brit. J. Radiol. 31, 361 (1958).

Epp, E.R., Boyer, A.L., Doppke, K.P., Underdosing of lesions resulting from lack of electronic equilibrium in upper respiratory air cavities irradiated by 10 MV x-ray beams, Int. J. Radiat. Oncol. Biol. Phys. 2, 613 (1977).

Fullerton, G.D., Sewchand, W., Payne, J.T., Levitt, S.H., CT determination of parameters for inhomogeneity corrections in radiation therapy of the esophagus, Radiology 124, 167 (1978).

Gerbi, B.J., Khan, F. M., Measurement of dose in the buildup region using fixed-separation plane-parallel ionization chambers, Medical Physics 17, 1 (1990).

Giese, R.A., McCullough, E.C., The use of CT scanners in megavoltage photon-beam therapy planning, Radiology 124, 133 (1977).

Gillin, M.T., Kline, R.W., Cox, J.D., Heterogeneity measurements and calculations in the absence of complete build-up, (Abstract) Proceedings of the 23rd Annual A.S.T.R. Meeting (1981).

Greene, D., Stewart, J.R., Isodose curves in non-uniform phantoms, Brit. J. Radiol. 38, 378 (1965).

Hettinger, G. Svensson, H., Photographic film for determination of isodose from betatron electron radiation, Acta. Radiol. 5, 74 (1967).

Hogstrom, K.R., Mills, M.D., Almond, P.R., Electron beam dose calculations, Phys. Med. Biol. 26, 445 (1981).

Holt, J.G., Laughlin, J.S., Moroney, J.P., The extension of the concept of tissue air ratios to high energy x-ray beams, Radiology 96, 437 (1970).

Jette, D, Bielajew, A., Electron dose calculation using multiple-scattering theory: Second-order multiple-scattering theory, Medical Physics 16, 5 (1989).

Jette, D., Lanzi, L.H., Pagnamenta, A., Rozenfeld, M., Bernard, D., Kao, M., Sabbas, A.M., Electron dose calculation using multiple-scattering theory: Thin planar inhomogeneities, Medical Physics 16, 5 (1989).

Johns, H. E., Cunningham, J.R., The Physics of Radiology, (4th ed.), Charles C. Thomas, Springfield, IL, 1983.

Karzmark, C.J., Dewbert, A., Loevinger, R., Tissue-phantom ratios - an aid to treatment planning, Brit. J. Radiol. 38, 158 (1965).

Khan, F.M., Moore, V.C., Levitt, S.H., Field shaping in electron beam therapy, Brit. J. Radiol. 49, 883 (1976).

Khan, F.M., The Physics of Radiation Therapy, William & Wilkins, Baltimore, MD, 1984.

Khan, F.M., Doppke, K.P., Hogstrom, K.R., Kutcher, G.J., Nath, R., Prasad, S.C., Purdy, J.A., Rozenfeld, M., Werner, B.L., Clinical electron-beam dosimetry: Report of AAPM Radiation Therapy Committee Task Group No. 25, Medical Physics 18, 73 (1991).

Loevinger, R., Karzmark, C.J., Weissbluth, M., Radiation dosimetry with high energy electrons, Radiology 77, 906 (1961).

Mayneord, W.V., Lamerton, L.F., A survey of depth dose data, Brit. J. Radiol. 14, 255 (1941).

McDonald, S.C., Keller, B.E., Rubin, P., Method for calculating dose when lung tissue lies in the treatment field, Medical Physics 3, 210 (1976).

McGinley, P.H., McLaren, J.R., Barnett, B.R., Small electron beams in radiation therapy, Radiology 131, 231 (1979).

Meli, J., Output factors and dose calculations for blocked x-ray fields, Medical Physics 13, (1986).

Mira, J.G., Fullerton, G.D., Ezekiel, J., Potter, J.L., Evaluation of computed tomography numbers for treatment planning of lung cancer, Int. J. Radiat. Oncol. Biol. Phys. 8, 1625 (1982).

Mohan, R., Chui, C., Miller, D., Laughlin, J.S., Use of computerized tomography in dose calculations for radiation treatment planning, CT: The Journal of Computed Tomography 5, 273 (1981).

Nilsson, B., Schnell, P.O., Build-up studies at air cavities measured with thin thermoluminescent dosimeters, Acta. Radiol. (Ther.) 15, 427 (1976).

Niroomand-Rad. A., Gillin, M.T., Kline, R.W., Grimm, D.F., Film dosimetry of small electron beams for routine radiotherapy planning, Medical Physics 13, 416 (1986).

Orton, C.G., Bagne, F., (eds), Practical Aspects of Electron Beam Treatment Planning, AAPM Publication, American Institute of Physics, New York, NY, 1978.

Orton, C.G., Mondalek, P.M., Spicka, J.T., Herron, D.S., Andres, L.I., Lung corrections in photon beam treatment planning: Are we ready? Int. J. Radiat. Oncolo. Biol. Phys. 10, 2191- 2199 (1984).

Orton, C.G., Herskovic, A., A proposal for universal introduction of lung corrections, Int. J. Radiat. Oncol. Biol. Phys. 10, 2383 (1984).

Parker, R.P., Hobday, P.A., Cassell, K.J., The direct use of CT numbers in radiotherapy dosage calculations for inhomogeneous media, Phys. Med. Biol. 24, 802 (1979).

Sontag, M.R., Battista, J.J., Bronskill, M.J., Cunningham, J.R., Implications of computed tomography for inhomogeneity corrections in photon beam dose calculations, Radiology 124, 143 (1977).

Sontag, M.R., Cunningham, J.R., The equivalent tissue-air ratio method for making absorbed dose calculations in heterogeneous medium, Radiology 129, 787 (1978).

Sundblom, L., Dose planning for irradiation of thorax with cobalt in fixed beam therapy, Acta Radiol. 3, 342 (1965).

Tatcher, M., A method for varying the effective angle of wedge filters. Radiology 97, 132 (1970).

Van Dyk, J., Battista, J.J., Rider, W.D., Half-body radiotherapy: The use of computed tomography to determine the dose to lung, Int. J. Radiat. Oncol. Biol. Phys. 6, 463 (1980).

Van Dyk, J., Keane, J.J., Rider, W.D., Lung density as measured by computed tomography: Implications for radiotherapy, Int. J. Radiat. Oncol. Biol. Phys. 8, 1363 (1982).

Van Dyk, J., Lung dose calculations using computerized tomography: Is there a need for pixel based procedures? Int. J. Radiat. Oncol. Biol. Phys. 9, 1035 (1983).

Wong, J.W., Henkelman, R.M., A new approach to CT pixel-based photon dose calculations in heterogeneous media, Medical Physics 10, 199 (1983).

Young, M.E.J., Gaylord, J.D., Experimental test of corrections for tissue inhomogeneities in radiotherapy, Brit. J. Radiol. 43, 349 (1970).

Zwicker, R.D., Shahabi, S., Wu, A., Sternick, E.S., Effective wedge angles for 6-MV wedges, Medical Physics 12, 347 (1985).

PROBLEMS

1. 1 Gy is the same as

    a)   1 rad
    b)   10 cGy
    c)   100 cGy
    d)   1 erg

2. Radiation dose is often determined using the following methods:

    a)   TLD
         photodynamic therapy
         ionization chambers

    b)   photographic film
         TLD *(thermo luminescant dosemeter)*
         ionization chambers

    c)   ionization chambers
         TLD
         film badges

3. The point of maximum electron equilibrium is referred to as

    a)   TAD
    b)   SFD
    c)   MEE
    d) D_{max}

4. A HVT is a way of expressing   *Half Value thickness*

    a)   the filtration of a beam
    b)   the dose
    c)   the quality of the beam *(or the hardness)*
    d)   the TAR

5. Dose rates in air express

    a)   the dose measured for a 10 x 10 cm field at a 10 cm depth in a
         phantom
    b)   the dose measured without a phantom and with a build-up cap *(air)*
         at a given distance
    c)   the dose measured without a phantom and without a build-up
         cap at a given distance

d)   the dose measured without a built-up cap for a 10 x 10 cm field at a given distance

6.   Dose rates

a)   decrease with increased field size and increase with increased distance

b)   increase with increased field size and decrease with decreased distance

c)   increase with increased field size and decrease with increased distance *(inverse sq law for distance)* $\left(\frac{SSD_1}{SSD_2}\right)^2$

7.   Increasing the distance from 80 cm to 90 cm causes the dose rate to change by $\left(\frac{80}{90}\right)^2 = 0.7901$

a)   0.8095
b)   0.8111
c)   0.6400
d)   0.7901

8.   Percentage depth dose is dependent on   *= energy, field size, SSD + composition of matter*

a)   SSD
      distance
      treatment time

b)   distance
      field size
      cGy/M.U.

c)   field size
      distance
      energy

d)   energy
      tissue density
      treatment time

9.   The correct match is represented by which option (1, 2, 3, or 4) below?

a)   the ratio of dose at a specified point in tissue or in a phantom to the dose at the same distance in the beam at a reference depth *= TPR*

b)   the ratio of the dose at a specified point in tissue or in a phantom to the dose at the same point when it is at the depth of maximum dose *(dmax) = TMR*

c)   the ratio of the dose at a specified point in a medium to the dose
      at the same point in free space— *an*

1) a) TAR   2) a) TPR   3) a) TMR   4) a) TPR
    b) TPR   b) TMR   b) TPR   b) TAR
    c) TMR   c) TAR   c) TAR   c) TMR

10.   The TAR at 5 cm depth for a 10 x 10 cm field, minus the TAR at 5 cm
      depth for a 0 x 0 cm field gives the

      a)   TMR
      b)   SAR
      c)   TPR
      d)   SMR

11.   In a fixed SSD technique, the dose is routinely normalized *ie you
      have 100% at:*

      a)   at the isocenter
      b)   at tumor depth
      c)   at D_{max} *for a single field or midplane for
             multiple field*
      d)   on the surface

12.   In an isocentric treatment technique, the dose is routinely
      normalized

      a)   at the isocenter / *midplane*
      b)   at the tumor depth
      c)   at D_{max}
      d)   on the surface

13.   The width of the penumbra *increases* with

      a)   decreased SSD
           decreased source-collimator distance
           decreased field size

      b)   decreased SSD
           increased source-collimator distance
           increased source size

      c)   increased SSD
           decreased source-collimator distance
           increased source size

d)   increased SSD
increased source-collimator distance
decreased source size

14.   Wedge angles refer to

a)   the angle of the actual wedge filter

this is correct b)   the angle at which an isodose curve at a specified depth is tilted as a result of the wedge being inserted in the beam

c)   the angle at which an isodose curve at a specified depth is tilted with respect to the central axis of the beam

15.   A guide for determining the needed electron beam energy (in MeV) is to

a)   divide the maximum tumor depth in centimeters by 3

b)   divide the 80% isodose line by 10 and then by the maximum tumor depth in centimeters

c)   multiply the maximum tumor depth in centimeters by 5 and then divide by 3

d)   multiply the maximum tumor depth in centimeters by 3 *because of rapid fall off?*

16. In a typical electron beam, which of the following statements is true?

a)   all of the isodose curves in the penumbra region bulge out, causing great difficulties in uniformly matching adjacent electron fields

b)   only the 50% to 90% isodose lines bulge out in the penumbra region, causing great difficulties in uniformly matching adjacent electron fields

c)   only the 10% to 50% isodose lines bulge out in the penumbra region, causing great difficulties in uniformly matching adjacent electron fields

d)   all of the isodose lines converge in the penumbra region, causing great difficulties in uniformly matching adjacent electron fields

SOLUTIONS

1.	c	9.	2
2.	b	10.	b
3.	d	11.	c
4.	c	12.	a
5.	b	13.	c
6.	c	14.	b
7.	d	15.	d
8.	c	16.	c

CHAPTER 4

DOSE CALCULATION FOR EXTERNAL BEAMS - PART I

The problems in this chapter assume that the reader has read and fully understand Chapter 3.

Some of the factors used in the dose calculations in this chapter may be eliminated depending on how the available data is presented. For example, it is customary to present the dose rate for a cobalt-60 unit for a 10 x 10 cm field and then have a table of area factors for other field sizes. An area factor is the ratio of the dose rate for a given field size to that of a reference field size, usually 10 x 10 cm. The dose rate for a reference field multiplied by the area factor for the treated field gives the dose rate for the treated field. On the other hand, the dose rates may have been measured and tabulated for a large number of field sizes, which eliminates the need for an area factor. Likewise, the cGy/M.U. may have been set so that one cGy is the same as one M.U. for a reference field, which again, is usually a 10 x 10 cm field.

In this text, the reference dose rate and cGy/M.U. (dose rate$_{ref}$ or cGy/M.U.$_{ref}$) are for a 10 x 10 cm field.

The two most commonly used techniques in treating patients are with a fixed source-surface distance (SSD) or a fixed source-axis distance (SAD). The SSD method requires moving the patient between treatment of each field to adjust the SSD so that it is the same for every field with obvious inconvenience, delay, and lack of precision. The methods used in calculating dose in the patient are different in these two techniques. Percentage depth dose, which requires that the source-surface distance be constant, is used in the SSD technique, while TAR, TPR, or TMR, which require a fixed SAD, is used in the SAD technique. The following text will give examples of dose calculation on the central axis for square fields using both methods.*

FIXED SOURCE-SURFACE DISTANCE TECHNIQUE

The technique using fixed SSD and percentage depth dose (%DD) is practical when single fields are used. Single fields are not recommended for deep-seated lesions because of the fall-off of dose with depth and the resulting dose gradient through the tissues. Whether one can use a single-field or multiple fields to treat a tumor must be determined for each situation. The criteria are

a) depth of maximum dose (surface or D_{max}
b) dose gradient throughout the tumor
c) availability of other alternatives

In this section, typical dose calculations are shown using a fixed source-surface distance and a variety of beam energies.

DOSE CALCULATION AT DEPTH OF MAXIMUM DOSE

Treatment of shallow lesions through a single field is sometimes desirable. The dose is then prescribed either at D_{max} or at an appropriate depth. Shallow lesions are best treated using beams of low penetrating power such as superficial, lower orthovoltage, or electron beams. Single field treatment, using higher energy beams, is considered in this text only for the purpose of dose calculation.

In the majority of instances, dose calculation consists of finding the required treatment time or of the number of monitor units needed to deliver the prescribed treatment. However, in some instances it is necessary to find what dose was delivered during a certain period of time or while a certain number of monitor units were given. This could happen, for example, when the treatment was interrupted prior to completion either because the patient became ill or because the machine failed. In these situations, it is necessary to determine what dose was in fact delivered. In the next few examples, we will calculate *both* the required treatment time, or M.U., and what dose was delivered during the treatment.

---

* All data tables used in the dose calculations are labelled A.1- A.8 and can be found in an appendix at the end of this volume (pages 337 - 344).

Superficial Beams

Consider the treatment of a 5 x 5 cm field using a beam with a HVT of 2 mm Cu. The SSD is 50 cm and the dose rate without the patient present, sometimes referred to as in air, is 68 cGy/min at 50 cm distance. The backscatter factor is 1.145.

To find the treatment time for the prescribed dose

$$\text{Time} = \frac{\text{prescribed dose}}{\text{dose rate in air} \times \text{backscatter}} \qquad (4.1)$$

The prescription is for 200 cGy at D_{max}, which in this case is the surface.

The treatment time is found from

$$\frac{200}{68 \times 1.145} = 2.57 \text{ min (2 min 34 sec)}$$

The dose rate at the surface in the above expression is found from

Dose rate at the surface = time x dose rate in air x backscatter factor   (4.2)

$$1 \text{ min} \times 68 \times 1.145 \text{ cGy} = 77.9 \text{ cGy/min}$$

Electron Beams

Consider the same treatment as in the above example, but this time with 6 MeV electrons. The SSD is 95 cm and the dose rate$_{ref}$ for a 10 x 10 cm field is 1.0 and for a 5 x 5 cm field it is 0.643. The prescription is 200 cGy at D_{max}, which is at 1.5 cm of depth for the 6 MeV electron beam.

To find the M.U. necessary to deliver the prescribed dose at D_{max}

$$\text{M.U.} = \frac{\text{prescribed dose}}{\text{cGy/M.U. (field}_{ref}) \times \text{cGy/M.U. (tx. field)}} \qquad (4.3)$$

To deliver 200 cGy at D_{max} the required M.U. would therefore be

$$\frac{200}{1.0 \times 0.643} = 311 \text{ M.U.}$$

The cGy/M.U. at D_{max} in the above expression is found from

cGy/M.U. = M.U. × cGy/M.U. (field$_{ref}$) × cGy/M.U. (tx. field)   (4.4)

$$1 \text{ M.U.} \times 0.643 \text{ cGy} = 0.643 \text{ cGy/M.U. at } D_{max}$$

Cobalt-60 Beams

Consider the same treatment as in the previous examples but using a cobalt-60 unit at 80 cm SSD. The dose rate$_{ref}$ at D_{max} is 114 cGy/min for a 10 x 10 cm field. The area factor for a 5 x 5 cm field is 0.92.

To find the treatment time necessary to deliver the prescribed dose at D_{max}

$$\text{Time} = \frac{\text{prescribed dose}}{\text{dose rate}_{ref} \times \text{ area factor}} \qquad (4.5)$$

To deliver 200 cGy at D_{max}, which for cobalt-60 is at 0.5 cm depth, the treatment time would be

$$\frac{200}{114 \times 0.92} = 1.91 \text{ min (1 min 55 sec)}$$

The dose rate at D_{max} in the above expression is found from

$$\text{Dose rate at } D_{max} = \text{time} \times \text{dose rate}_{ref} \times \text{area factor} \qquad (4.6)$$

$$1.0 \text{ min} \times 114 \times 0.92 = 104.9 \text{ cGy/min}$$

Linear Accelerator Beams

Consider the same treatment as in the previous examples but using a 4 MV photon beam at 80 cm SSD. The dose rate$_{ref}$ is 1.0 cGy/M.U. for a 10 x 10 cm field. The cGy/M.U. factor for a 5 x 5 cm field is 0.945.

To find the M.U. necessary to deliver prescribed D_{max} dose

$$\text{MU} = \frac{\text{prescribed dose}}{\text{cGy/M.U.}} \qquad (4.7)$$

To deliver 200 cGy at D_{max}, which for 4 MV is at 1 cm depth, the number of M.U. would be

$$\frac{200}{0.945} = 212 \text{ M.U.}$$

The dose rate at D_{max} in the above expression was found from

$$\text{Dose rate at } D_{max} = \text{M.U.} \times \text{cGy/M.U.} \qquad (4.8)$$

$$1 \text{ M.U.} \times 0.945 = 0.945 \text{ cGy/M.U.}$$

DOSE CALCULATION AT A DEPTH FOR A SINGLE FIELD

In the following examples, the dose prescribed for treatment of a tumor at 5 cm depth is calculated using the same variables as in the previous section except that the field size is increased to 8 x 8 cm.

Superficial Beams

Using a beam with a HVT of 2 mm Cu, 50 cm SSD and an 8 x 8 cm field the dose rate without the patient present is 68 cGy/min. Note that the dose rate without the patient present is the same as for the 5 x 5 cm field used in an earlier example. The backscatter factor, however, is 1.250, which is considerably higher than for the 5 x 5 cm field. The percentage depth dose at 5 cm depth for an 8 x 8 cm field at 50 cm SSD is 64.9%. For each 100 cGy delivered at D_{max}, the dose at 5 cm depth is 64.9 cGy.

The treatment time necessary to deliver the prescribed dose is found from

$$\text{Time} = \frac{\text{prescribed dose}}{\text{dose rate in air} \times \text{BSF} \times \text{\%DD}} \tag{4.9}$$

To deliver 200 cGy at 5 cm depth the treatment time would be

$$\frac{200 \times 100}{68 \times 1.250 \times 64.9} = 3.63 \text{ min (3 min 38 sec)}$$

As a check, we note that the dose delivered at a depth in the above example is

$$\text{Depth dose} = \text{time} \times \text{dose rate in air} \times \text{BSF} \times \text{\%DD} \tag{4.10}$$

$$3.63 \text{ min} \times 68 \times 1.250 \times 64.9/100 = 200 \text{ cGy}$$

which is correct.

Electron Beams

In this example, a 14 MeV electron beam is used. The SSD is 95 cm and the field size is 8 x 8 cm. The dose rate$_{ref}$ is 0.953 cGy/M.U. for a 10 x 10 cm field. The area factor for an 8 x 8 cm field is 0.995 and the percentage depth dose at 5 cm depth is 80%. (Note that the cGy/M.U. for the 14 MeV electron beam is different from that of the 6 MeV electron beam used in an earlier example, the area factors vary with field size, cones, and energies.)

The M.U. necessary to deliver the prescribed dose at depth is found from

$$\text{M.U.} = \frac{\text{prescribed dose}}{\text{cGy/M.U.} \times \text{area factor} \times \text{\%DD}} \tag{4.11}$$

To deliver 200 cGy at 5 cm depth (80% isodose line), the number of M.U. would be

$$\frac{200 \times 100}{0.953 \times 0.995 \times 80} = 264 \text{ M.U.}$$

The dose delivered at a depth in the above example is found from

$$\text{Depth dose} = \text{M.U.} \times \text{cGy/M.U.} \times \text{area factor} \times \%DD \qquad (4.12)$$

or

$$264 \text{ M.U.} \times 0.953 \times 0.995 \times 80/100 = 200 \text{ cGy}$$

Cobalt-60 Beams

Using a cobalt-60 unit at 80 cm SSD and an 8 x 8 cm field, 200 cGy is to be delivered at 5 cm depth. The dose rate$_{ref}$ for a 10 x 10 cm field is 114 cGy/min. The area factor is 0.985 for a 8 x 8 cm field and the percentage depth dose from Table A.1 is 77.4%. (Note that the dose rate is unchanged from the example of the previous cobalt-60 beam calculation but the area factor for this larger field is increased.)

The treatment time necessary to deliver the prescribed dose at a depth is found from

$$\text{Time} = \frac{\text{prescribed dose}}{\text{dose rate}_{ref} \times \text{area factor} \times \%DD} \qquad (4.13)$$

To deliver 200 cGy, the treatment time would be

$$\frac{200 \times 100}{114 \times 0.985 \times 77.4} = 2.30 \text{ min (2 min 18 sec)}$$

The dose delivered at a depth in the above example is found from

$$\text{Dose} = \text{time} \times \text{dose rate}_{ref} \times \text{area factor} \times \%DD \qquad (4.14)$$

$$2.30 \times 114 \times 0.985 \times 77.4/100 = 200 \text{ cGy}$$

Linear Accelerator Beams

Using a 4 MV photon beam at 80 cm SSD and an 8 x 8 cm field, 200 cGy is to be delivered at 5 cm depth. The cGy/M.U.$_{ref}$ is 1.0 for a 10 x 10 cm field and 0.99 for an 8 x 8 cm field. From Table A.2 the %DD is 81.8.

The M.U. necessary to deliver the prescribed dose at a depth is found from

$$\text{M.U.} = \frac{\text{prescribed dose}}{\text{cGy/M.U.} \times \%DD} \qquad (4.15)$$

To deliver 200 cGy, the required number of M.U. would be

$$\frac{200 \times 100}{0.99 \times 81.8} = 247 \text{ M.U.}$$

The dose delivered at a depth in the above example is found from

$$\text{Depth dose} = \text{M.U.} \times \text{cGy/M.U.} \times \%DD \qquad (4.16)$$

$$247 \text{ M.U.} \times 0.99 \times 81.8/100 = 200 \text{ cGy}$$

DOSE CALCULATION FOR PARALLEL OPPOSED BEAMS WITH EQUAL WEIGHTING

Parallel opposed beams are the most commonly used field arrangement. This technique is best suited for situations where reasonable dose uniformity throughout the target volume is desired. This section deals with the dose calculation of this and other multiple field techniques. Treatment techniques and field arrangements are discussed in Chapters 6 and 7 of *Treatment Planning and Dose Calculation in Radiation Oncology* (Bentel 1989). Superficial and electron beams are not suited for multiple-field arrangements, so the dose calculations in this section will be limited to that of cobalt-60 beams and linear accelerators.

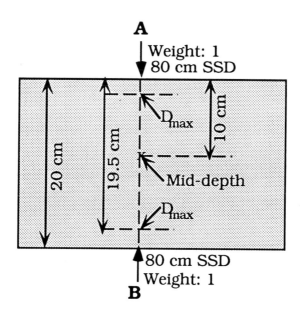

Fig. 4.1. Parallel opposed beams using 80 cm SSD and weighted equally.

Equal weighting implies equal dose somewhere. In a fixed SSD technique, it is customary to normalize the entrance dose of each field at D_{max} to 100% and to apply the weighting factor of each beam at this point. Weighting factors are usually expressed as ratios of the normalized dose at D_{max} from each field. Therefore, in an equally weighted parallel opposed field arrangement using a fixed SSD technique, the weighting would be 1 to 1 (Fig. 4.1).

Cobalt-60 Beams

In this example, it is assumed that 200 cGy is prescribed at mid-depth of a 20 cm thick patient. Two equally weighted, parallel opposed 15 x 15 cm fields are used at 80 cm SSD. The dose rate$_{ref}$ for a 10 x 10 cm field is 114 cGy/min. The area factor for a 15 x 15 cm field is 1.04 and the %DD at 10 cm depth from Table A.1 is 58.3.

The treatment time is found from

$$\text{Time} = \frac{\text{prescribed dose}}{\text{dose rate}_{ref} \times \text{area factor} \times \%DD} \qquad (4.17)$$

In this example, each field must deliver an equal D_{max} dose. Since all variables are identical for both fields, the tumor dose (T.D.) and the D_{max} dose will be the same for both fields.

The treatment time necessary to deliver 100 cGy at 10 cm depth is

$$\frac{100 \times 100}{114 \times 1.04 \times 58.3} = 1.45 \text{ min (1 min 27 sec)}$$

The D_{max} dose is found from

$$\text{Dose} = \text{time} \times \text{dose rate}_{ref} \times \text{area factor} \qquad (4.18)$$

so

$$1.45 \times 114 \times 1.04 = 172 \text{ cGy per field.}$$

Linear Accelerator Beams

Using the same example as above but with 4 MV photon beams, the calculation is very similar. The cGy/M.U. for a 15 x 15 cm field is 1.03 and the %DD from Table A.2 is 62.4.

The M.U. necessary to deliver 100 cGy at 10 cm depth is

$$\frac{100 \times 100}{1.03 \times 62.4} = 156 \text{ M.U.}$$

CALCULATING ENTRANCE AND EXIT DOSE FROM PARALLEL OPPOSED BEAMS WITH EQUAL WEIGHTING

Using the same treatment variables as in the previous cobalt-60 example, the total dose (entrance and exit) at the depth of D_{max} is calculated as follows.

Field A (Fig. 4.1) delivers 100% at D_{max}. Therefore, in the cobalt-60 treatment, using equation 4.18, the dose is 1.45 min x 114 cGy/min x 1.04, or 172 cGy. The %DD at 19.5 cm depth (the patient's thickness minus 0.5 cm, which is the depth of maximum dose for cobalt-60) from field B is only 31.3% of the D_{max} dose (Table A.1). Using equation 4.18, the exit dose from field B is 1.45 x 114 x 1.04 x 31.3%, which is 54 cGy.

The total dose at D_{max} is therefore 172 + 54 = 226 cGy. The dose can, in a similar manner, be calculated at any point on the central axis of parallel opposed fields.

Dose Ratios

In the previous example, it was found that the maximum dose was 226 cGy, while the midplane dose was 200 cGy.

The ratio of these two doses is found by

$$\text{Dose ratio} = \frac{\text{maximum dose}}{\text{midplane dose}} \qquad (4.19)$$

so the ratio of the entrance-exit dose and the midplane dose in the previous example is

$$\frac{226}{200} = 1.13$$

Multiplying the midplane dose by the ratio yields the maximum dose. If 4000 cGy is delivered at the midplane in the patient, the maximum dose is

$$4000 \times 1.13 = 4520 \text{ cGy}$$

DOSE CALCULATION FOR PARALLEL OPPOSED BEAMS WITH UNEQUAL WEIGHTING

Unequal weighting in a fixed SSD technique implies that a different dose is delivered at D_{max} of each field. The result is a higher dose in the tissue near the entrance of the favored field and a lower dose in the tissue near the entrance of the other field.

In the following example, a patient is treated for a parotid tumor using parallel opposed 10 x 10 cm fields and 80 cm SSD. The patient's thickness is 14 cm and the fields are weighted 2 to 1 favoring the right side. In this treatment, 4 MV photon beams are used, and the prescription is 200 cGy per fraction calculated at the patient's midline (Fig. 4.2).

The cGy/M.U. is 1.0 and the %DD at 7 cm depth from Table A.2 is 73.0%. Since the fields are identical and the dose is prescribed at the midline, the total M.U. required to deliver 200 cGy is found using equation 4.15.

$$\frac{200 \times 100}{1.0 \times 73.0} = 274 \text{ M.U.}$$

Two thirds of this dose is to be delivered from the patient's right side and one third from the left side, therefore

$$\text{Right side} \qquad \frac{2 \times 274}{3} = 183 \text{ M.U.}$$

$$\text{Left side} \qquad \frac{1 \times 274}{3} = 91 \text{ M.U.}$$

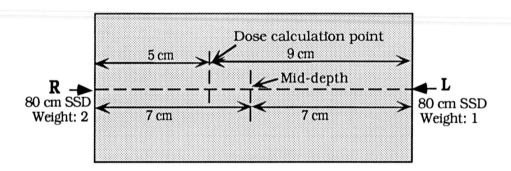

Fig. 4.2. Parallel opposed beams using 80 cm SSD and weighted 2 to 1 favoring the right side.

In the following example, the same treatment is given, but the dose is prescribed at 5 cm depth from the patient's right side (Fig. 4.2).

Using Table A.2, the %DD, from the patient's right side, at 5 cm depth, is 82.4% and from the left side, at 9 cm depth, it is 64.3%.

Since the D_{max} dose is weighted 2 to 1 and the tumor dose from each field is unknown, the combined M.U. required to deliver 200 cGy must be calculated first. The average %DD is found from

$$\frac{(82.4 \times 2) + 64.3}{3} = 76.4$$

The %DD from the right side is multiplied by two since the weighting from this side is such that the D_{max} dose is 200%.

The combined D_{max} dose is found from

$$D_{max} = \frac{\text{prescribed dose}}{\text{cGy/M.U.} \times \text{average \%DD}}$$
  (4.20)

so

$$\frac{200 \times 100}{1.0 \times 76.4} = 264 \text{ M.U.}$$

(cGy equals M.U. in this example since the cGy/M.U. is 1.0.)

Two thirds of this dose is delivered from the patient's right side and one third from the left side.

Right side: $\dfrac{2 \times 262}{3}$ = 175 M.U. (cGy at D_{max})

Left side: $\dfrac{1 \times 262}{3}$ = 87 M.U. (cGy at D_{max})

The tumor dose delivered from each side is found from

$$\text{Tumor dose} = \text{M.U.} \times \text{cGy/M.U.} \times \%DD$$
  (4.21)

so the tumor dose from the patient's right side is

$$175 \text{ M.U.} \times 1.0 \times 82.4\% = 144 \text{ cGy}$$

and the tumor dose from the patient's left side is

$$87 \text{ M.U.} \times 1.0 \times 64.3\% = 56 \text{ cGy}$$

CALCULATING ENTRANCE AND EXIT DOSE FROM PARALLEL OPPOSED BEAMS WITH UNEQUAL WEIGHTING

In an unequally weighted parallel opposed field arrangement, the dose at the depth of D_{max} of each field will be different.

Using the parameters in the previous example, the dose at D_{max} of each field is found as follows.

The right field (R) is weighted by a factor of 2 and the left field (L) is weighted by 1.

The dose at D_{max} of field R is found from

$$\text{Entrance + Exit dose} = (\text{M.U.}_R \times \text{cGy/M.U.}_R \times \%DD_R)$$

$$+ (\text{M.U.}_L \times \text{cGy/M.U.}_L \times \%DD_L) \qquad (4.22)$$

Via field R, 175 M.U. are delivered, and the cGy/M.U. is 1.0 and the %DD is 100. The %DD at 13 cm depth from L (patient's thickness minus depth of D_{max}) is 49.8% (Table A.2). Via field L, 87 M.U. are delivered, and the cGy/M.U. is 1.0. Using equation 4.22, the dose at D_{max} of field R is

$$(175 \times 1.0 \times 100/100) + (87 \times 1.0 \times 49.8/100) = 218 \text{ cGy}$$

The dose at D_{max} of field L is found by

$$\text{Entrance + Exit dose} = (\text{M.U.}_L \times \text{cGy/M.U.}_L \times \%DD_L)$$

$$+ (\text{M.U.}_R \times \text{cGy/M.U.}_R \times \%DD_R) \qquad (4.23)$$

The dose at D_{max} of field L is therefore

$$(87 \times 1.0 \times 100/100) + (175 \times 1.0 \times 49.8/100) = 174 \text{ cGy}$$

This shows a gradient of dose throughout the volume from a maximum of 218 cGy on the patient's right side to 174 cGy on the left side.

DOSE CALCULATION FOR MULTIPLE BEAMS WITH EQUAL WEIGHTING

Many treatment plans utilize multiple fields directed at a common target. Although such treatment plans are best delivered via isocentric techniques, for the purpose of this exercise, it is assumed to be delivered via a fixed SSD technique.

Composite isodose distributions are calculated and the dose is usually prescribed at an isodose line which encompasses the target volume. In this example, it is assumed that four equally weighted fields are used. Each field is 10 x 15 cm, the SSD is 80 cm, and a cobalt-60 unit is used to deliver the treatment. The dose rate$_{ref}$ at D_{max} for a 10 x 10 cm field is 114 cGy/min and the area factor is 1.035. The prescribed dose is 200 cGy at the 190% line (Fig. 4.3). Since the D_{max} dose is the same for all four fields and the combined %DD (190%) is the result of four 100% D_{max} doses, it is acceptable to assume that one fourth of 190% (47.5%) is delivered from each field. That, of course, is not true for all points along this isodose line.

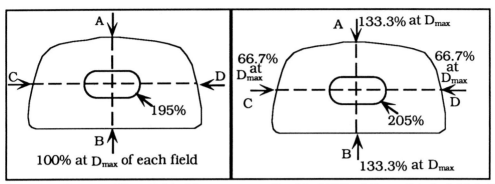

Fig. 4.3. Four equally weighted beams normalized to 100% at D_{max} of each field (left) result in a total %DD of 190% as indicated. The same field arrangement is used (right), but here two of the fields are weighted twice as heavily as the other two. The total %DD is 205% as indicated.

The average %DD in a multiple-field treatment plan can be found from

$$\frac{\text{total \%DD (isodose line)}}{\text{number of 100\% } D_{max} \text{ doses}} \qquad (4.24)$$

The required treatment time per field can be found from one of two methods:

1) $$\text{Treatment time per field} = \frac{\text{prescribed dose}}{\% \text{ isodose line} \times \text{dose rate} \times \text{area factor}} \qquad (4.25)$$

$$\frac{200 \times 100}{190 \times 114 \times 1.035} = 0.89 \text{ min/field (53 sec)}$$

or

2) $$\text{Treatment time per field} = \frac{\text{prescribed dose per field}}{\text{average \%DD} \times \text{dose rate} \times \text{area factor}} \qquad (4.26)$$

$$\frac{50 \times 100}{47.5 \times 114 \times 1.035} = 0.89 \text{ min /field (53 sec)}$$

The D_{max} dose per field is found from either

$$D_{max} \text{ dose} = \frac{\text{total prescribed dose}}{\text{isodose line}} \quad or \quad \frac{\text{dose per field}}{\text{average \%DD}} \qquad (4.27)$$

so

$$\frac{200 \times 100}{190} = 105 \text{ cGy} \quad or \quad \frac{50 \times 100}{47.5} = 105 \text{ cGy}$$

DOSE CALCULATION FOR MULTIPLE BEAMS WITH UNEQUAL WEIGHTING

In the next variation of the previous example the same treatment is delivered but it is assumed that two fields are weighted twice as heavily as the other two. The prescribed dose is 200 cGy at the 205% line (Fig. 4.3). The total D_{max} dose for all fields combined is still 400% but it is now distributed so that two fields are given one third each and the other two one sixth each of the combined D_{max} dose.

The combined D_{max} dose required for this treatment is found from

$$\text{Total } D_{max} \text{ dose} = \frac{\text{prescribed dose}}{\text{average \%DD}} \tag{4.28}$$

The average %DD is found from

$$\text{Average depth dose} = \frac{\text{isodose line}}{\text{number of 100\% } D_{max} \text{ doses}} \tag{4.29}$$

so

$$\frac{205}{4} = 51.3\%$$

and the combined D_{max} dose is

$$\frac{200 \times 100}{51.3} = 390 \text{ cGy}$$

$$\text{Two fields will receive } \frac{1 \times 390}{3} = 130 \text{ cGy each}$$

$$\text{Two fields will receive } \frac{1 \times 390}{6} = 65 \text{ cGy each}$$

In this particular example, the total %DD is higher than in the plan using equal weighting because the two fields with the heavier weighting deliver a higher %DD than the other two fields.

In the following example, a slightly different approach is used.

A patient is treated for carcinoma of the pancreas using a three-field technique. The anterior field is 12 x 8 cm with a small corner of the field blocked out. The right and left lateral fields are 8 x 8 cm and a 30° wedge is used in each field. All fields are treated at 80 cm SSD using a 4 MV photon beam. The anterior field is weighted by a factor of 2 and each lateral field by a factor of 1 (Fig. 4.4).

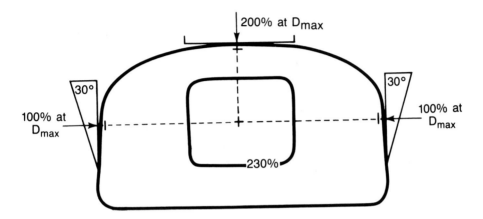

Fig. 4.4. A three-field technique with anterior field weighted twice as heavily as each lateral field. The combined %DD is 230%, which results from a total D_{max} dose of 400%.

Field	Anterior	Rt Lateral	Lt Lateral
SSD	80 cm	80 cm	80 cm
Beam energy	4 MV	4 MV	4 MV
Field size	12 x 8 cm	8 x 8 cm	8 x 8 cm
Eq. sq. field	9.5 cm^2	8 cm^2	8 cm^2
Isodose line	230%	230%	230%
Weighting f.	2.0	1.0	1.0
Tray factor	0.96	1.0	1.0
Wedge factor	1.0	0.71	0.71
cGy/M.U.	0.995	0.98	0.98

The prescribed dose is 200 cGy along the 230% isodose line. The treatment plan was calculated by entering 200% at D_{max} of the anterior field and 100% for each of the lateral fields. The average %DD is therefore 230/4 or 57.5% of each 100% D_{max} entrance dose. The combined D_{max} dose is therefore

$$\text{Combined } D_{max} \text{ dose} = \frac{\text{prescribed dose}}{\text{average } \%DD} \qquad (4.30)$$

$$\frac{200 \times 100}{57.5} = 348 \text{ cGy}$$

Two fourths or one half of this dose is to be delivered via the anterior field

or
$$\frac{1 \times 348}{2} = 174 \text{ cGy}$$

One fourth of the dose at D_{max} is to be delivered via each of the lateral fields

$$\frac{1 \times 348}{4} = 87 \text{ cGy}$$

The M.U. per field necessary to deliver the prescribed dose using correct weighting is found by

$$\text{M.U.} = \frac{\text{dose rate at } D_{max}}{\text{cGy/M.U.} \times \text{tray factor} \times \text{wedge factor}} \qquad (4.31)$$

The number of M.U. from the anterior field is therefore

$$\frac{174}{0.995 \times 0.96 \times 1.0} = 182 \text{ M.U.}$$

This field has no wedge so the wedge factor is 1.0 and could be omitted.

The number of M.U. needed for each of the lateral fields is therefore

$$\frac{87}{0.98 \times 1.0 \times 0.71} = 125 \text{ M.U.}$$

These fields had no block-supporting tray, so the tray factor is 1.0 and could also be omitted. Transmission factors for beam attenuators which intercept only a portion of a field (bars on the treatment couch, etc.) should be used with caution. Tissue under the section of the field that is not intercepted by the attenuator will receive a higher dose, which could result in irreversible injury.

The method used in accomplishing desired weighting becomes very important in calculation of the average %DD at the prescribed isodose line. The average %DD is found by dividing the %DD of the isodose line by the number of 100% D_{max} doses and not by the number of fields.

In the first example of the two plans with unequal weighting, the isodose distribution was for four fields calculated with a combined D_{max} dose of 400%. Two fields were weighted twice as heavily as the other two, meaning that of the 400%, two sixths or one third (133%) was given via each of the two favored fields and one sixth (66.6%) was delivered via each of the other two fields. In the second example, the isodose distribution was calculated using three fields with a combined D_{max} dose of 400%. One field was weighted twice as heavily as each of the other two fields. In this case the anterior field received one half of 400% or 200% and the other two fields were given 100% each. In the second case, the same isodose distribution would be achieved if the anterior field was given a D_{max} dose of 100% and each of the lateral fields 50% each. Each isodose line would be reduced by one half because the total weighted %DD at D_{max} was reduced by one half from 400% to 200%. In this case, the dose would be prescribed to the 115% isodose line and from equation 4.24, the average %DD would be 115/2, or 57.5%. Other differences between the two examples are the slight difference in field sizes in the second example and the addition of beam attenuators such as a block-supporting tray and wedges.

DOSE CALCULATION FOR TREATMENTS AT AN EXTENDED DISTANCE

In this example, it is assumed that a single field is used to treat a 6 x 40 cm field at 100 cm SSD. The prescribed dose is 200 cGy at D_{max} using a cobalt-60 unit. The dose rate$_{ref}$ for a 10 x 10 cm field is 114 cGy at 80 cm SSD. The area factor for a 6 x 40 cm field is 1.03. The dose decreases inversely with the square of the distance so it is necessary to find the inverse square factor (ISF) of the distance at which the equipment was calibrated (80 cm + the reference depth) and the distance at which the treatment is given (SSD + reference depth). In this example, the calibration was at 80.5 cm from the source and the dose is to be calculated at D_{max}, which is 100.5 cm from the source.

Using equation 3.1, the inverse square factor is found by

$$\left(\frac{80.5}{100.5}\right)^2 = 0.6416$$

To find the treatment time, necessary to deliver the prescribed dose at an extended distance

$$\text{Time} = \frac{\text{prescribed dose}}{\text{dose rate} \times \text{area factor} \times \text{ISF}} \qquad (4.32)$$

So to deliver 200 cGy at D_{max} using 100 cm SSD, the treatment time would be

$$\frac{200}{114 \times 1.03 \times 0.6416} = 2.65 \text{ min (2 min 39 sec)}$$

To verify that the inverse square factor was applied correctly, we will do the same calculation, but now *without* the inverse square factor, to make sure that the treatment time just calculated for the larger SSD is in fact longer than at the "normal" SSD. Therefore, to deliver the same treatment at the "normal" SSD, the treatment time is

$$\frac{200}{114 \times 1.03} = 1.70 \ (1 \text{ min } 42 \text{ sec})$$

which is shorter as we expected.

The preceding section can be summarized in one large calculation formula as follows

$$\text{M.U. (time)} = \frac{\text{prescribed dose}}{(\%DD/100) \ (cGy/M.U.(\text{dose rate}_{ref})) \ (Tr.f.) \ (wdg.f) \ (ISF)} \qquad (4.33)$$

FIXED SOURCE-AXIS DISTANCE TECHNIQUE

Dose calculations for treatments using a fixed SAD (often referred to as "SAD treatments") are primarily used for isocentric treatment techniques, but are also well suited for dose calculations at extended distances since TARs, TPRs, and TMRs are independent of distance. An isocentric technique is impractical when a single field is used, so this section is limited to dose calculations for parallel opposed fields (which can often be carried out very conveniently by SAD methods) and for multiple-field arrangements (which are particularly suited for the SAD method).

DOSE CALCULATION FOR PARALLEL OPPOSED BEAMS WITH EQUAL WEIGHTING

Parallel opposed fields are best treated using an isocentric technique. Since the dose throughout the volume is relatively uniform, it is customary to place the isocenter at mid-depth between the two entry points. This requires measurement of the patient's thickness, or diameter, in the direction of the beam at the central axis. The isocenter is then set by subtracting one half of the patient's diameter from the SAD. In a patient whose diameter is 22 cm, using a therapy machine with a 100 cm SAD, the SSD would be (100 - 11 cm) = 89 cm. Rotating the gantry 180°, would result in 89 cm SSD for the opposing field as well.

Cobalt-60 Beams

In this example, we assume a treatment delivered via equally weighted parallel opposed fields using a cobalt-60 machine. The fields are 17 x 17 cm and the patient's diameter is 18 cm. The dose rate$_{ref}$ without the patient present for a 10 x 10 cm field is 109 cGy/min. The area factor for a 17 x 17 cm field is 1.056. The tissue-air ratio at 9 cm depth is 0.799 (Table A.3). The prescription is for 200 cGy to be delivered at mid-depth.

The treatment time is found from

$$\text{Time} = \frac{\text{prescribed dose}}{\text{dose rate}_{ref} \times \text{area factor} \times \text{TAR}} \qquad (4.34)$$

Since these fields are identical and equally weighted, the calculation for the two fields is the same. The treatment time necessary to deliver 100 cGy at 9 cm depth is

$$\frac{100}{109 \times 1.056 \times 0.799} = 1.09 \text{ min } (1 \text{ min } 5 \text{ sec})$$

Linear Accelerator Beams

In this example, we assume a treatment is delivered via equally weighted parallel opposed beams using 10 MV photons. The patient's diameter is 24 cm, the SAD is 100 cm, and the fields are 17 x 17 cm (Fig. 4.5). The cGy/M.U. at D_{max} is 1.03 and the TMR from Table A.5 at 12 cm depth is 0.813.

The number of M.U. is found from

$$\text{M.U.} = \frac{\text{prescribed depth dose}}{\text{cGy/M.U.} \times \text{TAR}} \tag{4.35}$$

To deliver 100 cGy at 12 cm depth

$$\frac{100}{1.03 \times 0.813} = 119 \text{ M.U.}$$

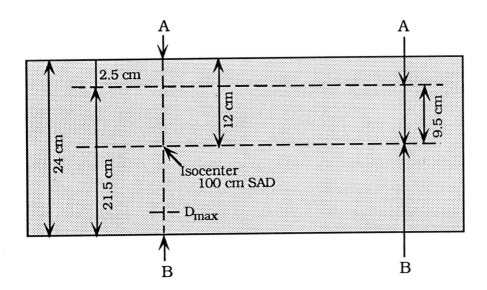

Fig. 4.5. Parallel opposed fields using an isocentric technique. The dose is calculated at the isocenter (100 cm SAD) and at D_{max}.

CALCULATING ENTRANCE AND EXIT DOSE FROM PARALLEL OPPOSED BEAMS WITH EQUAL WEIGHTING

Using the parameters in the previous example the entrance and exit doses are calculated as follows:

Field A (Fig. 4.5) delivers 100 cGy at the isocenter (12 cm depth). The TMR at D_{max} (2.5 cm depth) is 1.0. The distance at this point is 100 cm minus 9.5 cm (Fig. 4.5) or 90.5 cm. The dose is higher at this point by the inverse square factor at this distance. Using equation 3.1. the inverse square factor is

$$\left(\frac{100}{90.5}\right)^2 = 1.2210$$

(Note that the reference point in this calculation is at the isocenter while in a fixed SSD technique the reference point typically is at D_{max}.)

The dose at a point on the central axis is found from

$$\text{Dose} = \text{M.U.} \times \text{cGy/M.U.} \times \text{TMR (TAR or TPR)} \times \text{ISF} \qquad (4.36)$$

The dose at D_{max} of field A is then

$$119\,\text{M.U.} \times 1.03 \times 1.0 \times 1.2210 = 150\,\text{cGy}$$

The cGy/M.U. at this distance would be slightly less than 1.03 because the field is smaller, but the shorter distance to the collimator causes somewhat more scatter at this point. In this example, we assumed that these factors cancel and that the cGy/M.U. is the same at 90.5 and at 100 cm except for the effect of the inverse square factor. The dose at the same point from field B is found from using equation 4.36.

The TMR for field B is 0.616 at 21.5 cm depth (Table A.5).

The distance from field B to this point is 9.5 cm longer than to the isocenter so it is (100 + 9.5) 109.5 cm.

Using equation 3.1 the inverse square factor for field B is

$$\left(\frac{100}{109.5}\right)^2 = 0.834$$

Using equation 4.36 the dose delivered from field B is

$$119 \times 1.03 \times 0.616 \times 0.834 = 63\,\text{cGy}$$

The dose at D_{max} is 150 cGy from field A and 63 cGy from field B which gives a total dose of 213 cGy, a 6.5% higher dose than at mid-depth.

CALCULATING DOSE FROM PARALLEL OPPOSED BEAMS WITH UNEQUAL WEIGHTING

In an isocentric technique it is customary to normalize the dose at the isocenter and weight the beam at this point. In this example, where two parallel opposed 4 MV fields are used to treat a right parotid tumor (Fig. 4.6) it is assumed that the isocenter is in the patient's midline. The SAD is 80 cm and the fields are 9 x 14 cm. The beams are weighted 2 to 1 from the patient's right meaning that two thirds of the prescribed dose at the isocenter is delivered via the right field and one third via the left field. The patient's diameter is 13 cm and the cGy/M.U. without the patient present at 80 cm distance is 1.01. From Table A.4 the TAR at 6.5 cm depth is 0.892. The prescription is for 180 cGy to be delivered at the isocenter (Fig. 4.6A).

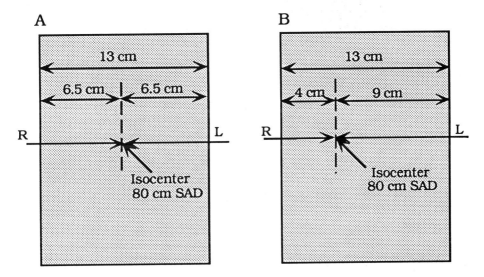

Fig. 4.6. Parallel opposed fields using an isocentric technique with the isocenter in the midplane of the patient (A) and at 4 cm depth in tissue (B). The beams are weighted 2 to 1 favoring the right field in both arrangements.

The M.U. necessary to deliver this treatment can be found from

$$\text{M.U.} = \frac{\text{fraction of prescribed dose}}{\text{cGy/M.U.} \times \text{TAR}} \qquad (4.37)$$

Since the dose at the isocenter is different for these two fields, they are calculated separately. The M.U. to be set for the right field would be

$$\frac{2 \times 180}{3 \times 1.01 \times 0.892} = 133 \text{ M.U.}$$

The M.U. to be set for the left field would be

$$\frac{1 \times 180}{3 \times 1.01 \times 0.738} = 80 \text{ M.U.}$$

In the following example the same treatment is to be delivered, but the isocenter is moved to 4 cm depth from the right side (Fig. 4.6B). The weighting, the field size, and the SAD remain unchanged. The TAR from Table A.4 at 4 cm depth is 0.977 and at 11 cm depth, 0.738. The cGy/M.U. is 1.01.

The M.U. necessary to deliver two thirds of the prescribed dose (180 cGy) through the patient's right field at the isocenter is, using equation 4.37

$$\frac{2 \times 180}{3 \times 1.01 \times 0.977} = 122 \text{ M.U.}$$

The M.U. necessary to deliver one third of the prescribed dose through the left field is

$$\frac{1 \times 180}{3 \times 1.01 \times 0.738} = 80 \text{ M.U.}$$

The calculated number of M.U. decreased from the right side and increased from the left side when compared with the previous example. Shifting the isocenter farther away from the midplane and suitably weighting the beams could result in the same M.U. from both fields.

In the next example, a tumor in the posterior aspect of the right lung is treated via parallel opposed oblique fields using 4 MV photon beams (Fig. 4.7). The fields are 10 x 10 cm and the SAD is 80 cm. The depth from the anterior skin surface to the isocenter is 23 cm and from the posterior skin surface it is 7 cm. The TAR at 23 cm depth is 0.410 and at 7 cm depth it is 0.866 (Table A.4). The fields are weighted 2 to 1 favoring the right posterior oblique (RPO) field. The cGy/M.U. is 1.0. The prescribed dose is 300 cGy at the isocenter.

The M.U. necessary to deliver two thirds of the prescribed dose from the right posterior oblique field using equation 4.37 is

$$\frac{2 \times 300}{3 \times 1.0 \times 0.866} = 231 \text{ M.U.}$$

The M.U. necessary to deliver one third of the prescribed dose from the left anterior oblique (LAO) field is

$$\frac{1 \times 300}{3 \times 1.0 \times 0.410} = 244 \text{ M.U.}$$

In this situation, the field with the lower weighting requires a larger number of M.U. than the field with the higher weighting, due to the greater depth of the isocenter.

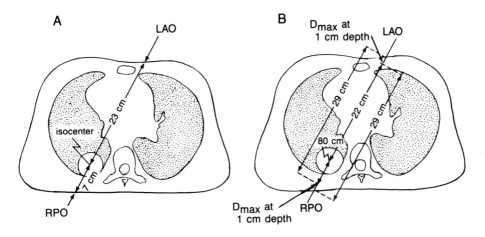

Fig. 4.7. Oblique parallel opposed beams used in treatment of a posterior lung lesion. The dose is calculated at the isocenter (A) and at D_{max} of each field (B).

CALCULATING ENTRANCE AND EXIT DOSE FOR PARALLEL OPPOSED BEAMS WITH UNEQUAL WEIGHTING

The entrance and exit doses at D_{max} of each field are calculated as follows:

A. DOSE AT DEPTH OF MAXIMUM DOSE, RPO FIELD

Entrance Dose
The entrance dose of the RPO field is found by using equation 4.36. The M.U. delivered via the RPO field is 231. The TAR at D_{max} is 1.0 and, using equation 3.1, the inverse square factor is

$$\left(\frac{80}{80-6}\right)^2 = 1.1687$$

The entrance dose of the RPO field is therefore

$$231 \text{ M.U.} \times 1.0 \times 1.1687 = 270 \text{ cGy}$$

<u>Exit Dose</u>

The exit dose of the LAO field is found by using equation 4.36. The M.U. delivered via the LAO field is 244, the TAR at 29 cm (Fig. 4.7B) is 0.305, and the inverse square factor is

$$\left(\frac{80}{80+6}\right)^2 = 0.8653$$

The exit dose from the LAO field at D_{max} of the RPO field is therefore

$$244 \text{ M.U.} \times 1.0 \times 0.305 \times 0.8653 = 64 \text{ cGy}$$

The total dose at D_{max} of the RPO field is then 270 cGy plus 64 cGy which is 334 cGy.

B. DOSE AT DEPTH OF MAXIMUM DOSE, LAO FIELD

<u>Entrance Dose</u>

The entrance dose of the LAO field is found from equation 4.36. The M.U. delivered via the LAO field is 244, the TAR at D_{max} is 1.0, and using equation 3.1, the inverse square factor (Fig. 4.7B) is

$$\left(\frac{80}{80-22}\right)^2 = 1.9025$$

Using equation 4.36 the entrance dose at D_{max} of the LAO field is

$$244 \times 1.0 \times 1.0 \times 1.9025 = 464 \text{ cGy}$$

<u>Exit Dose</u>

The exit dose of the RPO field is also found from equation 4.36. The M.U. delivered via the RPO field is 231, the TAR at 29 cm depth (Fig. 4.7B) is 0.305, and the inverse square factor is

$$\left(\frac{80}{80+22}\right)^2 = 0.6151$$

Using equation 4.36, the exit dose of the LAO field is

$$231 \times 1.0 \times 0.305 \times 0.6151 = 43 \text{ cGy}$$

The total dose at D_{max} of the LAO field is therefore (464 + 43) 507 cGy.

In tabular form, the doses delivered by each field at each point are as follows

Dose Calculation Point	RPO field	LAO field	Total Dose
	M.U. 231	M.U. 244	
Isocenter	200 cGy	100 cGy	300 cGy
D_{max}, RPO	270 cGy	64 cGy	334 cGy
D_{max}, LAO	43 cGy	464 cGy	507 cGy

It is obvious from this example that when the isocenter is offset away from mid-depth, the weighting factor must be carefully selected to avoid very high doses in either D_{max} region. In this example, equal weighting would further increase the dose at D_{max} in the anterior oblique field and decrease the dose at D_{max} of the posterior oblique field. Increasing the weighting factor on the posterior oblique field would reduce the difference.

A general rule for selecting the weighting factor is to find the ratio of the TAR of each field and apply a similar ratio to the weighting factor. To achieve optimal dose uniformity between the two entrance points, the field with the highest TAR should be favored.

DOSE CALCULATION FOR MULTIPLE BEAMS WITH EQUAL WEIGHTING

Treatment plans consisting of multiple fields are best delivered using an isocentric technique. The dose is customarily normalized at the isocenter, and the dose is prescribed to an isodose line encompassing the target volume.

In this example, a patient is treated via a four-field technique using a 4 MV linear accelerator. The isocenter is at 80 cm and each field is 10 x 15 cm. The prescribed dose is 200 cGy at the 95% isodose line (Fig. 4.8). The cGy/M.U. is 1.025 for each field and the dose is normalized to 100% at the isocenter. The TAR for fields A and B is 0.793 and for fields C and D, it is 0.645.

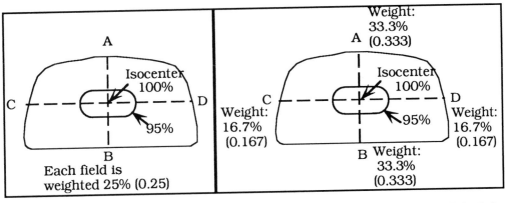

Fig. 4.8. Isocentric four-field technique using (left) equal weighting and (right) weighted 2 to 1.

The M.U. necessary to deliver this treatment is found from

$$M.U. = \frac{\text{prescribed dose per field}}{\text{cGy/M.U.} \times \text{TAR} \times \text{isodose line}/100}$$ (4.38)

Using equation 4.38, the M.U. necessary to deliver the prescribed dose from fields A and B is

$$\frac{50}{1.025 \times 0.793 \times 0.95} = 65 \text{ M.U. per field}$$

and the M.U. necessary to deliver the prescribed dose from fields C and D is

$$\frac{50}{1.025 \times 0.645 \times 0.95} = 80 \text{ M.U. per field}$$

The difference in the number of M.U. is due to the difference in the TAR. All other factors are the same for all fields.

DOSE CALCULATION FOR MULTIPLE BEAMS WITH UNEQUAL WEIGHTING

In this example, the same field arrangement is assumed, but fields A and B are weighted by a factor of 2 and fields C and D are weighted by a factor of 1 (Fig. 4.8). In this plan, the dose is normalized to 100% at the isocenter. Fields A and B are weighted by a factor of 0.333 (one third) and fields C and D by 0.167 (one sixth). One third of 200 cGy is delivered at the isocenter from each of fields A and B and one sixth of the prescribed dose is delivered via each of fields C and D.

The M.U. necessary for each field to deliver the prescribed dose is found from

$$M.U. = \frac{\text{fraction of the prescribed dose}}{\text{cGy/M.U.} \times \text{TAR} \times \text{isodose line}/100}$$ (4.39)

Using equation 4.39, the M.U. necessary from each of fields A and B is

$$\frac{1 \times 200}{3 \times 1.025 \times 0.793 \times 0.95} = 86 \text{ M.U. per field}$$

and the M.U. necessary from each of fields C and D is

$$\frac{1 \times 200}{6 \times 1.025 \times 0.645 \times 0.95} = 53 \text{ M.U. per field}$$

The effect of beam attenuators is calculated precisely as in other techniques and will therefore not be included here.

The calculation formula for an SAD technique is very similar to that of a fixed SSD technique and is summarized as follows:

$$\text{MU (time)} = \frac{\text{prescribed dose}}{\text{(TAR, TPR, TMR) (isod./100) (cGy/MU) (dose rate}_{ref}\text{) (area f.) (tr.f.) (wdg f.)}} \quad (4.40)$$

DOSE CALCULATION FOR TREATMENTS AT AN EXTENDED DISTANCE

In some situations, it is necessary to treat patients at extended distances in order to accommodate large fields. It is then somewhat uncertain how the dose is affected. The dose can, for example, change due to the increased distance between the collimator and the calculation point and also because of scatter from the floor and walls of the treatment room. Actual measurements of dose under these conditions are highly recommended. If time and conditions do not permit actual measurements to be made prior to treatment, it is possible to calculate the dose with reasonable confidence using TAR or TMR methods.

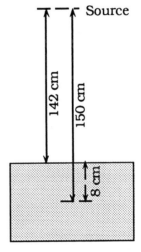

Fig. 4.9. Diagram of treatment at an extended distance.

In this example, the lower half-body of a patient is to be treated at 142 cm SSD (Fig. 4.9). The patient's thickness is 16 cm and the maximum collimator opening is used. The treatment is delivered using a cobalt-60 unit with a dose rate$_{ref}$ of 109 cGy/min at 80 cm distance when the patient is not present. The area factor for the maximum collimator opening is 1.07. The maximum field size for which TARs are available at this energy is 35 x 35 cm (Table A.3).

Though the maximum collimator opening on this machine produces a field size at 150 cm which is much greater than 35 x 35 cm, it is reasonable to use the 35 x 35 cm TAR value (0.935 at 8 cm depth) because the beam flashes over the sides of the patient and the irradiated area is therefore elongated. In any event, the TAR varies very slowly with area when the field is large (as do area factors, cGy/M.U., and %DD), particularly at higher energies. For example, the TAR for cobalt-60 (8 cm depth) increases only 6.5%, from 0.852 to 0.907, (Table A.3) when the field area is more than doubled from 20 x 20 cm to 30 x 30 cm; the same field change for 10 MV photons (Table A.5) gives less than 1% increase in TAR (0.906 to 0.910). The exact field size chosen in our present problem is therefore not critical.

The treatment time necessary to deliver the prescribed treatment can be found from

$$\text{Time} = \frac{\text{prescribed dose}}{\text{dose rate}_{ref} \times \text{area f.} \times \text{TAR} \times \text{ISF}} \tag{4.41}$$

The treatment time necessary to deliver 300 cGy per field can be found from

$$\frac{300}{109 \times 1.07 \times 0.935 \times 0.2844} = 9.67 \text{ min (9 min 40 sec)}$$

where 0.2844 is the inverse square factor for a point 8 cm beyond the new SSD of 142 cm, that is, for a point 150 cm from the source:

$$\left(\frac{80}{150}\right)^2 = 0.2844$$

REFERENCE

Bentel, G.C., Nelson, C.E., Noell, K.T., *Treatment Planning and Dose Calculation in Radiation Oncology*, Pergamon Press, Inc. Elmsford, NY, 1989.

PROBLEMS

SSD TECHNIQUE

DOSE CALCULATION AT DEPTH OF MAXIMUM DOSE

1. **Superficial beam**
   A skin lesion is to be treated using a superficial beam. The prescription is for 300 cGy per fraction. The field size is 7 x 8 cm and the SSD is 50 cm. The HVT is 2.5 mm Cu and the backscatter factor is 1.123. The dose rate at 50 cm SSD without the patient present is 57 cGy/min. What is the required treatment time? (Give the answer in minutes and seconds.)

2. **Electron beam**
   An 8 MeV electron beam is used to deliver 300 cGy at D_{max}. The field size is 8 x 8 cm and the SSD is 100 cm. The dose rate$_{ref}$ is 1.0 cGy/M.U. for a 10 x 10 cm field. The cGy/M.U. for an 8 x 8 cm field is 0.872. What M.U. setting should be set to deliver this treatment?

3. **Cobalt-60 beam**
   A cobalt-60 beam is used to deliver 200 cGy at D_{max}. The field size is 10 x 12 cm and the SSD is 80 cm. The dose rate$_{ref}$ for a 10 x 10 cm field at D_{max} is 112.7 cGy/min. The area factor for a 10 x 12 cm field is 1.02. What treatment time is needed to deliver this treatment? (Give the answer in minutes and seconds.)

4. **Linear accelerator**
   A 4 MV photon beam is used to deliver 200 cGy at D_{max}. The field size is 15 x 15 cm and the SSD is 80 cm. The dose rate$_{ref}$ is 1 cGy/M.U. for a 10 x 10 cm field. The cGy/M.U. for a 15 x 15 cm field is 1.037. What M.U. setting should be used to deliver this treatment?

DOSE CALCULATION AT DEPTH FOR A SINGLE BEAM

5. **Superficial beam**
   350 cGy is prescribed at 3 cm depth. The field size is 3 x 4 cm and the SSD is 50 cm. A 3 mm Cu HVT beam is used and the dose rate in the absence of the patient at 50 cm is 63.4 cGy/min. The backscatter factor is 1.094 and the %DD at 3 cm depth is 78%. What is the treatment time necessary to delivery this treatment? (Give the answer in minutes and seconds.)

6. **Electron beam**
   250 cGy is prescribed at 3.5 cm depth using a 14 MeV electron beam. The field size is 6 x 8 cm and the SSD is 100 cm. The dose rate$_{ref}$ is 1.0

for a 10 x 10 cm field and 0.898 for a 6 x 8 cm field. The %DD at 3.5 cm is 92%. How many M.U. should be set to deliver this treatment?

7. Cobalt-60 beam
180 cGy is prescribed at 4.5 cm depth using a cobalt-60 beam. The field size is 8 x 8 cm and the SSD is 80 cm. The dose rate$_{ref}$ at D_{max} for a 10 x 10 cm field is 109.3 cGy/min. The area factor for an 8 x 8 cm field is 0.973. What is the treatment time required to deliver this treatment? (Give the answer in minutes and seconds.) Use Table A.1 for %DD.

8. Linear accelerator
100 cGy is prescribed at 5 cm depth to be delivered using a 4 MV photon beam. The field size is 12 x 12 cm and the SSD is 80 cm. The cGy/M.U.$_{ref}$ is 1.0 for a 10 x 10 cm field and it is 1.027 for a 12 x 12 cm field. What M.U. setting should be used to deliver this treatment? Use Table A.2 for %DD.

DOSE CALCULATION FOR PARALLEL OPPOSED FIELDS

9. Cobalt-60 beam
180 cGy is prescribed in the midplane of the brain. Parallel opposed lateral cobalt-60 fields are used. The lateral diameter of the head is 14 cm. The field size is 17 x 23 cm and the SSD is 80 cm. The dose rate$_{ref}$ for a 10 x 10 cm field is 107.3 cGy/min and the area factor is 1.047. What treatment time is required per field to deliver this treatment? (Give the answer in minutes and seconds.) Use Table A.1 for %DD.

10. Linear accelerator
200 cGy is prescribed at the midplane of the lung. Parallel opposed anterior and posterior 4 MV photon beams are to be used. The field size is 13 x 13 cm and the SSD is 80 cm. The AP diameter of the patient's chest is 21 cm. The cGy/M.U.$_{ref}$ is 1.0 for a 10 x 10 cm field and for a 13 x 13 cm field it is 1.022. What M.U. setting per field is necessary to deliver this treatment? Use Table A.2 for %DD.

CALCULATING ENTRANCE AND EXIT DOSE FROM PARALLEL OPPOSED EQUALLY WEIGHTED BEAMS

11. Giving 120 M.U. through each field in the treatment delivered in Problem #10, what will the dose be at a) mid-depth and at b) D_{max} of either of the two parallel opposed fields? Use Table A.2 for %DD.

12. Giving 120 M.U. through field 1 and 240 M.U. through field 2 in the treatment in Problem #10, what will the total dose be at a) midplane, b) D_{max} of Field 1, and c) D_{max} of field 2?

13. 150 cGy is prescribed at 3 cm depth from the right side of the brain. Parallel opposed cobalt-60 fields are used. The field size is 8 x 8 cm and the SSD is 80 cm. The fields are weighted 2 to 1 favoring the patient's right side. The lateral diameter of the head is 15 cm. The dose rate$_{ref}$ for a 10 x 10 cm field is 105.6 cGy/min and the area factor for an 8 x 8 cm field is 0.985. What will the treatment time be for a) the right field and b) the left field? (Give the answers in minutes and seconds.) Use Table A.1 for %DD.

14. A three-field treatment plan is used to treat a brain tumor. Each field is 6 x 6 cm and the SSD is 80 cm. A 4 MV photon beam is used for all fields. 180 cGy is prescribed to the 206% isodose line. The fields are equally weighted. The cGy/M.U. $_{ref}$ for a 10 x 10 cm field is 1.0 and for a 6 x 6 cm field it is 0.956. A 30° wedge is used in two of the three fields. The wedge factor is 0.81. What M.U. setting should be used in a) the unwedged field, and b) the two wedged fields?

15. 200 cGy is prescribed at D$_{max}$ in a spine field which is 6 x 30 cm at 80 cm SSD. The cGy/M.U.$_{ref}$ for a 10 x 10 cm field is 1.0 at D$_{max}$ (81 cm) and for a 6 x 30 cm field it is 1.026 at D$_{max}$ (81 cm). Due to the length of the field, the treatment must be delivered at 90 cm SSD. What M.U. setting is necessary in order to deliver this treatment?

SAD TECHNIQUE

16. Cobalt-60 beam
190 cGy is prescribed at the midplane of the arm. Parallel opposed cobalt-60 beams are used. The field size is 6 x 12 cm and the SAD is 80 cm. The dose rate$_{ref}$ is 112.6 cGy/min at 80 cm for a 10 x 10 cm field and the area factor for a 6 x 12 cm field is 0.995. The diameter of the arm is 9 cm. The isocenter is at mid-depth in the arm. What is the required treatment time for each field? (Give the answer in minutes and seconds.) Use Table A.3 for TAR.

17. Linear accelerator
200 cGy is prescribed at the midplane of the pelvis. Parallel opposed 10 MV photon beams are used. The field size is 17 x 17 cm and the SAD is 100 cm. The cGy/M.U.$_{ref}$ is 1.0 for a 10 x 10 cm field and 1.085 for a 17 x 17 cm field. The diameter of the pelvis is 25 cm. The isocenter is at the mid-depth of the pelvis. What M.U. setting should be used for each field in order to deliver this treatment? Use Table A.5 for TAR.

18. From the treatment delivered in Problem #17, find the maximum entrance and exit dose.

19. 180 cGy is prescribed to the 95% isodose line in a four-field isocentric treatment plan. All fields are equally weighted and 4 MV photon

beams are used. The field sizes are 8 x 8 cm and the SAD is 80 cm. The cGy/M.U.$_{ref}$ is 1.0 for a 10 x 10 cm field and 0.98 for 8 x 8 cm field. The depth of the isocenter is 10 cm for fields A and B and 16 cm for fields C and D. What is the M.U. setting is required for each field? Use Table A.4 for TAR.

20.   200 cGy is prescribed to the 98% isodose line in a treatment plan using parallel opposed isocentric fields. The field sizes are 9 x 10 cm and the SAD is 100 cm. A 10 MV photon beam is used. Field A is weighted twice as much as field B. The isocenter is at 5 cm depth in field A and at 15 cm depth in field B. The cGy/M.U.$_{ref}$ for a 10 x 10 cm field is 1.0 and for a 9 x 10 cm field it is 0.995. What is the M.U. needed for each field to deliver the treatment, and what is the D$_{max}$ dose (entrance and exit) of field A and of field B? Use Table A.4.

SOLUTIONS

1. ~~6 min 15 sec~~ 4' 41"

2. 344 M.U.

3. 1 min 45 sec

4. 193 M.U.

5. 6 min 28 sec

6. 303 M.U.

7. 2 min 7 sec

8. 118 M.U.

9. 1 min 7 sec/field

10. 164 M.U.

11. Midplane dose: 147 cGy
    D_{max} dose: 163 cGy

12. a) 220 cGy
    b) 203 cGy
    c) 286 cGy

13. Right side: 1 min 18 sec
    Left side: 39 sec

14. a) Unwedged field: 91 M.U.

    b) Wedged fields: 113 M.U./field

15. 246 M.U.

16. 57 sec

17. 115 M.U.

18. 216 M.U.

19. A&B: 65 M.U.
    C&D: 87 M.U.

20. a) Field A: 146 M.U.
       Field B: 114 M.U.

    b) D_{max}, Field A: 210 cGy
       D_{max}, Field B: 210 cGy

CHAPTER 5

DOSE CALCULATION FOR EXTERNAL BEAMS - PART II

In Chapter 4, dose calculations on the central axis for square fields were explained. In this chapter, dose calculations on and off the central axis and for rectangular and irregularly shaped fields will be explained. As was evident in Chapter 4, tabulated values are usually available only for square fields. In clinical practice, the problem arises of finding data for rectangular and irregular fields. In this chapter, some methods to solve these problems will be shown.

THE CONCEPT OF EQUIVALENT SQUARE FIELDS

In a *very* small field (which we can represent as a 0 x 0 cm field, although that is only an abstraction as was previously explained), the dose is effectively due to primary radiation only. As the field size is increased, the scattered radiation resulting from photons interacting with the medium causes the absorbed dose to increase. The amount of scattered radiation is greater at a larger depth than at D_{max}, causing the percentage depth dose to increase with larger field sizes. Since the higher energy photons are scattered more predominantly in a forward direction, the percentage depth dose increases with increased area and is less pronounced for the higher energy beams than for the lower energy beams (page 67, Chapter 3).

EQUIVALENT SQUARE METHOD

The shape of the field, not just its area in square centimeters, also affects the percentage depth dose. In the two fields shown in Fig. 5.1, for example, the total area is the same. However, the percentage depth dose in field B is smaller than in field A because radiation scattered from the distal portions of field B is less likely to reach the center of the field where the percentage depth dose is observed than is the scattered radiation from field A where the area is symmetrically arranged around the calculation point.

Several authors (Jones 1949, Day 1950,1961, Batho 1956) have shown that percentage depth dose data for rectangular fields can be approximated by an equivalent square method.

Using Table A.6, a 6 x 20 cm field is equivalent to a 9 x 9 cm field. The percentage depth dose for a 9 x 9 cm field could therefore be used when calculating dose for the 6 x 20 cm field.

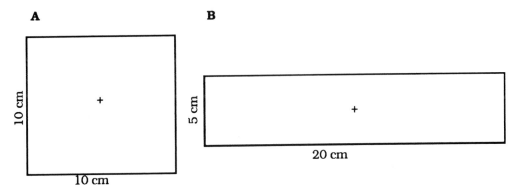

Fig. 5.1. The areas in (A) and (B) are the same but the field in (B) contributes less scatter than (A) at the calculation point (+) because of the elongated shape.

AREA/PERIMETER METHOD

Another method, developed by Sterling (Sterling 1964) is to equate a rectangular field with a square field if they have the same area/perimeter (A/P).

Since the area (A) of the rectangular field is a x b and its perimeter (P) is 2a + 2b (two sides plus two ends), we have

$$A/P = \frac{a \times b}{2(a+b)} \tag{5.1}$$

where a is the field width and b is the field length.

Consider for example a 6 x 20 cm field

$$A/P = \frac{6 \times 20}{2(6 + 20)}$$

so
$$\frac{120}{52} = 2.3$$

To find the A/P for a square field, where a = b, we have

$$A/P = \frac{a^2}{4^a} = \frac{a}{4} \qquad\qquad (5.2)$$

In a square field of side 9 cm, for example,

$$A/P = \frac{9}{4} = 2.25$$

We found, then, that A/P for a 6 x 20 cm field and for a 9 x 9 cm square field are very nearly the same, so tabulated data for a 9 x 9 cm field (equivalent field) can therefore be used to find the values for a 6 x 20 cm field.

Although this method is widely used in clinical practice, caution must be used in applying it.

CLARKSON'S METHOD

Tabulated data customarily refer to the central axis of square fields, and as we have just seen, can also be applied to rectangular fields but can not be used to estimate the dose on the central axis of an irregularly shaped field (Fig. 5.2) or at points away from the central axis of any field. For these situations, the dose may be estimated by finding the primary and scatter component of the dose separately and adding them together, a method originally introduced by Clarkson (Clarkson 1941). This method is best accomplished using TAR and SAR tables or TMR and SMR tables.[*]

The TAR or TMR for a 0 x 0 cm field represents the primary component of a beam. The TAR or TMR for a given field size includes both the primary and the scattered dose. The difference between the two represents the scatter component or scatter-air ratio in the case of TAR and scatter-maximum ratio (SMR) in the case of TMR. Both SAR and SMR have been previously defined in Chapter 3 (page 66).

---

[*] All data tables used in the dose calculations in this chapter are labelled A.1-A.8 and can be found in an appendix at the end of this volume (pages 337 - 344).

Scatter-air ratio and SMR tables published in the literature are usually tabulated for circular fields only. It is, however, possible to find the equivalent square field from these tables.

Using Table A.3, it is found that the TAR for a 10 x 10 cm cobalt-60 field at 10 cm depth is 0.701 and the TAR at the same depth for a 0 x 0 cm field is 0.534. The scatter component is therefore found from

$$0.701 - 0.534 = 0.167$$

From Table A.7 it is found that a circular field with a radius of 5.65 (100 cm^2) at a depth of 10 cm has an interpolated SAR value of 0.174. The difference is a result of the fact that the tabulated values for SARs and SMRs for circular fields correspond to square or rectangular fields having the same scatter rather than the same area.

Fractional SARs and SMRs.

The scatter of any field can be estimated by using segments of circular fields. If a circular field is divided into 15° segments (a convenient choice since 15° goes into 360° a whole number [24] of times), the SAR due to one such segment is one twenty-fourth of the SAR due to the whole circle. In this method, radii separated by 15°, that is, 24 segments, are measured from the calculation point to the field margins. The SARs or SMRs for each radius are found and are then divided by 24 to give the fractional value. The fractional SARs or SMRs for the 24 segments are summed and are then added to the TAR or TMR for a 0 x 0 cm field (TAR$_0$ or TMR$_0$) at the same depth. The sum gives the TAR or TMR value for the calculated field. An alternate method is to find the SAR for each radius, then divide by the number of radii to find the average SAR. The result will be the same as in the method just described.

TABLE 5.1

SCATTER-AIR RATIO CALCULATION AT THE CENTRAL
AXIS OF THE FIELD IN FIGURE 5.2

Cobalt-60

Radius No	Length (cm)	Fractional SAR	Radius No	Length (cm)	Fractional SAR
1	4.7	0.0013	13	10.0	0.0024
2	10.5	0.0025	14	10.5	0.0025
3	11.5	0.0027	15	9.5	0.0023
4	10.5	0.0025	16	7.5	0.0019
5	8.5	0.0022	17	5.5	0.0015
6	4.5	0.0012	18	4.0	0.0011
7	4.5	0.0012	19	4.5	0.0012
8	4.7	0.0013	20	6.5	0.0017
9	8.5	0.0022	21	8.5	0.0022
10	10.0	0.0024	22	10.5	0.0025
11	10.5	0.0025	23	11.5	0.0027
12	10.5	0.0025	24	10.5	0.0025

SAR = **0.049**

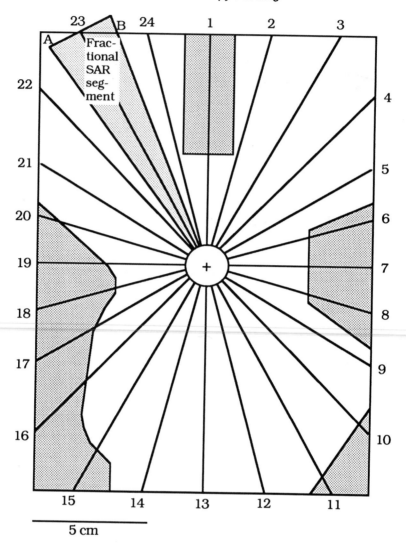

Fig. 5.2. An irregularly shaped field illustrating the calculation point (+) and 24 radii used in calculating the SAR (Table 5.1). A small triangle of the field lies outside SAR segment 23 at (A). This is, however off-set by a small triangle outside the field, which is included in the SAR segment at (B).

The fractional SARs or SMRs can also be used to estimate the equivalent square of a rectangular or irregularly shaped field. For example, Table 5.1 shows that the field in Fig. 5.2 yields an SAR of 0.049 at D_{max} using a cobalt-60 beam and 80 cm SSD (Table A.3). The TAR at D_{max} for a 0 x 0 cm field is 1.0. Adding 0.049 to 1.0 yields a TAR of 1.049. From Table A.3 a TAR value of 1.049 at D_{max} is given for a 15 x 15 cm field. The irregularly shaped field in Fig. 5.2 therefore has the same scattering properties as a 15 x 15 cm square field and %DD and TAR tables for this field may be used.

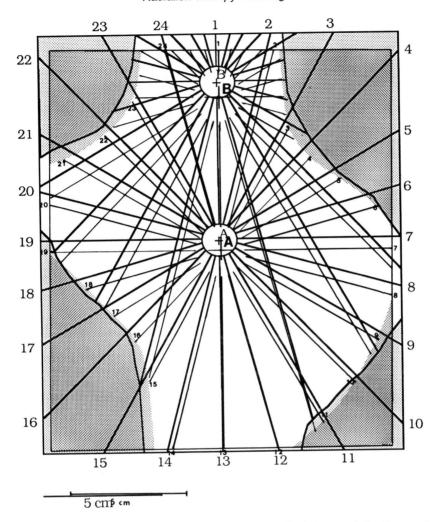

Fig. 5.3 An irregularly shaped field indicating two calculation points; the central axis (A) and an off-axis point (B) with 24 radii used in calculating the SAR (Table 5.2).

CALCULATING DOSE ON THE CENTRAL AXIS

As another example, the field in Fig. 5.3 is to be treated using a 4 MV photon beam at 80 cm SAD. The prescription is for 100 cGy at 8 cm depth. The TAR for a 0 x 0 cm field at 8 cm depth is 0.690 (Table A.4) and the SAR, using Table A.8, is 0.191 (Table 5.2) so the TAR for this field at 8 cm depth is (0.690 + 0.191) 0.881. The cGy/M.U. for this field is 1.03. The M.U. required to deliver this treatment is found from

$$M.U. = \frac{\text{prescribed dose}}{(TAR_0 + SAR) \times cGy/M.U. \times \text{tray factor}} \qquad (5.3)$$

TABLE 5.2

SCATTER-AIR RATIO CALCULATION FOR THE FIELD IN FIGURE 5.3

----

4 MV Photons

	Point A			Point B			
Radius No	Length (cm)	Frac-tional SAR **D 8 cm**	Radius No	Length (cm)	Frac-tional SAR **D 8 cm**	Frac-tional SAR **D 7 cm**	Frac-tional SAR **D 5 cm**
1	8.5	0.0086	1	2.0	0.0029	0.0028	0.0026
2	9.0	0.0089	2	2.0	0.0029	0.0028	0.0026
3	6.0	0.0071	3	2.0	0.0029	0.0028	0.0026
4	5.5	0.0067	4	3.0	0.0042	0.0041	0.0037
5	6.0	0.0071	5	3.0	0.0042	0.0041	0.0037
6	7.0	0.0078	6	2.5	0.0036	0.0035	0.0032
7	7.5	0.0081	7	2.5	0.0036	0.0035	0.0032
8	7.5	0.0081	8	2.5	0.0036	0.0035	0.0032
9	8.0	0.0084	9	3.0	0.0042	0.0041	0.0037
10	8.0	0.0084	10	10.0	0.0093	0.0088	0.0075
11	8.5	0.0086	11	13.0	0.0100	0.0095	0.0080
12	9.0	0.0089	12	15.0	0.0105	0.0099	0.0083
13	8.5	0.0086	13	15.0	0.0105	0.0099	0.0083
14	9.0	0.0089	14	13.0	0.0100	0.0095	0.0080
15	7.0	0.0078	15	10.5	0.0094	0.0089	0.0076
16	5.5	0.0067	16	10.0	0.0093	0.0088	0.0075
17	5.5	0.0067	17	8.5	0.0086	0.0083	0.0070
18	6.0	0.0071	18	4.5	0.0058	0.0056	0.0049
19	7.0	0.0078	19	3.5	0.0048	0.0046	0.0042
20	8.0	0.0084	20	3.5	0.0048	0.0046	0.0042
21	8.0	0.0084	21	3.5	0.0048	0.0046	0.0042
22	7.0	0.0078	22	3.0	0.0042	0.0041	0.0037
23	7.5	0.0081	23	2.0	0.0029	0.0028	0.0026
24	8.0	0.0084	24	2.0	0.0029	0.0028	0.0026
		SAR = **0.191**			SARs = **0.140**	**0.134**	**0.117**

So, for this treatment, the required M.U. is

$$\frac{100}{(0.690 + 0.191) \times 1.03 \times 0.96} = 115 \text{ M.U.}$$

CALCULATING DOSE AT AN OFF-AXIS POINT

To estimate the dose at points away from the central axis, the method used is similar to the one described above for a central axis point calculation. The exception being the need for the application of an off-axis ratio.

Off-Axis Ratio

Flattening filters are used in the beam of linear accelerators to flatten the isodose curves across a field at a specified depth. This, however, frequently causes the dose to be higher away from the central axis, particularly at shallow depths (see Fig. 5.4 and page 70, Chapter 3). Isodose charts for cobalt-60 beams, on the other hand, demonstrate a lower dose in the periphery of the field. Such non-uniformity of dose across a beam must be considered in dose calculations away from the central axis of the beam. To estimate the dose at such points, the variation of dose across the beam or the off-axis ratio (OAR) at appropriate depth must be known.

The OAR is defined as

$$OAR = \frac{\%DD \text{ at the off-axis point}}{\%DD \text{ on the central axis}} \qquad (5.4)$$

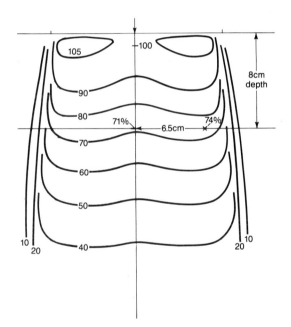

Fig. 5.4. The %DD is found on the central axis (71%) and at the off-axis point at the same depth (74%).

The most practical method to estimate the OAR is to find the %DD along the central axis at the depth under consideration and the %DD off the central axis of the beam at the same depth and at the appropriate distance away from the central axis using an isodose chart measured for the actual beam and for appropriate field size.

For example, the %DD in Fig. 5.4 at the off-axis point is 74 and at the same depth along the central axis it is 71. The OAR is therefore 74/71 = 1.042, that is, the dose at the off-axis point is 4.2% higher than the dose at the same depth on the central axis. Few departments have isodose charts plotted for every field size and distance so some assumptions must be made. For example, to find the OAR for an SAD technique using an isodose chart plotted for an SSD technique, the assumption is made that the shape of the individual isodose curves does not change very much with distance. Interpolation between individual isodose lines and for different field sizes also causes uncertainties in the estimation of the OAR. More elaborate methods of calculating the OAR, have been described (Chui 1986).

Calculating dose at an off-axis point with a flat surface

The dose at an off-axis point is best estimated by considering the primary dose and the scatter separately. The SAR is determined as previously described, but the axis from which the radii originate is placed at the off-axis calculation point (Fig. 5.3). In this example, the SAR for a 4 MV photon beam at B is found by using Table A.8 and is 0.140 at 8 cm depth (Table 5.2). The TAR_0 value at 8 cm depth from Table A.4 is 0.690, so the TAR at this point is $0.690 + 0.140 = 0.830$. Using an isodose chart for a 17 x 17 cm field at 80 cm SSD, the %DD at a point 6.5 cm from the central axis at 8 cm depth is 74 and on the central axis it is 71, so the OAR is $74/71 = 1.042$ (Fig. 5.4). The field in Fig. 5.3 is given 115 M.U. which delivers 100 cGy at 8 cm depth on the central axis. The dose at the off-axis point is found from

$$\text{Dose} = \text{M.U.} \times \text{cGy/M.U.} \times (TAR_0 + SAR) \times OAR \times \text{tray factor} \qquad (5.5)$$

so in this field, the dose at 8 cm depth, assuming that the patient skin surface is flat (Fig. 5.5), is

$$115 \times 1.03 \times (0.690 + 0.140) \times 1.042 \times 0.96 = 98 \text{ cGy}$$

The dose at the off-axis point and at the central axis are practically the same. The higher dose due to the overflattening of the beam is offset by less scatter at the off-axis point.

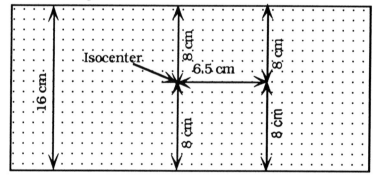

Fig. 5.5. An illustration of the geometry of off-axis point calculation using a flat contour.

Calculating dose at an off-axis point when the surface is not flat

In the previous example, the surface of the patient was assumed to be flat, that is, the SSD is the same at the central axis and at the off-axis point. In the following example the same field is treated as in the previous example, but the patient's irregular surface results in a 3 cm vertical air gap (Fig. 5.6).

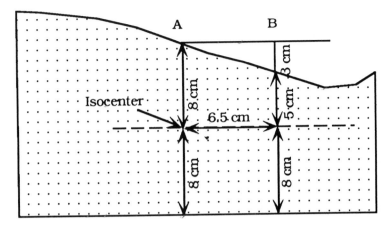

Fig. 5.6. Diagram of the geometry when calculating dose on a slanting surface.

In this isocentric treatment, the SAD is, of course, the same at B (Fig. 5.6), however, the depth is reduced from 8 cm to 5 cm. The TAR_0 value at 5 cm depth using a 4 MV photon beam is 0.835 (Table A.4) and the SAR at the same depth is 0.117 (Table 5.2). Using the same treatment as in the previous example but with an OAR of 1.0595 (89/84) at 5 cm depth, the dose in B is found using equation 5.5, so

$$115 \times 1.03 \times (0.835 + 0.117) \times 1.0595 \times 0.96 = 115 \, cGy$$

The dose at B in this example is considerably higher than in the previous example when the overlying surface was flat. This is primarily due to a decreased amount of attenuating tissue overlying the calculation point in B (Fig. 5.6).

Calculating dose at an off-axis point at a different depth - SAD technique

In an isocentric treatment technique, it is not necessary to know what the source-surface distance is since TARs, TPRs, SARs, and SMRs are independent of distance. It is, however, necessary to know the relationship between the dose-calculation point and the isocenter. This is because dose rates, cGy/M.U., etc., are customarily specified on the central axis of the beam. Figure 5.6 demonstrates the relationship of the dose-calculation point to the isocenter. In the next example, the dose from parallel opposed anterior and posterior fields using an isocentric technique is calculated to the spinal cord (Fig 5.7).

In this example, the spinal cord is at 7 cm depth from the anterior surface and at 5 cm depth from the posterior surface. The treatment field in Fig. 5.3 is used again with an identical opposed field. The patient's thickness at the central axis (Fig. 5.3A) is 16 cm and at the off-axis point (Fig. 5.3B) the thickness is (7 + 5) 12 cm. Vertical air gaps are present in both fields (Fig. 5.7), that is, the patient's surface is not flat. The dose-calculation point

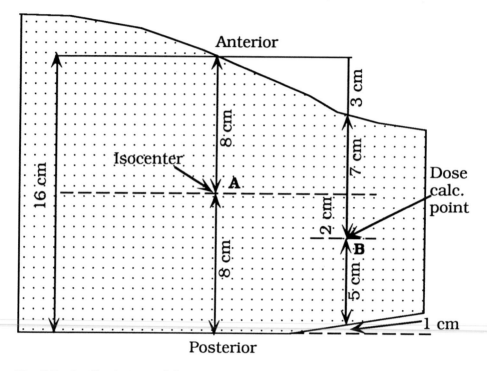

Fig. 5.7. An illustration of the geometry of an off-axis calculation at a depth different from the isocenter. The sum of the SSDs and the patient's thickness is the same on the central axis and along a vertical axis through point B.

lies 2 cm posterior of the isocenter; thus, an inverse square factor must be included in the calculation (page 58, Chapter 3).

The inverse square factor for the anterior field is $\left(\frac{80}{82}\right)^2$ or 0.9518

and for the posterior field it is $\left(\frac{80}{78}\right)^2$ or 1.0519

The TAR$_0$ at 7 cm depth is 0.734 (Table A.4) and the SAR is 0.134 (Table 5.2). The OAR at 7 cm depth is 1.053 (79.5/75.5).

The dose to the spinal cord from the anterior field is found from

$$\text{Dose} = \text{M.U.} \times \text{cGy/M.U} \times (\text{TAR}_0 + \text{SAR}) \times \text{OAR} \times \text{tray factor} \times \text{ISF} \quad (5.6)$$

that is

$$115 \times 1.03 \times (0.734 + 0.134) \times 1.053 \times 0.96 \times 0.9518 = 99 \text{ cGy}$$

The TAR_0 at 5 cm depth is 0.835 (Table A.4) and the SAR is 0.117 (Table 5.2). The OAR at 5 cm depth is 1.0595.

Using equation 5.6 the dose to the spinal cord from the posterior field is

$$115 \times 1.03 \times (0.835 + 0.117) \times 1.0595 \times 0.96 \times 1.0519 = 121 \text{ cGy}$$

In this example, the OAR was estimated at the depth of the off-axis point, and the assumption was made that the change in OAR, caused by the slant of the patient's surface contour, is negligible.

Calculating dose at an off-axis point at a different depth - SSD technique

In an SSD technique it is necessary to know the actual SSD at the dose-calculation point since the %DD used in this dose-calculation method is expressed as a percentage of the dose at D_{max} and depends on the distance.

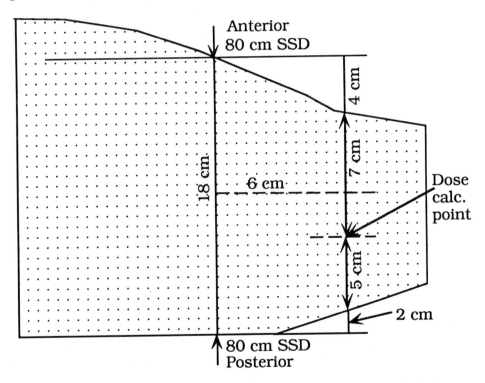

Fig. 5.8. Diagram of off-axis calculation point in a SSD treatment technique.

To illustrate this point, the next example deals with a fixed SSD technique in the treatment of a lung tumor via parallel opposed fields. The spinal-cord dose is to be calculated at a point 6 cm from the central axis using a cobalt-60 beam at 80 cm SSD (Fig. 5.8). The patient's thickness at the central axis is 18 cm. The treatment time is 1.22 min/field, the dose rate is 114 cGy/min, and the area factor is 1.032 for each field. No beam-shaping block is used, thus no transmission factor for block-supporting tray is included in the calculation. The spinal cord is at 7 cm depth from the anterior surface and the vertical air gap at this point is 4 cm. The OAR is 0.953 and the SAR for this field is found to be the same as for a 12 x 12 cm field. The %DD at 7 cm depth is 69.7 (Table A.1). The dose at an off-axis point using a fixed SSD technique is found from

$$\text{Dose} = \text{time (or M.U.)} \times \text{dose rate}_{(ref.)} \times \text{area f.} \times \%DD \times OAR \times ISF \quad (5.7)$$

The inverse square factor from equation 3.1 is $\left(\dfrac{80.5}{84.5}\right)^2 = 0.9076$

Using equation 5.7, the dose to the spinal cord from the anterior field is

$$1.22 \times 114 \times 1.032 \times (69.7/100) \times 0.953 \times 0.9076 = 86.5 \text{ cGy}$$

The spinal cord is at 5 cm depth from the posterior surface and the vertical air gap is 2 cm.

The inverse square factor from equation 3.1 is $\left(\dfrac{80.5}{82.5}\right)^2 = 0.9521$

The OAR is assumed to be the same as for the anterior field (0.953). The %DD at 5 cm depth is 79.2 (Table A.1).

Using equation 5.7, the spinal cord dose from the posterior field is

$$1.22 \times 114 \times 1.032 \times (79.2/100) \times 0.953 \times 0.9521 = 103 \text{ cGy}$$

Note in Fig. 5.8 that the sum of the patient's thickness and the SSDs at the central axis and at the off-axis point are the same. The anterior and posterior SSD at the central axis is 80 cm and the patient's thickness is 18 cm. The sum is 178 cm. At the off-axis point, the anterior SSD is 80 + 4 cm and the posterior SSD is 80 + 2 cm. The patient's thickness is 7 + 5 cm. The fact that the sum (84 + 82 + 12 cm) also is 178 cm is a simple check on the accuracy of the measurements.

In the preceding off-axis calculations, a vertical air gap was present. In some situations, the patient's contour may cause the SSD to be shorter than at the central axis. The dose-calculation procedure remains unchanged in that situation.

CALCULATING SARs WHEN THE RADII ARE INTERCEPTED BY A BLOCKED AREA

In many irregularly shaped fields, a radius from the calculation point to the extreme field margins may pass across a blocked area. This is a special situation which must be considered in a special way. Consider the field in Fig. 5.9 where radii numbers 16–21 pass through and extend beyond the blocked area. In this situation, the SAR value for the entire length (A to P) of the radius is first found. Then the SAR value for the part of the radius to the far edge of the block is subtracted (B to P) and the SAR value for the part to the near edge of the block (C to P) is added. Table 5.3 shows how the SAR is calculated using 4 MV photon data (Table A.8) for the field in Fig. 5.9.

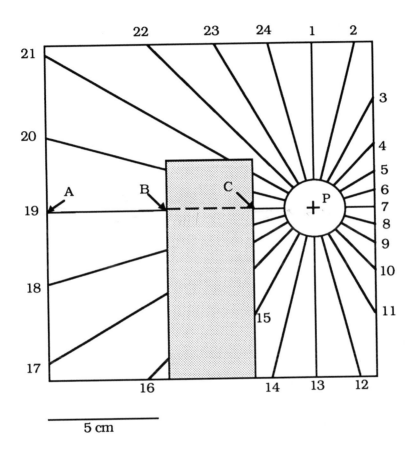

Fig. 5.9. An irregular shaped field where several radii extend beyond a blocked area (shaded). The SAR was calculated at P.

This method assumes that no primary dose is transmitted through the block and that no scatter is produced by the tissue under the block. In a typical situation, a small amount of primary dose is in fact transmitted, giving rise to some scattered dose under the block.

TABLE 5.3

SCATTER-AIR RATIO CALCULATION FOR THE FIELD IN FIGURE 5.9

----

4 MV Photons

Radius No	Length(cm)	Fractional SAR
1	7.5	0.0020
2	7.5	0.0020
3	5.5	0.0015
4	4.0	0.0011
5	3.0	0.0008
6	3.0	0.0008
7	3.0	0.0008
8	3.0	0.0008
9	3.0	0.0008
10	4.0	0.0011
11	5.0	0.0014
12	8.0	0.0022
13	7.5	0.0020
14	8.0	0.0022
15	5.5	0.0015
16	10.5; 9.5; 4.0	0.0027 - 0.0025 + 0.0011 = 0.0013
17	14.0; 8.0; 3.0	0.0030 - 0.0022 + 0.0008 = 0.0016
18	13.0; 7.0; 3.0	0.0029 - 0.0019 + 0.0008 = 0.0018
19	12.0; 6.5; 3.0	0.0028 - 0.0018 + 0.0008 = 0.0018
20	12.5; 7.0; 3.0	0.0029 - 0.0020 + 0.0008 = 0.0017
21	14.0; 5.0; 3.0	0.0030 - 0.0014 + 0.0008 = 0.0024
22	11.0	0.0028
23	9.0	0.0024
24	8.0	0.0022

SAR = **0.039**

CALCULATING DOSE UNDER A BLOCK

In some situations, calculation of the dose under a block or outside a field is necessary. Although shielding blocks are intended to reduce the dose to underlying organs, some transmission is unavoidable. This primary dose, with the addition of scattered radiation from the surrounding irradiated volume, are the two components which contribute dose under a block. Dose outside the field consists of scatter only.

Figure 5.10 illustrates a large abdominal field treated via a 4 MV photon beam and with a 5 HVT shielding block over each kidney. The dose to the left kidney was calculated at 9 cm depth. As in the equivalent square field calculation, 24 radii separated by 15° were drawn from the dose calculation point under the block to the periphery of the field. Since the calculation point is under a block, all radii pass through a blocked segment. The fractional SARs are found by using the same method as described previously. For example, the entire length of radius 20 in Fig. 5.10 is 18 cm and the fractional SAR (0.278/24) is 0.0116 (Table A.8). The distance from the calculation point to the far edge of the right kidney block is 11 cm and the fractional SAR (0.239/24) 0.0100 is subtracted. The distance from the calculation point to the near edge of the right kidney block is 7.5 cm and the SAR, which is added, is (0.200/24) 0.0083. The distance from the calculation point to the edge of the left kidney block is 2 cm and the fractional SAR, which is subtracted, is (0.069/24) 0.0029, leaving a total SAR value for this radius of (0.0116 - 0.0100 + 0.0083 - 0.0029) 0.0070. The fractional SARs for each radius are similarly found and are then added together to give the SAR of the field under consideration. The SAR at the calculation point in Fig. 5.10 was found to be 0.119 (Table 5.4).

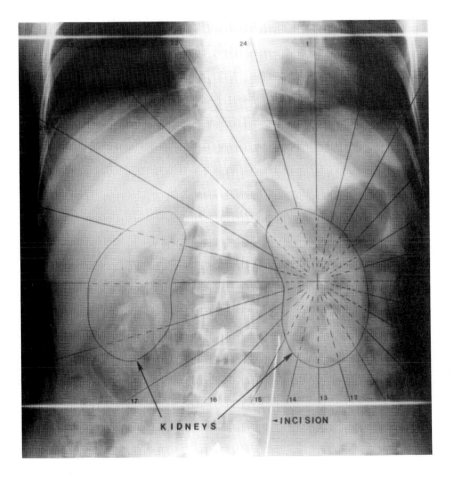

Fig. 5.10. Simulation film of an upper abdominal field; 5 HVT shielding blocks over the contrast-enhanced kidneys. Since radiographs are enlarged images of the patient, all measurements must be reduced to actual size.

TABLE 5.4

SCATTER-AIR RATIO CALCULATION FOR THE FIELD IN FIGURE 5.10

---

4 MV Photons

Radius No	Length (cm)	Fractional SAR
1	13.0; 3.5	0.0105 - 0.0048 = 0.0057
2	13.5; 3.0	0.0106 - 0.0043 = 0.0063
3	13.0; 3.0	0.0105 - 0.0043 = 0.0062
4	9.0; 3.0	0.0092 - 0.0043 = 0.0049
5	7.5; 2.5	0.0083 - 0.0035 = 0.0048
6	6.5; 2.5	0.0076 - 0.0035 = 0.0041
7	6.5; 2.5	0.0076 - 0.0035 = 0.0041
8	6.5; 3.0	0.0076 - 0.0043 = 0.0034
9	7.5; 3.0	0.0083 - 0.0043 = 0.0040
10	9.0; 3.5	0.0092 - 0.0048 = 0.0044
11	7.5; 4.0	0.0083 - 0.0055 = 0.0028
12	6.5; 4.5	0.0076 - 0.0060 = 0.0016
13	6.5; 4.5	0.0076 - 0.0060 = 0.0016
14	6.5; 4.5	0.0076 - 0.0060 = 0.0016
15	7.5; 3.5	0.0083 - 0.0048 = 0.0035
16	9.0; 2.5	0.0092 - 0.0035 = 0.0057
17	12.5; 2.0	0.0104 - 0.0029 = 0.0075
18	18.0; 12.0; 8.5; 2.0	0.0116 - 0.0102 + 0.0089 - 0.0029 = 0.0074
19	17.5; 12.5; 8.0; 2.0	0.0115 - 0.0104 + 0.0086 - 0.0029 = 0.0068
20	18.0; 11.0; 7.5; 2.0	0.0116 - 0.0100 + 0.0083 - 0.0029 = 0.0070
21	20.0; 2.5	0.0118 - 0.0036 = 0.0082
22	19.0; 4.0	0.0117 - 0.0055 = 0.0062
23	15.5; 4.0	0.0112 - 0.0055 = 0.0057
24	14.0; 4.0	0.0108 - 0.0055 = 0.0053

SAR = **0.119**

The primary dose delivered to a point under the block is found from

$$\text{Primary dose} = \text{M.U.} \times \text{cGy/M.U.} \times \text{OAR} \times \text{TAR}_0 \times \text{tray f.} \times \text{block f.} \quad (5.8)$$

The patient received 94 M.U., the cGy/M.U. was 1.06, and the off-axis ratio was 1.05. The TAR for a 0 x 0 cm field at 9 cm depth from Table A.4 is 0.655. The transmission through the shielding block is assumed to be 3% and through the block supporting tray 96%.

Using equation 5.8 the primary dose is therefore

$$94 \times 1.06 \times 1.05 \times 0.655 \times 0.96 \times 0.03 = 1.97 \text{ cGy}$$

The scatter at the same point is found from

$$\text{Scatter} = \text{M.U.} \times \text{cGy/M.U.} \times \text{tray factor} \times \text{SAR} \quad (5.9)$$

so in this patient the scatter is

$$94 \times 1.06 \times 0.96 \times 0.119 = 11.38 \text{ cGy}$$

The total dose at the center of the left kidney during the treatment of this field is the sum of the primary (1.97) and scatter (11.38) contributions, that is,

$$1.97 + 11.38 = 13.35 \text{ cGy}$$

The dose delivered at the patient's midplane on the central axis of each field is 85 cGy.

It should, however, be emphasized that the point in the left kidney selected for this dose calculation is farther from the irradiated volume than other segments of the kidneys and thus receives a lower dose.

CALCULATING DOSE FOR A ROTATION THERAPY TREATMENT

In rotation therapy techniques, the axis of rotation is placed in the tumor, and the therapy unit moves around the patient. The dose calculation method is the same whether the treatment machine makes a complete circle around the patient or a partial circle. The SAD remains constant, but the thickness of tissue which lies between the source and the isocenter varies as the patient's contour changes. For the purpose of dose calculation, the treatment can be considered as multiple stationary isocentric fields. In this example, radii are drawn in 15° intervals from the isocenter to the patient's external surface and the fractional TAR values are added (Fig. 5.11). For the purpose of calculating the dose, this TAR is then considered as in a stationary isocentric treatment.

The prescription is for 200 cGy to be delivered at the isocenter while the machine rotates 360° around the patient. The dose rate$_{ref}$ at the axis without the patient is 109 cGy/min, and the area factor for this field is 0.975.

The TAR (Table 5.5) for a 6 x 6 cm cobalt-60 beam used in the rotation treatment illustrated in Fig. 5.11 is found to be 0.530 from interpolated values in Table A.3. Using equation 4.34, the required treatment time is therefore

$$\frac{200}{109 \times 0.975 \times 0.530} = 3.55 \text{ min (3 min 33 sec)}$$

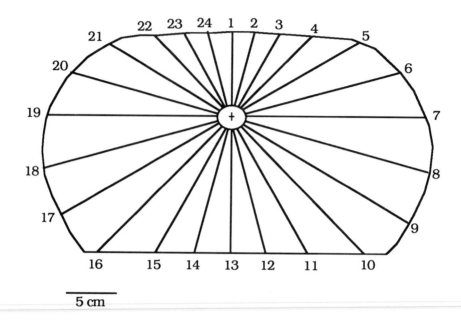

Fig. 5.11. In a rotation treatment, the fractional TARs are found for each radius (TAR/24) and are then added together.

TABLE 5.5

TISSUE-AIR RATIO CALCULATION
FOR THE 360° ROTATION IN FIGURE 5.11

Cobalt-60   6 x 6 cm Field

Radius No	Length (cm)	Fractional TAR	Radius No	Length (cm)	Fractional TAR
1	8.0	0.030	13	12.0	0.024
2	8.0	0.030	14	12.5	0.023
3	9.0	0.029	15	14.0	0.021
4	11.0	0.026	16	17.0	0.018
5	13.5	0.022	17	18.5	0.016
6	16.0	0.019	18	18.5	0.016
7	17.5	0.017	19	17.5	0.017
8	18.5	0.016	20	16.0	0.019
9	18.5	0.016	21	13.5	0.022
10	17.0	0.018	22	11.0	0.026
11	14.0	0.021	23	9.0	0.029
12	12.5	0.023	24	8.0	0.030

TAR = **0.528**

Since the dose rate from a cobalt-60 machine is relatively constant, the speed (degrees/min) with which the machine must rotate is determined by dividing the number of degrees in the rotation by the treatment time in minutes. In this cobalt-60 treatment, the machine must complete 360° in 3.55 minutes in order to deliver the prescribed dose at the isocenter.

The degrees/min can be found from

$$\frac{\text{number of degrees}}{\text{treatment time}} \qquad (5.10)$$

The degrees/min in this treatment is therefore

$$\frac{360°}{3.55} = 101.4°/\text{min}$$

Since the dose rate per time unit can be changed in a linear accelerator, the degrees/M.U. or, in some treatment units, the M.U./degree must be set.

It is always a good precaution to do a trial rotation without the patient present before the actual treatment begins, to verify that the number of degrees and the treatment time, or M.U., is correct. It is also a good practice to manually rotate the machine 360° around the patient before leaving the treatment room to make sure that accidental collisions will not occur during the treatment.

REFERENCES

Batho, H.F., Theimer, O., Theimer, R., A consideration of equivalent circle method of calculating depth doses for rectangular x-ray fields, J. Can. Assn. Radiol. 7, 1951 (1956).

Chui, C.S., Mohan, R., Off-center ratios for three-dimensional dose calculations, Medical Physics 13, 409, (1986).

Clarkson, J.R., A note on depth dose in fields of irregular shape, Brit. J. Radiol. 14, 265 (1941).

Day, M.J., A note on the calculation of dose in x-ray fields, Brit. J. Radiol. 23, 368 (1950).

Day, M.J., The equivalent field method for axial dose determination in rectangular fields, Brit. J. Radiol. Suppl. 10, 77 (1961).

Jones, D.E.A., A note on back-scatter and depth doses for elongated rectangular x-ray fields, Brit. J. Radiol. 22, 342 (1949).

Sterling, T.D., Perry, H., Katz, L., Derivation of a mathematical expression for the percentage depth dose surface of cobalt-60 beams and visualization of multiple field dose distributions, Brit. J. Radiol. 37, 544 (1964).

PROBLEMS

1. The %DD at a given depth

    a) increases with higher beam energies
    b) increases with lower beam energies
    c) beam energy doesn't matter

2. The amount of backscatter

    a) increases with lower beam energies
    b) increases with higher beam energies
    c) beam energy doesn't matter

3. Find the equivalent square for a 8 x 24 cm field using the area/perimeter method.

    $$2\left(\frac{area}{\ell+w}\right) = 12^2\, cm$$

4. Subtracting the SMR from the TMR for a 10 x 10 cm field will give the

    Scatter Max Ratio   Tissue Max Ratio

    a) TAR
    b) scatter dose
    c) TPR
    d) primary dose

5. Subtracting the TAR for a 0 x 0 cm field from the TAR for a 10 x 10 cm field will give the

    a) TAR for a 0 x 0 cm field
    b) scatter dose for 10 x 10 a cm field
    c) primary dose for 10 x 10 a cm field
    d) TMR for a 10 x 10 cm field

6. The OAR is the

    a) ratio of the dose at a given depth along the central axis and the dose at a point off the central axis at the same depth

    b) ratio of the dose at a given depth at a point away from the central axis and the dose at a point along the central axis at the same depth

    c) ratio of the dose at a point at a given depth off the central axis and the dose on an isodose curve at the same depth

7. A patient is receiving treatment to a lung tumor via parallel opposed 4 MV photon beams. The patient's diameter at the central axis of the beam is 20 cm. The treatment is isocentric and the field size is 12 x 18 cm at 80 cm SAD. 123 M.U. is delivered via each field. The cGy/M.U. for this field is 1.09. The dose in the spinal cord needs to be calculated at a point 7 cm cephalad from the central axis. The patient's diameter at this point is only 15 cm because of the slope of the anterior chest surface. The spinal cord is at 5 cm from the posterior surface and 10 cm from the anterior surface. The OAR for the posterior beam is 1.07 and for the anterior it is 1.035. What is the dose in the spinal cord? Use Table A.4 for TAR. There are no blocks and no wedges in this treatment.

8. Find the SAR at D_{max} at "+" in the field in Fig. 5.12. (Diagram is only one half of full size.) Use Table A.8 for SARs.

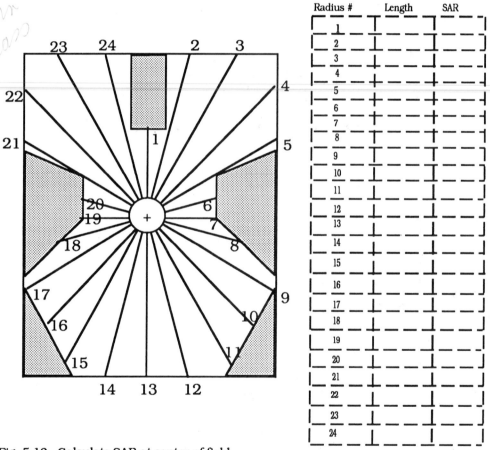

Fig. 5.12. Calculate SAR at center of field.

9. Calculate the dose to the kidney at "+" under a 5 HVT block in Fig. 5.13. A 4 MV photon beam was used. The OAR at point "+" is 1.025 and the cGy/MU is 1.07. 100 M.U. were delivered to one field only. The SSD was 80 cm and the depth was 12 cm. The tray factor is 0.96. (Dimensions are only one half of full size.)

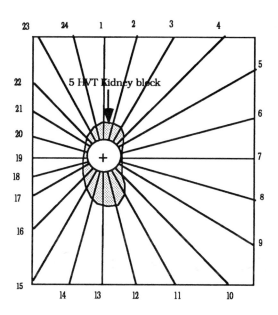

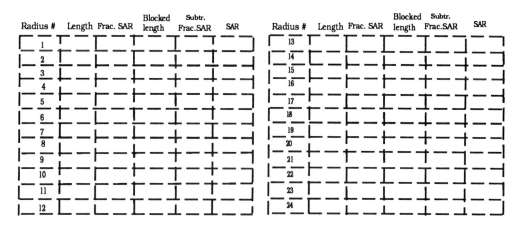

Fig. 5.13. Calculate under the kidney block. Use table to record length of each radius and fractional SARs. (Dimensions are only one half of full size.)

10. A patient with the contour in Fig. 5.14 (diagram is only one half of full size) is to be treated via a 360° rotation using an 8 x 8 cm cobalt-60 beam. The dose rate$_{ref}$ is 112.3 cGy/min for a 10 x 10 cm field and the area factor is 0.98. 200 cGy is prescribed at the isocenter. What is the required treatment time? (Give the answer in minutes and seconds.)

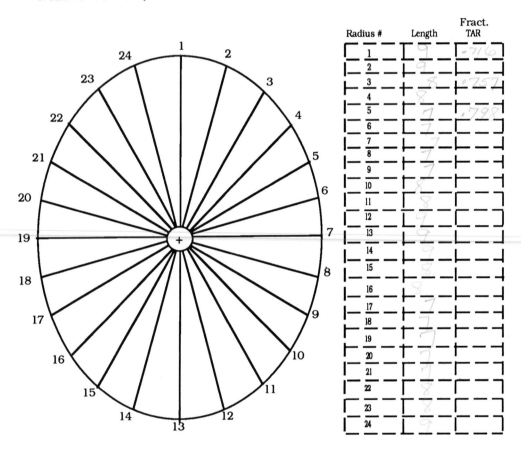

Radius #	Length	Fract. TAR
1	9	.716
2	9	
3	8	.757
4		
5	7	.798
6	7	
7		
8	7	
9	7	
10	8	
11	8	
12	9	
13	9	
14	9	
15	9	
16	8	
17	7	
18	7	
19	7	
20	7	
21	7	
22	8	
23	8	
24	9	

Fig. 5.14. Find the TAR for the contour (L) and use table to record fractional TARs.

11. In the above problem, how many degrees/minute must be set on the machine to deliver the prescribed dose while the machine rotates once through 360°?

SOLUTIONS

1. a

2. a

3. 12 cm^2

4. d

5. b

6. b

7. 255 cGy

8. 0.046

9. 14 cGy

10. 2 min 29 sec

11. 144.8 degrees/minute

CHAPTER 6

PROBLEMS ENCOUNTERED IN RADIATION THERAPY TREATMENT PLANNING

In radiation oncology treatment planning, many problems are not obvious to the beginner. The purpose of this section is to alert the planner to some of these not-so-obvious problems.

PATIENT POSITIONING PROBLEMS

The angle at which the beam impinges on the patient can be set either by changing the gantry or collimator orientation or by changing the patient's position with respect to the beam, which can be achieved either by changing the patient's position on the treatment couch or by changing the position of the couch with respect to the beam. In a kyphotic patient, for example, it would be difficult to place the patient in a position such that the axis of the torso is perpendicular to the vertical beam. Instead, the desired patient-beam relationship can be achieved by turning the couch 90° and then angling the gantry until the incident beam is perpendicular to the axis of the patient's torso (Fig. 6.1).

COMFORT

The first consideration in patient positioning should be patient comfort and safety during the treatments. A patient in an uncomfortable position is more likely to move during the treatment, and as a result, a portion of

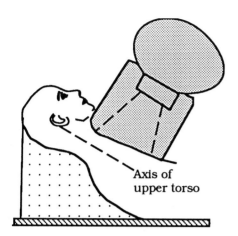
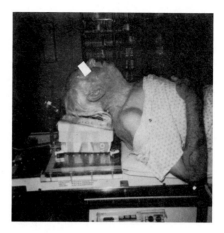

Axis of
upper torso

Fig. 6.1. In a kyphotic patient it may be necessary to turn the treatment couch 90° and then rotate the gantry until the beam is perpendicular to the patient's upper torso.

the target could be moved out of the beam while normal tissues which are not to be treated might inadvertently move into the beam.

A triangular pillow under the patient's knees will relax the back and make the patient feel more comfortable. This position changes the curvature of the lumbar spine and must be reproduced during the treatments. Allowing the patient to cross the legs will cause marks on the lateral aspect of the pelvis to change with respect to internal anatomy and should therefore be avoided. A rigid support, which fixes the separation of the patient's legs, can be made of styrofoam, and when used for patients being treated to the abdomen, pelvis, and lower extremities, will help reproduce the position (Fig. 6.2).

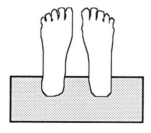

Fig. 6.2. A foot support helps in reproducing the patient's leg separation during the treatments.

Most treatment couches are quite narrow and do not provide a comfortable resting place for the patient's arms. Removable arm supports of thin plexiglass may be added to the width of the couch. The plexiglass may be anchored by placing part of it under the patient's body. Such arm supports should be used with caution if the chest is treated as they may cause patient-beam misalignment. An alternative arrangement can be made by placing a large sheet of plexiglass, wide enough to extend about 6 inches beyond the couch on each side, across the treatment couch under the chest to eliminate patient rotation. The use of arm supports effectively increases the width of the couch and may therefore prevent the head of the machine from clearing when lateral or rotational fields are used.

USE OF "BELLY BOARD"

Patients treated in the prone position are more difficult to make comfortable and the position is therefore more difficult to maintain. A prone patient may be more comfortable with a pillow under the ankles to allow the knees to be bent during the treatments. Some patients are more comfortable holding the arms above the head while in the prone position. The degree of arm elevation and the side to which the head is turned are important to daily reproduction of the relation between the skin marks and the underlying anatomy.

A belly board, sometimes used in an effort to displace the small bowel out of pelvic fields (Shanahan 1990), may also be more comfortable for prone patients, especially those treated during the immediate postsurgical period. In some patients, the addition of compression on the anterior surface of the lower pelvis promotes the desired small bowel displacement. The position of the patient on a belly board must be carefully reproduced and the exact location of the compression is also very important to the reproducibility (Fig. 6.3). Adequate support must be provided to allow the patient maximum relaxation during the treatment. The use of a belly board is also discussed in Chapter 7 (pages 171-175).

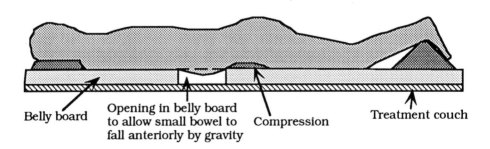

Belly board   Opening in belly board   Compression   Treatment couch
                 to allow small bowel to
                 fall anteriorly by gravity

Fig. 6.3. A prone patient may be more comfortable on a belly board which minimizes pressure on the abdomen.

In some patients, it is better to achieve small bowel or bladder sparing by treating the patient with a full bladder. The level of bladder fullness must then be reproduced for every treatment. Giving the patient a couple of glasses of water or a soft drink 1 hour before the treatment might be necessary if the patient forgets to hold the urine.

Elderly patients, very sick patients, and postsurgery patients are often limited as to what position they can tolerate. For them, compromises may have to be made in terms of positioning. For example, a patient who would be better treated in the prone position but is unable to tolerate this position due to postsurgical discomfort may have to be treated in the supine or decubitus position.

RESTRAINT

Elderly patients who are confused and patients with compromised coordination must be strapped to the treatment couch during the treatment and must be very closely supervised via closed-circuit television to prevent serious accidents from happening during the treatment.

TREATING A PATIENT IN A SITTING POSITION

A patient with superior vena cava obstruction may not be able to breathe while lying down and may have to be treated in an upright position. Such patients are often unable to get out of bed and can be treated while in bed with the head of the bed elevated. Until the patient's condition permits conventional positioning, treatment through a single anterior high-energy photon field may be the best solution. A patient sitting in bed may be helped by providing a foot board for support. This will prevent the patient from slipping down in the bed thus causing target-beam misalignment. Some patients may also benefit from having a firm support behind their back to help maintain the position during the treatment.

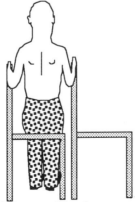

Fig. 6.4. A patient treated in a sitting position is more comfortable and can maintain the position longer if an arm rest is provided.

Most treatment equipment is designed to facilitate treatment of patients lying on a treatment couch, and it is not as simple to treat a sitting patient. The patient's position is difficult to reproduce and it is usually difficult to work at normal treatment distances. If the patient can sit sideways on a chair, both an anterior and a posterior field may be used without the beam traversing the chair back. The patient can rest one arm on the back of the chair and the other arm on the back of a second chair placed beside him on the other side (Fig. 6.4).

REPRODUCIBILITY

In addition to giving primary consideration to patient safety and comfort, the reproducibility of the setup must be maintained from the simulation to the treatment and from day to day in later treatments. The relationship between marks made on the patient's skin surface and the underlying internal anatomy must remain unchanged from the simulation to the treatment. Small discrepancies in the patient-beam alignment between the simulation and the treatment may appear trivial but can cause serious errors and should therefore be minimized. For example, the surface of some simulation couches are rigid while the couch in the treatment room may have an opening to allow a posterior field to be treated without the beam's traversing the treatment couch. A thin mylar sheet stretched across the opening or an insert consisting of a tennis-racket type net, will sag under the patient's weight, disturbing the relationship between skin marks and internal anatomy that existed during simulation. The integrity of these special couch supports must therefore be maintained and they may need to be replaced frequently. There are also some reasons for small changes in the patient-beam relationship which can not be eliminated, for example, respiration.

The practice of pulling the patient's clothing away from the treatment area, rather than having the patient undress for the treatment, creates rolls of clothing under the patient on either side of the treatment area. These rolls of clothing may not be in precisely the same place for each treatment and may be of various sizes depending on what kind of clothing the patient wears on a given day. Variation in the rolled-up clothing under the patient will change the curvature of the spine and the patient's position is then not precisely reproduced. Having the patient undress for each treatment eliminates this inconsistency.

The elevation of the patient's arms above the head, routinely used for treatment of breast carcinoma, Hodgkin's disease, and lateral fields in the thorax, must be very carefully reproduced for each treatment session. Positioning devices, such as Alpha Cradles®,* are essential to comfortable and reproducible patient positioning. An Alpha Cradle® with built-in handles for the patient to hold on to during the treatments helps the patient

---

* Smithers Medical Products, Inc., 391 Geneva Avenue, Tallmadge, Ohio 44278

to relax and also to maintain the raised-arm position without straining (Bentel 1990, 1991).

Changes of the patient's weight during a course of treatment and changes in swelling or tumor size during the course of treatment may cause changes in the position of skin marks with respect to the underlying anatomy. New positioning and restraining devices, in addition to resimulation of the treatment fields, may be required to ensure continuous correct patient-beam alignment when weight changes occur.

As shown in the previous sections, the position of the patient during the radiation treatment is not a trivial matter but requires rather serious consideration.

DOSE DISTRIBUTION IN MULTIPLE LEVELS

IRREGULAR CONTOUR

In general, treatment plans are generated in only one transverse plane within an often large treatment volume. This plane usually contains the central axis of the treatment fields. In most situations, it is adequate to view the dose distribution in this plane only because from previous experience we know that it will look similar in other transverse planes parallel to the first. There are, however, situations when further planning should be carried out, for example, when the patient's contour within the treatment fields varies more than a couple of centimeters, causing the dose to be different from that calculated in the principal plane. Typical examples would be in the treatment of the chest, either through anterior and posterior or oblique fields, treatment of breast carcinoma through tangential fields, and in treating the pelvis of an obese patient through anterior and posterior fields (Fig. 6.5).

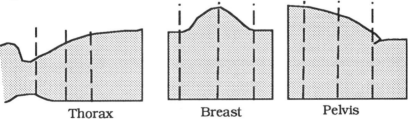

Thorax   Breast   Pelvis

Fig. 6.5. Examples of irregular contours where isodose distributions may be needed in more than one level.

Another examples of an irregular patient contour occurs in the treatment of the head and neck region. Even though smaller fields are usually used in this site, the dose variation within a treated area is quite unpredictable. As an example, the lateral diameter of the patient's neck varies a great deal, both in the transverse and the coronal planes, causing the dose to be inhomogeneous even when opposed lateral fields are used (Fig. 6.6). Calculation of isodose distributions in multiple planes should therefore be considered in such a case.

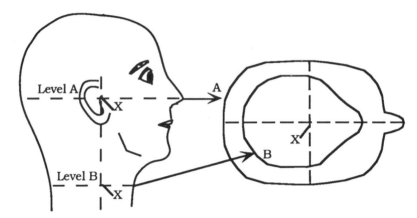

Fig. 6.6. Contours in the head and neck area show the changes in patient contour in both the axial plane and in the cephalad/caudal direction.

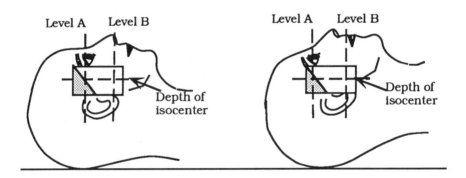

Fig. 6.7. In many situations, the thickness of tissue overlying the isocenter varies in the sagittal direction of the patient. Thus, the dose may vary along the anterior surface of the patient's face as in the left example above. When the patient's neck is extended, as on the right, the depths change further.

VARIATIONS IN THE DEPTH OF THE ISOCENTER

In isocentric techniques, where the dose is usually normalized at the isocenter, changes in the depth of the isocenter will have the same effect on the dose distribution as a change in the weighting of the beam (page 94, Chapter 4 and page 184, Chapter 7). As an example, when an anterior field is used in the treatment of maxillary antrum tumors, the presence of the nose causes dose variations within the anterior field. Extension of the chin, sometimes necessary in these patients, will also cause the depth of the isocenter* in a three-field technique to vary greatly (Fig. 6.7). A typical plan is shown on page 261 of *Treatment Planning and Dose Calculation in Radiation Oncology* (Bentel 1989). Similarly, in treating the neck of a kyphotic patient through anterior and posterior fields, the dose inhomogeneity will be accentuated by variations in depth of the isocenter (Figs. 6.8 and 6.9).

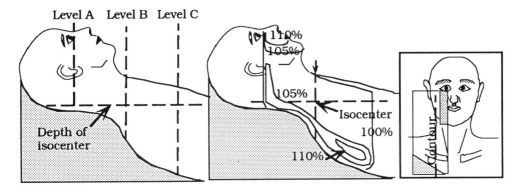

Fig. 6.8. Parallel opposed anterior and posterior fields in a kyphotic patient will result in undesirable dose inhomogeneities, and some normal tissues are difficult to shield. Only in contour (B) is the isocenter at mid-depth in the patient.

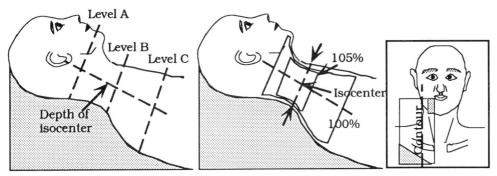

Fig. 6.9. Turning the couch 90° and then rotating the gantry until the beam is perpendicular to the axis of the torso (see also Fig. 6.1) improves dose uniformity, and shielding normal tissues becomes possible. The plane of the isocenter is in the patient's mid-depth at all three contours.

WEDGES

The problem of dose variation at other levels within a treatment, as previously described, is accentuated when wedges are used in the plan. This

---

* The isocenter is defined as a *point* around which the source rotates, but in this context it is represented by the axis that gantries rotate around.

is particularly important when the treatment fields are shaped so that the radiation goes through a thinner section of the wedge in a plane other than the plane on which the dose distribution is viewed. If the patient's tissue is also thinner at that point, a very hot spot could result, but it would be hidden to the casual observer unless a dose distribution was also displayed at such a level (Fig. 6.10).

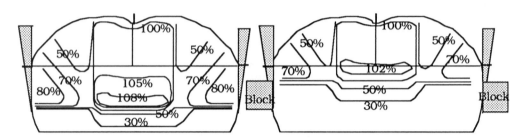

Fig. 6.10. An isodose distribution in a single plane is insufficient when a field is shaped so that the beam travels through a thinner part of a wedge in another plane. The high dose under the thinner part of the wedge (left) is not evident in the central axis plane (right).

PATIENT POSITIONING

Some of the problems described above can be eliminated by adjusting the patient's position or by causing the radiation beam to enter the patient at an unconventional angle. For example, an obese patient may be positioned prone to cause the anterior surface of the abdomen to be flattened against the couch top. In most patients, the posterior surface is fairly flat and less mobile than the anterior surface. This position is therefore preferable for marking of setup lines and it improves treatment-field reproducibility. This is discussed in more detail in Chapter 7 of *Treatment Planning and Dose Calculation in Radiation Oncology.*

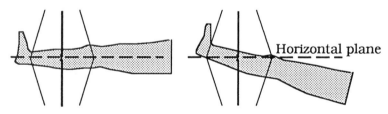

Fig. 6.11. An extremity should be perpendicular to the beam to give the best dose uniformity.

When treating an extremity through parallel opposed fields, the extremity should be elevated until its axis is parallel with the axis of gantry rotation, that is, the extremity should be at right angles to the direction of the beam (Fig. 6.11). With the patient in the supine position and using parallel opposed anterior and posterior fields, the extremity should be horizontal. When oblique opposed beams are used, the center of the extremity should still be parallel with the axis of the gantry rotation so that the treatment distance to the center of the extremity is the same everywhere within the treated segment.

TREATMENT DOCUMENTATION

Port films are often reviewed without the treatment chart or other details of the patient's history nearby. A short note on the simulation film giving the patient's diagnosis and any particular information about surgical margins, etc., would be helpful to a reviewer who is unfamiliar with the case. It is also good practice to mark incisions, palpable nodes, etc., with lead markers during the simulation procedure and to label them on the radiograph (Fig. 6.12).

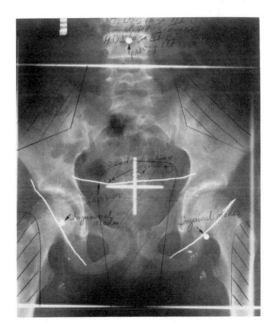

Fig. 6.12. Lead markers on scars, incisions, palpable nodes, and other important reference points during the simulation procedure are very useful for later reference. A statement of the diagnosis and a short note about the patient on the simulation film are also very helpful when films are reviewed.

MOVING THE PATIENT'S TREATMENT TO ANOTHER MACHINE

Treatment machines sometimes break down or require preventive maintenance but patient treatments must continue. If the treatment is moved to a treatment machine with different geometry and beam energy, the changeover may require that a change be made in the field size and it may also require resimulation.

In many instances, only recalculation of the dose will be necessary. If customized beam-defining blocks are used, these may need to be recut for the new treatment machine. This is a simple procedure if the treatment distance remains the same and only the target-to-tray distance is different on the new machine. However, if the treatment distance is different, the film distance will have to be adjusted accordingly on the block-cutting equipment when the new blocks are constructed. For example, if the simulation film from which the blocks were originally cut was taken with 80 cm source-axis distance (SAD) and the patient is changed to a machine with 100 cm SAD, 20 cm must be added to the original target-film distance (TFD) when the blocks are cut for the new machine. If the reverse is the case, 20 cm must be subtracted from the original TFD when the blocks are recut.

$$\frac{80}{TFD_x} = \frac{100}{TFD_{original}}$$

TREATMENT ERRORS

This section will focus on *errors* that sometimes occur in dose calculations, or in the setup of a patient's treatment rather than on the *uncertainties* associated with dose delivery. Human errors will occasionally occur in every radiation therapy department and a system needs to be in effect to deal with such a problem.

Treatment errors can be divided in to two groups; failure to deliver the prescribed dose and failure to treat the intended volume of tissue. Errors in dose delivery can be caused by a) error in table look-up, b) error in dose calculation, c) error in measurements of the patient's dimensions, or d) treatment machine malfunction. Errors of these types are often small and through a rigid quality assurance program can be detected before a second or third treatment is delivered.

More serious errors, both in terms of dose and dose distribution, occur when a wedge is omitted from the beam, or is inserted in the wrong orientation. In Chapter 3 (page 72), we learned that wedges, while altering the shape of the isodose curves, also attenuate the beam. The attenuation depends on the wedge angle and the beam energy but can be as high as 50%: if a wedge with 50% attenuation is inadvertently omitted, then, not only is the dose distribution altered, but the *amount* of dose on the central axis is doubled. The changes in the dose distribution caused by the omission of a wedge with a steep angle is more severe than if a wedge with a smaller angle is omitted. When a wedge is inserted but the orientation is reversed, the dose on the central axis is unchanged, but the error in the dose distribution is obviously significant.

Errors in wedge orientation may be counteracted by using a wedge with a steeper angle in the correct orientation during the next few treatments but that will, of course, deliver a somewhat different dose distribution and consideration must therefore be given to the effect that this will have on the tissues within the field. A good "rule of thumb" to bear in mind is that omission of a 30° wedge during only one of 30 treatments results in a 1° change in the slope of the isodose curve in this field. The slope of the isodose curve is 30° whether we give one or 30 treatments so by leaving the wedge out during one treatment the effect will be one thirtieth, or in this case 1° (about 3%). Similarly, the omission of a 30° wedge during 5 of 10 treatments will result in a 15° (or 50%) change in the slope of the isodose curve.

Another serious error is caused when a beam-shaping block is inadvertently omitted, inserted with the wrong orientation, or is inserted in the wrong field. Unlike dose-delivery errors, these types of errors are usually not repeated during multiple treatments, and are more difficult to detect unless portal verification films are taken during delivery of each dose fraction. The impact of field-placement errors is similar to that of errors in dose delivery, in that some segment of the target may have been outside the irradiated area and thus received no dose.

The course of action when an error is discovered should be based on the magnitude of the error and its relative proportion of the entire treatment course. For example, was 185 rather than the prescribed 180 cGy delivered, or was 300 rather than 150 cGy delivered; did the error occur during 1 of 20 treatments or was it during 2 of 5? Consideration should also be given to the radiosensitivity of the normal tissues which received the wrong dose and to the effect in these organs which can be expected from the error.

The philosophy of how to correct dose errors varies among physicians. While some think that the error in dose should be corrected during the following one or two treatments depending on the magnitude of the error, others think that unintentionally deviating from the prescribed dose one day does not justify making the same deviation in the opposite direction, now intentionally, one more day. Each situation must be considered individually and modifications must be made by the physician only.

ADJACENT FIELDS

One of the most frequently occurring problems is that of gaps between adjacent fields. It is also the cause for most concern by radiation oncologists, particularly when the gap occurs over the spinal cord. Although the creation of a gap is dealt with in the same way in all parts of the body, this section will only address the problem of field gaps over the spinal cord.

It is commonly assumed that the beam-defining light represents the intersection of the 50% isodose line with the patient's skin (Fig. 6.13) and the physicist will usually ensure that it is set in this way (see also page 70, Chapter 3). It is also assumed that the patient's surface is perfectly flat and in most instances it is not. Therefore, when actually setting up the fields on the patient, consideration must be given to the shape of the patient's contour at the field junction (Keys 1990).

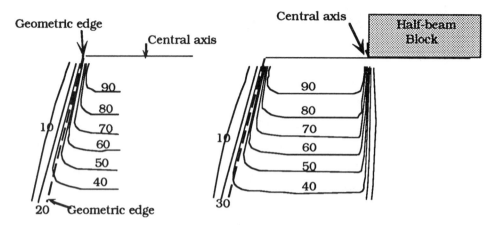

Fig. 6.13. The intersection of the 50% isodose line and the patient's skin surface is usually the geometric edge of the beam (light field). When a half-beam block is used in the beam, the effect of divergence at the block margin is removed, but the penumbra, although improved, still remains.

CREATING A FIELD GAP BY CUSTOMIZED BEAM SHAPING

It is almost always assumed that the field edges of the two adjacent fields are defined by the collimator and, thus, are perfectly straight. In such a situation, we can calculate the necessary gap by using simple geometry (Chapter 6 in *Treatment Planning and Dose Calculation in Radiation Oncology*). However, with increasing frequency these field edges are created by customized blocks. For example, in a mantle field, the field margin is usually defined by the collimator; however, in the adjacent para-aortic field it is not unusual to have the margin defined by a customized block (Fig. 6.14). This often occurs when the para-aortic field must extend into the previously irradiated mantle field to include the spleen which usually lies within the region shielded by the left lung block in the mantle field. In the patient's midline, where the mantle field was unshielded, the para-aortic field must be shaped to create the necessary gap. This block must be made so that a straight line is formed perpendicular to the spinal cord.

In this situation in which the field margins of the previously treated fields were defined by the collimator and the gap must be created by a customized blocks in the new fields, it is difficult to define precisely where the block must be drawn on the simulation film. Calculation of the necessary gap, using the distance from the central axis of the new field to where the field gap will be, should give the necessary gap on the skin surface. Placing a lead marker at this point on the anterior surface would indicate where the customized block needs to be placed. If both the previous and the new fields are treated while the patient is supine, the anterior and posterior fields will be identical and both beam-shaping blocks can be produced from the same radiograph.

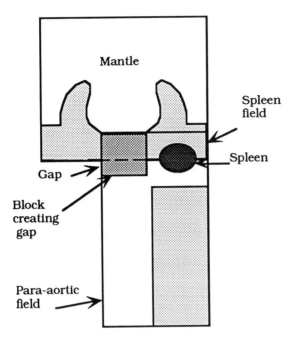

Fig. 6.14. Anterior mantle and para-aortic fields where the separation between them is defined with a customized block. The spleen, in this case, lies under the lung block previously used in the mantle field.

Another situation when the margin might be formed by a block rather than by the collimator edge is in patients with lung carcinoma, where the necessary shape of the field would require a block across the spinal cord. Any field edge across the spinal cord should form a straight line so that simple geometry is maintained for field matching if the patient returns for additional treatment to an adjacent area (Fig. 6.15).

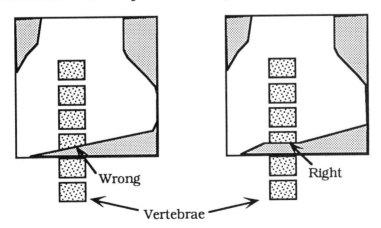

Fig. 6.15. Beam shaping across the spinal cord should always be made straight across the spine to facilitate subsequent field matching.

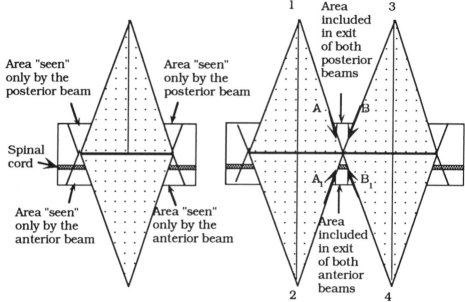

Line A and A₁ should demarcate the same anatomical reference since A includes what A₁ excludes.

Fig. 6.16. Left: The same length of spinal cord is not included in the anterior and the posterior field because the fields are identical at the patient's mid-depth and the spinal cord lies farther posterior. Right: A typical field matching situation where the patient's position is the same for all four fields. For a perfect geometric match, lines A and A₁ should "see" the same point of the spinal cord in this set up and lines B and B₁ should "see" the same point. The geometric edges of all four fields coincide at the patient's mid-depth.

WHEN THE PATIENT'S POSITION IS DIFFERENT

As has previously been mentioned, both in this text and in *Treatment Planning and Dose Calculation in Radiation Oncology*, the ideal situation for field matching is when the patient's position is the same for all fields considered in the field matching (Fig. 6.16). However, in many instances where field matching is required, the patient's position may not be the same for all fields. In this situation, the safest method is to consult simulation or port films of the previously treated fields and determine which segment of the spinal cord has been treated and then to set up the new fields without including the same segment again. This might mean that the anterior and posterior fields, if opposed fields are needed, will not be identical. This is because the spinal cord lies closer to the posterior surface. To include the same segment of the spinal cord in the two fields, the anterior field must be smaller on the skin surface than the posterior field (Fig. 6.17).

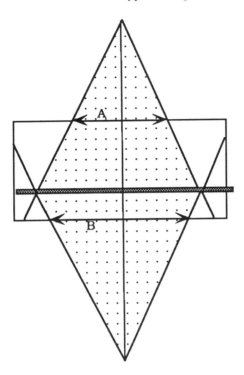

Fig. 6.17. The anterior field (A) is smaller on the anterior surface than the posterior (B) on the posterior surface when both "see" the same length of the spinal cord. This is because the spinal cord lies farther posterior (at a longer distance from the anterior surface) where the beam has spread more.

ADDING A SINGLE FIELD ADJACENT TO AN AREA PREVIOUSLY TREATED THROUGH OPPOSED FIELDS

Patients previously treated through parallel opposed anterior and posterior fields are usually patients with lung carcinoma treated in the supine position. They often return with metastatic disease in the spine or a spinal-cord compression requiring immediate intervention. If the compression is at least more than one vertebral body away from the previously treated segment of the spinal cord, then a routine gap calculation, given in detail on page 150 of *Treatment Planning and Dose Calculation in Radiation Oncology,* can be used. Even if only a posterior field is contemplated, the supine position should be strongly considered in order to maintain optimal geometry in the gap region.

USING A HALF-BEAM BLOCK

To minimize the gap between the previously treated fields and the new field, the central axis of the new field should be set as close as possible to the edge of the previously treated field, and then a half-beam block be inserted to block out the previously treated area (Figs. 6.13 and 6.18). This eliminates any beam spread of the new field into the previously treated area and thus minimizes the size of the untreated area. This technique may be advantageous in situations where the spinal-cord compression is very close to the previously treated segment of the spinal cord.

Some patients present with spinal-cord compressions in more than one site. When two sites are close to one another, even if the patient does not have any symptoms from disease in this segment, in most instances, it is best to include this region as well, because it is possible that microscopic disease is already present. From a field-matching viewpoint, it is almost impossible to match fields safely and treat the small segment between them later on.

SHIFTING THE LOCATION OF THE GAP

The disadvantage of treating two adjacent areas sequentially rather than concurrently is that one can not "feather" the field edges in anticipation of a future field matching problem.

In patients in whom adjacent fields are treated concurrently or in planned sequence, the field margins are often shifted to "smear out" the dose gradient between the adjacent areas. Such instances would be, for example, in the treatment of the entire central nervous system where all fields are usually treated concurrently and in the treatment of Hodgkin's disease where the planned fields are treated sequentially but with a planned break between treatment courses. Careful dose documentation must be kept with respect to the region affected by the gap shift because very high dose areas can be unintentionally created (Bentel 1990).

TATTOOS AS FIELD MARKERS

Tattoos on the patient's skin to indicate the precise position of treatment fields must be used with caution. As the patient's weight changes so do these tattoos with respect to underlying anatomical landmarks. Changes in tumor size, swelling, and in the case of a child, growth will also change the relative position of the tattoos and the underlying anatomy. Therefore, tattoos must be used with caution, particularly if some time has passed between the placement of the tattoos and the subsequent treatment when these marks may become important.

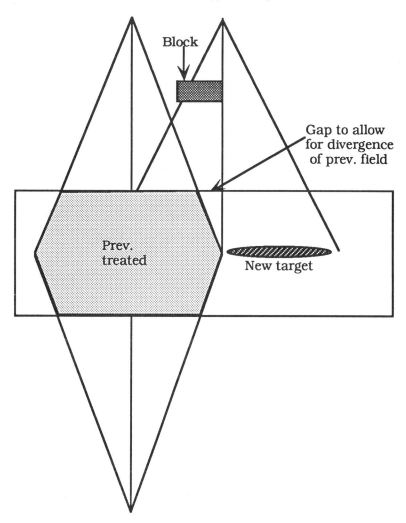

Block

Gap to allow
for divergence
of prev. field

Prev.
treated

New target

Fig. 6.18. Using a half-beam block when the new treatment field lies close to previously treated area reduces the size of the gap needed between the fields.

COMMUNICATION PROBLEMS

One often-encountered problem is the differences in terminology among the staff. Confusion and error can be reduced by proper use of the technical terms of radiation oncology; though terms are inherently precise, careless use of terminology can lead to serious errors.

In treatment planning, for example, it is more important to outline the target volume (often symbolized by TV) than the tumor volume (also symbolized by TV) because the former is always larger than the latter. In most situations, it is necessary for the treatment-planning staff to know the size and location of the *target* so that it can be included in the final plan. For a subsequent boost, the target and the tumor volumes may be synonymous. The dosimetrist is often presented with CT images or simulation films where the "TV" is outlined. The dosimetrist plans the fields so that this volume is covered, only to learn later that the physician also wanted to treat a large margin surrounding the area marked TV, now intended to signify the target volume. A new plan must be made to include this "TV" (target volume). If everyone would agree on proper terminology, symbols, and abbreviations before a great deal of effort is spent on planning the treatment, everyone would benefit, including the patient, and embarrassing moments would be prevented.

The term "given dose" was once in common use to describe surface or D_{max} doses. The expression given dose is too vague and leads to ambiguities unacceptable in modern radiation oncology. Is the given dose delivered by one field on the surface, at a depth, at a depth on the central axis, at an isodose curve; is it the minimum tumor dose, or perhaps the maximum tumor dose? With modern sophisticated methods of determining dose at practically any point in tissue, given dose has given way to terminology which more clearly describes dose. The reporting of doses must be accompanied by a description of where the dose was delivered using current methods of determination. There must be no ambiguity as to what dose was delivered and where.

In describing simple anatomical landmarks, careless use of proper terminology can cause major errors in beam position. For example, giving instructions to the simulator technologist to place a lead marker on the "bony canthus" is ambiguous. The canthus is the angle at *either* end of the eyelids, so there are two canthi, distinguished as the temporal or outer canthus, and the nasal or inner canthus (Dorland 1985). Not only can the two canthi be confused with each other, but the outer canthus is sometimes confused with the lateral bony ridge of the orbit, resulting in an error of as much as 0.75 cm in field placement with obvious consequences (Fig. 6.19).

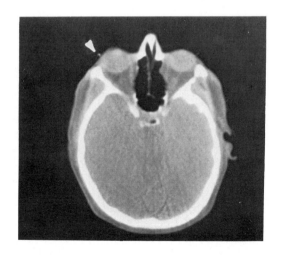

Fig. 6.19. The lateral bony ridge of the orbit and the lateral canthus of the eye (arrow) are usually separated by approximately 0.75.

The physician may sometimes use terminology unfamiliar to technologists. Occasionally, to avoid any embarrassment of asking, other staff just guess at the physician's intentions and the desired result may not be reached.

A vertical beam direction is, to many individuals, synonymous with an anterior field because of the conventional supine patient position. However, when the patient's position is changed (prone or decubitus), the vertical beam direction becomes a posterior or lateral field (Fig. 6.20). The field positions are usually described with respect to the patient and not with how the treatment machine happens to be positioned. It is not unusual to hear someone refer to a vertical beam as an anterior field regardless of the patient's position. Such very simple misunderstanding could lead to serious errors in treatment delivery. In communicating the intended field arrangement among the staff, it is critical that everyone understand and carry out the prescribed treatment with proper patient-beam arrangement.

In a growing number of treatments, not only are the gantry and collimator angled, but also the treatment couch. Gantry angles are customarily expressed from 0° to 360°, while collimator and couch angles usually are expressed from 0° to 90°. Gantry angles are not uniform between treatment machines and different manufacturer may have different systems of defining gantry angles. Since there is little or no need to turn the collimator or couch more than 90° to either side, the problem of expressing the angle is simpler. However, there is a serious problem of defining in which direction these angles are; for example, whether the couch is turned 10° to the left or to the right, positive or negative, and is it with respect to the patient or to the gantry? The expression "kicking the couch out" is much too general in modern radiation therapy. Specific instructions as to the direction in which the couch is to be turned and the documentation of the number of degrees are vital in safely relaying the information from the simulation room to the treatment room.

With the advent of three-dimensional treatment planning and the ability to rotate and view CT and MRI images in practically any plane, a common language becomes paramount to the communication and understanding among the many individuals involved in the planning and delivery of a course of treatments. Describing different beam angles or the planes in which we view the patient's anatomy can be very confusing. The precision in delivering radiation therapy which we are capable of with the use of very sophisticated tools must not be compromised by misunderstandings or ambiguities. Sailer et al. have proposed a uniform language for describing planes in which three-dimensional treatment plans are viewed (Goitein 1990, Sailer 1990).

With the growing number of new modalities and the rapid development and application of three-dimensional treatment planning systems, the need for a common language is paramount. The conventions, for example, by which gantry, collimator, and couch angles are described vary among institutions and may even vary among the staff within one institution. As a result, the confusion may lead to errors in treatment delivery and when discussions among the staff as to what is what, are carried on in front of the patient, as the case may be in the simulator room or treatment room, the patient quickly loses confidence in the staff's abilities.

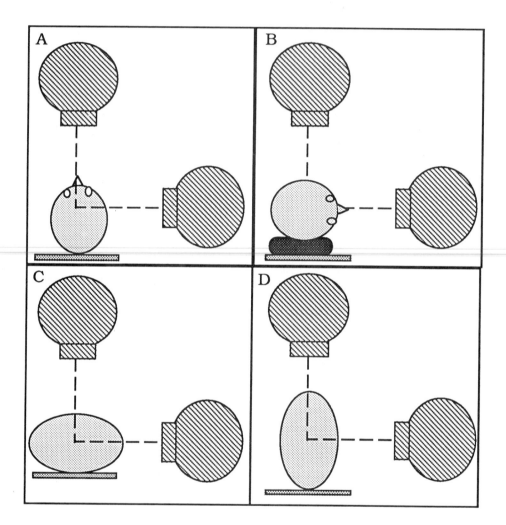

Fig. 6.20. A vertical beam is not always an anterior field. Field description should always be made with respect to the patient and not the machine.

REFERENCES

Bentel, G.C., Nelson, C.E., Noell, K.T., <u>Treatment Planning and Dose Calculation in Radiation Oncology</u>, Pergamon Press, Inc. Elmsford, NY, 1989.

Bentel, G.C., Positioning and immobilization device for patients receiving radiation therapy for carcinoma of the breast, <u>Medical Dosimetry</u> 15, 3 (1990).

Bentel, G.C., Positioning and immobilization of patients undergoing radiation therapy for Hodgkin's disease, <u>Medical Dosimetry</u> 16, 111 (1991).

<u>Dorland's Illustrated Medical Dictionary</u> (26th ed.), W.B. Saunders, Philadelphia, PA, 1985.

Sailer, S. L., Bourland, D., Rosenman, J. G., Sherouse, G. W., Chaney, E. L., Tepper, J. E., 3-D beams need 3-D names, <u>Int. J. Radiat. Oncol. Biol. Phys.</u> 19, 797 (1990).

Goitein, M., Oblique sections need 3-D names also, <u>Int. J. Radiat. Oncol. Biol. Phys.</u> 19, 821 (1990).

Keys, R., Grigsby, P. W., Gapping fields on sloping surfaces, <u>Int. J. Radiat. Oncol. Biol. Phys.</u> 18, 1183 (1990).

Shanahan, T.G., Mehta, M.P., Bertelrud, K.L., Buchler, D.A., Frank, L.E., Gehring, M.A., Kubsad, S.S., Utrie, P.C., Kinsella, T.J., Minimization of small bowel volume within treatment fields utilizing customized "Belly Boards," <u>Int. J. Radiat. Oncol. Biol. Phys.</u> 19, 469 (1990).

PROBLEMS

1. A patient's head position should be made comfortable by

    a) using the softest head support possible
    b) placing a head support of the right height under the head
    c) using regular bed pillow under the head

2. The patient's head position when treating a vertex field should be

    a) with the chin extended as much as possible
    b) with the chin tucked down on the chest
    c) the head position doesn't matter

3. To treat a vertex field, we may have to turn the

    a) couch 90° and the gantry until desired angle is achieved
    b) collimator and the couch
    c) gantry and the collimator only

4. When treating an extremity, the axis must be

    a) parallel with the treatment couch
    b) elevated until it is horizontal
    c) perpendicular to the beam

5. Dose distributions in multiple levels may be necessary when the following area is treated

    a) the pelvis of a thin patient
    b) the breast of a large patient
    c) the brain of an obese patient

6. Treatment fields should always be shaped so that the beam edge

    a) crosses the spinal cord at an angle
    b) crosses perpendicular to the spinal cord
    c) with respect to the spinal cord doesn't matter

7. In port films of parallel opposed isocentric fields of a lung tumor, the

    a) anterior field will appear to treat a longer segment of the spinal cord than the posterior field

b) posterior field will appear to treat a longer segment of spinal cord than the anterior field

a) two fields will appear to treat the same segment of spinal cord

8. To minimize the gap between two adjacent fields

   a) a posterior field alone can be used
   b) an anterior field alone can be used
   c) a half-beam block can be used

9. When adjacent areas must be treated it is best to

   a) calculate the gap necessary between the fields to prevent an overlap
   b) set a 2 cm gap between all fields
   c) rely on tattoos to prevent an overlap

10. A common language in radiation therapy is important to

    a) prevent the patients from understanding what we do
    b) prevent errors and misunderstandings
    c) promote swift and correct actions

SOLUTIONS

1.	b		6.	b
2.	b		7.	a
3.	a		8.	c
4.	c		9.	a
5.	b		10.	b

CHAPTER 7

TREATMENT PLANNING PROBLEMS IN VARIOUS SITES; SPECIAL SITUATIONS

There are many situations in radiation therapy that require special consideration of the patient's size, shape, or condition. This chapter will offer some solutions to various technical dilemmas encountered in different disease sites.

PELVIS

The majority of patients receiving radiation therapy for malignancies in the pelvis are treated in the supine position. There are, however, some benefits in treating them in the prone position, primarily to minimize the volume of small bowel within the treatment fields. Vicryl mesh, a full bladder, and the use of a belly board are some of the methods used to move the small bowel anteriorly and cephalad out of the radiation field (page 148, Chapter 6). The benefits of the prone position, vicryl mesh, and a full bladder have been previously described in *Treatment Planning and Dose Calculation in Radiation Oncology* (Bentel 1989) and will therefore not be discussed further in this section.

A belly board (page 148, Chapter 6) is an insert which fits over the treatment couch and has an opening which eliminates the pressure of the hard treatment couch on the abdomen of the prone patient and thus permits the small bowel to be displaced by gravity (Shanahan 1990). The small bowel is confined inside the peritoneal cavity and is protected by the abdominal muscles (Fig. 7.1). In patients with good abdominal muscle tone,

171

the effect of gravity on the small bowel is thought to be less than in patients with poor tone. Alhough flabby tissue folds, often seen in obese patients, fall into the opening in the belly board (Fig. 7.2), it is a misconception to believe that the small bowel falls anteriorly. Thin patients benefit as much from the belly-board position as do obese patients. The absence of abdominal pressure caused by the table top is advantageous in practically all cases.

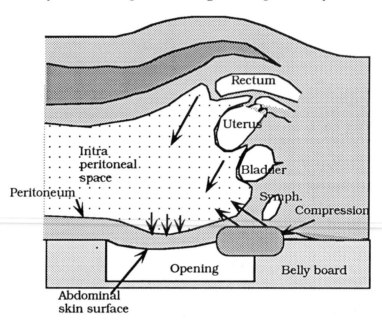

Fig. 7.1. The small bowel is contained within the peritoneum and may fall anteriorly by gravity when the patient is prone on a belly board. In some patients, compression on the lower pelvis may help push the small bowel more cephalad.

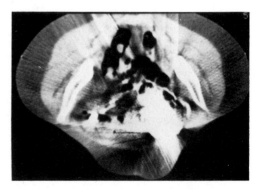

Fig. 7.2. In obese patients, the contour is increased because fatty tissue folds fall into the opening in the belly board. A three-field rather than a four-field technique should be used.

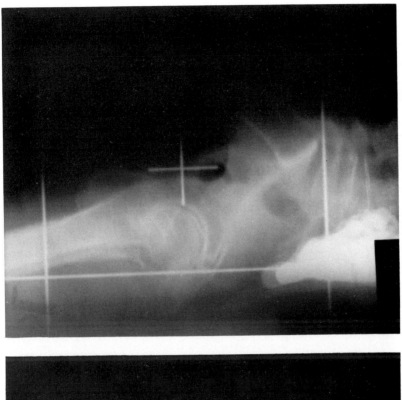

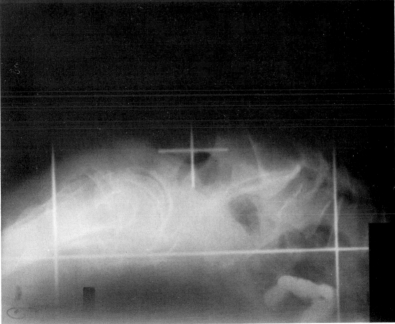

Fig. 7.3. A prone patient without (upper) and with (lower) a compression roll. Some shift of the small bowel is observed in this very thin patient.

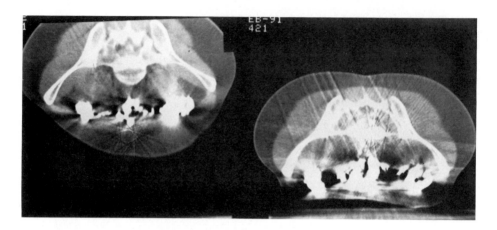

Fig. 7.4. CT images with (left) and without (right) the belly board show a small displacement of the bowel contrast in the patient in Fig. 7.3.

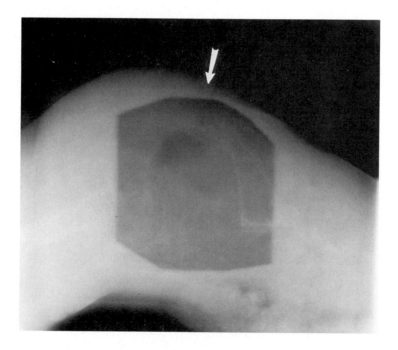

Fig. 7.5. A compression roll under the patient changes the patient's position so that the anterior and posterior fields include a larger volume of the abdomen. By turning the couch 90° and then the gantry, as shown on page 147, Chapter 6, for a kyphotic patient, the volume of normal tissue in the abdomen can be minimized.

The use of a belly board in very obese patients should be limited to patients being treated through a three-field technique (described in Chapter 7 of *Treatment Planning and Dose Calculation in Radiation Oncology*), because flabby tissue folds tend to fall into the opening in the belly board causing the patient's thickness to be excessive (Fig. 7.2). An anterior treatment field, for example, would pass through a large thickness of attenuating normal tissue before reaching the target and should therefore be omitted. In a thin or moderately obese patient, either a three- or a four-field technique could be used while the patient is on a belly board.

In some patients, placement of a compression roll under the lower abdomen may help to push the small bowel out of the pelvis. Determination of which technique is more beneficial in each situation can only be made through comparison of lateral radiographs taken with the patient in each position 1 to 2 hours after the swallowing barium contrast (Figs. 7.3, 7.4, and 7.5).

Very obese patients present other difficult problems. The tendency of flabby skin folds to move over underlying tissues causes field marks on the skin to be unreliable. Peniculus, formed by skin folds in the lower abdomen, can be the cause of undesirable skin reaction due to lack of skin sparing in the creases between the folds. The rubbing of two skin surfaces against each other causes irritation and inhibits healing of the injury. This problem becomes less apparent with higher energy radiation beams where the maximum dose lies at a greater depth, but must still be given proper consideration. Some patients can, with their hands, pull the skin folds up to eliminate creases. Straps and tape can be used to accomplish a similar result. Both methods of eliminating skin creases are unsatisfactory because the patient's thickness may vary from treatment to treatment. Because of slippage or non-uniform taping, it can even vary during the treatment, thus resulting in uncertainty of the delivered dose. As in all other instances, it is important that the contour on which the dose calculations are made truly represents the size and the shape of the patient in treatment position.

Many of the problems just described can be reduced by treating the patient in the prone position without a belly board, particularly if sparing of the small bowel is not of paramount concern. In the prone position, the abdomen is flattened against the hard treatment couch and thus the patient's thickness is consistent; it is also reduced in many patients. The patient's posterior skin surface is usually quite flat and provides a more reliable surface on which to mark the treatment fields. Skin folds can be avoided in the prone patient by having the patient pull up the skin folds while getting into the prone position.

In the treatment of rectal carcinoma, it is not unusual to use lateral fields that of necessity "flash over" the patient's posterior skin surface, resulting in decreased skin sparing (Fig. 7.6). When such a patient is treated in the supine position, it is necessary to include the top of the couch in the treatment field. Scattering off the couch will further reduce the skin-sparing effect. Furthermore, in the supine patient, the buttocks are pushed together, reducing skin sparing in the crease between the buttocks (Fig.7.7). The resulting reaction can be very painful and uncomfortable, and the injury is often exacerbated because the two skin surfaces constantly rub against each other. As a result, the healing process is often protracted and the patient can be incapacitated for a long time. Placing the patient in the prone position would spread the buttocks apart thus improving the skin sparing in the crease. The treatment fields would no longer include the treatment couch so the problem of scattering from the couch is eliminated.

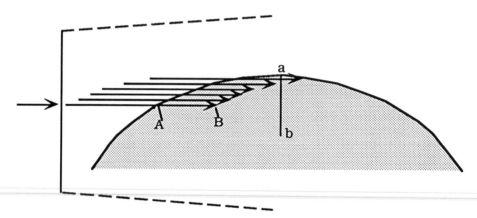

Fig. 7.6. When a radiation beam flashes over skin surfaces, the skin-sparing effect is reduced. The distance from A to B is the depth of the maximum dose (D_{max}). Therefore, maximum dose occurs at the tip of each arrow, and as we can see, this is very close to the skin surface near the "summit" of this rounded contour. In the midline, equilibrium occurs at the tip of the topmost arrow, that is, at a much shallower depth than if the beam entered vertically downwards.

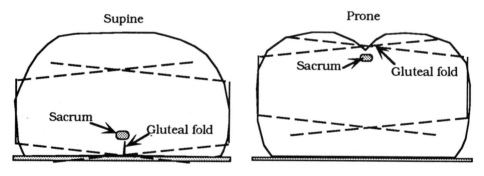

Fig. 7.7. When lateral fields need to be very far posterior, scatter off the couch reduces skin sparing when the patient is supine (left). The buttocks are also pushed together and there is no skin sparing. Placing the patient in the prone position (right) eliminates the scatter off the couch and spreads the buttocks.

The use of anterior and posterior pelvic fields alone should be limited to patients in whom no benefit would be gained by the addition of lateral fields. This would occur in patients in whom lateral fields encompass the entire patient thickness. However, it is important to remember that although at some point the entire patient thickness is included in the lateral fields, some normal tissue sparing can be achieved by shaping these fields to the target in the "beam's-eye view" (Fig. 7.8). For example, segments of small bowel which lie within the anterior and posterior fields can often be spared by the lateral fields thus reducing the dose within the segment. (See *Treatment Planning and Dose Calculation in Radiation Oncology*, Chapter 7.)

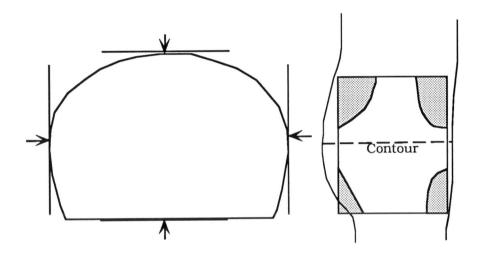

Fig. 7.8. Although it appears as if no tissue is spared in the lateral fields at the central-axis level (left), through beam shaping, normal tissues are spared in the lateral fields at other levels.

If it is necessary to include the perineal surface in the treatment fields, consideration must be given to the decreased skin sparing when the radiation beam travels parallel with the skin surface. Lateral fields, which include the perineal surface, provide no skin sparing at all since the beams will travel through one of the thighs before reaching the perineum. The most caudal part of the perineum will often receive a higher dose than intended because the thickness decreases as the perineum slopes caudal (Fig. 7.9). Consideration must also be given to the dose and lack of skin sparing in the male genitalia which, of necessity, are partly included in the anterior and posterior fields.

To reduce some of the problems just described, the couch can be turned 90° with respect to its normal 0° position and then the gantry turned to avoid or minimize the dose to the male genitalia (Fig. 7.10). An electron field can be added to adequately treat the perineum.

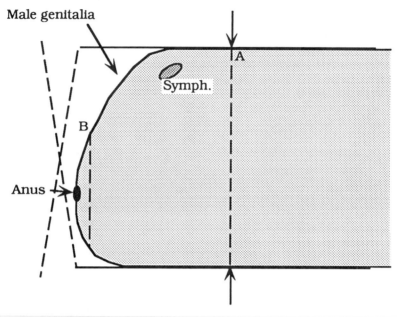

Fig. 7. 9. The patient's sagittal contour varies in thickness causing higher dose at B, where the thickness is less, than at A. When a beam flashes over the perineum (or any other surface), skin sparing is reduced (See also Fig. 7.6).

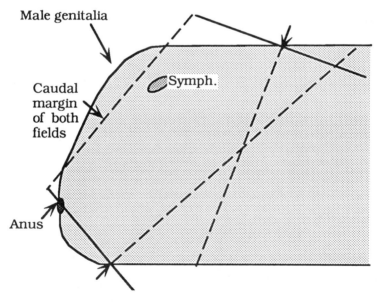

Fig. 7.10. In some patients it is possible to turn the couch 90° and then rotate the gantry until the beam includes the anus but avoids the genitalia. A separate electron field can be used to treat the perineal incision.

When extremely obese patients are treated, an isocentric technique may not be possible because the clearance between the patient's skin surface and the collimator of the machine is inadequate. Electron contamination, mainly due to secondary electron scatter from the collimator, reduces the skin-sparing effect when the distance between the collimator and the patient's skin surface is too short. A distance of 15 to 20 cm is recommended to keep the surface dose within acceptable levels in most high-energy radiation beams (Johns 1952, Richardson 1954, Khan 1973). The risk of a collision with the patient or the treatment couch is also increased when the clearance is decreased (page 35, Chapter 2).

The factors to consider in deciding whether to use an isocentric technique or not are: a) the importance of an isocentric technique in the particular patient, b) the amount of dose delivered through the field, and c) the actual distance between the collimator and the patient's skin surface. The first depends on how critical the precision of field reproducibility is, how generous the margins are around the target, and the level of cooperation by the patient.

Low pelvic tumors, such as in the uterine cervix, vagina, and the prostate gland, should be marked with a gold seed so that the inclusion of the lower margin of the tumor can be verified on simulation films. This is particularly important when the field size is reduced for a boost (higher dose to a smaller volume).

ABDOMEN

WHOLE ABDOMEN

Whole-abdominal irradiation is used with increasing frequency in the management of gynecologic conditions such as ovarian and endometrial malignancies, where it is intended to deliver therapeutic doses to the entire peritoneal surface and to intraperitoneal metastasis. Generally speaking, whole-abdominal irradiation involves the use of anterior and posterior fields with shielding of dose-limiting organs. Due to the domelike shape of the diaphragm, which separates the abdominal cavity from the thoracic cavity, it is impossible to treat the entire abdominal cavity without also treating a considerable volume of lung (Chapter 7 in *Treatment Planning and Dose Calculation in Radiation Oncology*). The beams must therefore be shaped to include as much as possible of the abdominal cavity while minimizing the amount of lung parenchyma in the radiation field. Other difficulties involve the constant motion of the diaphragm with respiration and the presence of radiosensitive organs, primarily the kidneys and the liver, within the abdominal cavity. Willett et al. have suggested gated irradiation, a technique in which the treatment is delivered while the patient is holding the breath (Willett 1987). The irradiation is interrupted at short intervals while the patient is taking in a new breath.

Kidney and liver doses can be kept below tolerance levels by partially shielding these organs when treating the entire abdominal cavity. Such organ protection can be achieved either by fully blocking the organs once the tolerance dose is reached or by using shielding blocks which allow only partial transmission of the radiation beam during the entire treatment course. The choice will depend on the prescribed dose to the abdominal cavity and must be tailored to the specific situation.

In practically all of these patients, blocks used to shield kidneys and liver will also shield possible tumor sites. Therefore, in patients where it is urgent to treat the entire abdomen, it might be advantageous to deliver the initial treatment without any shielding. When tolerance doses have been reached, 5 HVT shielding (which only transmits about 3% of the dose) can be added in segments of both fields to prevent excessive doses from being delivered to the kidneys and liver. This method of shielding may also be selected for treatment of patients where it is uncertain whether the planned course of treatment can be completed because of the hematologic picture, the patient's general condition, or the level of patient compliance.

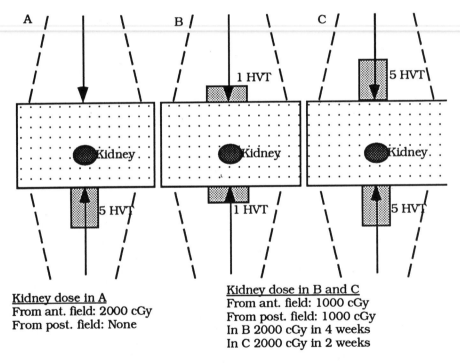

Kidney dose in A
From ant. field: 2000 cGy
From post. field: None

Kidney dose in B and C
From ant. field: 1000 cGy
From post. field: 1000 cGy
In B 2000 cGy in 4 weeks
In C 2000 cGy in 2 weeks

Fig. 7.11. Diagram illustrating different kidney-shielding methods. In (A) a 5 HVT shield is placed in the posterior field only. In (B) a 1 HVT shield is used in both fields while in (C), 5 HVT shields are used in both fields following the delivery of 2000 cGy in the kidney. The dose in the unshielded area is 4000 cGy delivered in 4 weeks. The dose in the kidney in (A) is 2000 cGy in 4 weeks with a dose gradient throughout the shielded area. In (B) the kidney dose is 2000 in 4 weeks with uniform dose distribution in the shielded area, and in (C) the kidney dose is 2000 cGy in *2 weeks*.

Other options include use of a 5 HVT shield in one field only during a portion of the treatment course. This would cause most of the dose to be delivered through one field only, resulting in a dose gradient throughout the shielded organ. (See beam weighting in *Treatment Planning and Dose Calculation in Radiation Oncology* and page 95, Chapter 4 and page 184, Chapter 7 of this text.) Using a partial transmission block in both fields during a portion of the treatment would deliver uniform dose throughout the organ. The dose distribution and the biological effect will be different in these methods because of the weighting of the beams and also because of the fractionation schema in which the dose is delivered (Fig. 7.11).

Rosenthal et al. found that a larger section of the anterior abdomen was shielded by using posterior kidney blocks because of the divergence of the block edges (Rosenthal 1990). While anterior kidney blocks will shield a smaller section of the abdominal cavity, they offer less effective kidney shielding because of the greater depth of the kidneys below the anterior surface. Rosenthal et al. concluded that posterior kidney blocks were preferable over anterior. A section of the treatment can also be delivered through lateral fields in which the kidneys can be shielded. In all of these options, a section of the abdominal cavity is unavoidably shielded.

Careful beam shaping of whole-abdominal fields should be carried out in an attempt to minimize the volume of irradiated bone marrow, thus reducing the risks of bone marrow depression.

PANCREAS

The prognosis for patients with carcinoma of the pancreas is dismal and the delivery of cancerocidal doses of ionizing radiation is limited by the tolerance of adjacent normal organs, primarily the kidneys and the liver. Both the target and the normal organs in the vicinity of the pancreas must therefore be precisely localized. Pancreatic tumors are best localized through magnetic resonance imaging (MRI) or computerized tomography (CT) studies while the patient is in the treatment position. These imaging methods show the position not only of the pancreas and the tumor, but also of the kidneys, the liver, and the spinal cord with respect to the target. Placement of metallic clips in the tumor bed during prior surgery will increase the confidence with which the target is radiographically localized.

The dose in the kidneys can be maintained below tolerance levels by treating the pancreas through an anterior and two lateral fields only. A posterior field would deliver a higher dose to the kidney(s) and the spinal cord than to the anteriorly located pancreas. In a three-field technique the kidney(s) and the spinal cord would receive exit dose from the anterior field only. (See Chapter 7 of *Treatment Planning and Dose Calculation in Radiation Oncology*.) The dose to the liver can be reduced by increasing the weighting of the anterior and left lateral field. Depending on the size of the fields and the precise position of the kidneys with respect to the target, a small fraction of the total dose may be delivered from a posterior field.

PELVIS AND PARA-AORTIC LYMPH NODES

Treatment of the pelvis and para-aortic lymph nodes in one field is often complicated by the need for different dose fractionation in the two sites. The fraction size to the pelvis is often 180 cGy/fraction while to the para-aortic lymph nodes, it is 150 cGy/fraction to reduce small bowel toxicity. A four-field technique can be used to treat both areas, but an attenuator which transmits about 83% (150/180) of the pelvic dose must be used in the segments of the fields that cover the para-aortic lymph nodes. Another method is to treat all fields until 150 cGy is delivered in the para-aortic region and then reduce the size of the fields to encompass only the pelvis and deliver another 30 cGy. This method requires longer setup time and is quite complicated. A simpler method is to deliver 150 cGy to the para-aortic lymph nodes through anterior and posterior opposed fields and then deliver the additional 30 cGy through lateral fields to the pelvis only. As in all other off-axis dose calculations, the patient's thickness, the off-axis factor, and the effect of the field size and shape must be considered when the amount of beam attenuation is calculated.

PELVIS AND INGUINAL LYMPH NODES

Treatment of the pelvis and inguinal lymph nodes is described in *Treatment Planning and Dose Calculation in Radiation Oncology* (p.169). Another technique, recently described by Kalend (Kalend 1990) consists of a large anterior field which encompasses the pelvis and the inguinal lymph nodes, and a posterior field covering the pelvis only. The desired dose to the inguinal lymph nodes is delivered through the anterior field. A beam attenuator is used in the segment of the anterior field which is opposed by the posterior fields. The amount of beam attenuation is calculated so that the midpoint of the pelvis receives the same dose from the anterior and the posterior field. The anterior beam attenuator is fabricated with bevelled edges that extend slightly out into the inguinal section of the field to compensate for the divergence of the posterior field. The width of the bevelled section depends on the thickness of the patient, that is, the amount of divergence of the posterior field and the slope of the bevelled edge depend on the penumbral width of the posterior beam.

When a four-field technique is used to treat the pelvis, the inguinal nodes are sometimes boosted via anterior electron fields. This is a very difficult and risky method because of the difficulties associated with matching the edges of electron and photon fields. Furthermore, matching the dose fall-off at depth of an electron beam with that of the isodose lines from a four-field technique is an almost impossible task. This type of complex field matching must be carefully planned in advance, for example, the shape of the lateral photon fields must have the shape of the dose profile (cross plot) of the selected electron beam (Fig. 7.12).

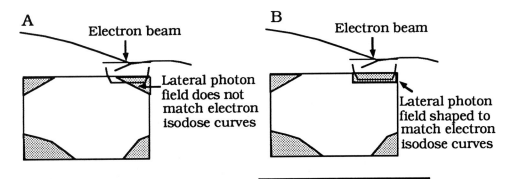

Fig. 7.12. Matching an inguinal electron field with the isodose lines from a four-field technique is very difficult, particularly if the lateral fields are not shaped to match the electron isodose curves (A). Compensators are needed in the electron beams to tilt the isodose curves so that they match the photon isodose curves. The lateral photon fields must be shaped to match the electron beam isodose curves (B).

THORAX

LUNG

Patients with carcinoma of the lung usually require treatment of the primary tumor, bilateral hilar nodes, and in some cases, bilateral supraclavicular nodes also. Anterior and posterior fields will best cover this large target while minimizing the volume of lung parenchyma within the irradiated fields. The disadvantage of using anterior and posterior fields is the dose gradient within the fields resulting from the slope of the patient's chest from the caudal to the cephalad margins of the anterior field. The dose in the spinal cord near the cephalad margin of the fields is of particular concern because it is consistently higher than the calculated central axis dose. The precise dose difference depends on the varying patient thickness at the central axis of the fields and near the cephalad margin, the beam profile (or off-axis ratio) at the depth of the spinal cord, and the energy of the radiation beam.

As with practically all tumors in the chest, the spinal-cord tolerance limits the dose that can be delivered through anterior and posterior fields. A boost dose is often necessary after a spinal-cord dose of 4400 to 4600 cGy has been delivered through the larger anterior and posterior fields. Some physicians prefer to deliver the boost dose via smaller anterior and posterior fields but with the spinal cord shielded. Unfortunately, in many patients, the spinal-cord shield will also shield tumor, thus compromising target coverage.

Opposed oblique or lateral fields are often utilized to deliver the boost treatment in patients with small residual tumors in the hilum. The boost can be delivered through oblique fields angled approximately 30° off the vertical axis. In general, smaller angles causes a smaller volume of normal lung parenchyma to lie within the fields.

The practice of setting up oblique fields without a patient contour and treatment plan can result in the depth of the isocenter being different for the two opposed fields, leading to the same effect on the dose as that of weighted beams (Fig. 7.13). When equal weighting is used in parallel opposed fields where the isocenter is at mid-depth, the maximum dose, which with lower energy beams can be 10% to 20 % higher than at the midplane dose, will occur in the entrance/exit region of each field. If the isocenter is not at the same depth in the two fields, the effect will be the same as weighting the beams: the maximum dose (in the shallow tissues of the field) increases as the isocenter depth increases. This high dose can be reduced by increasing the weighting of the opposite field.

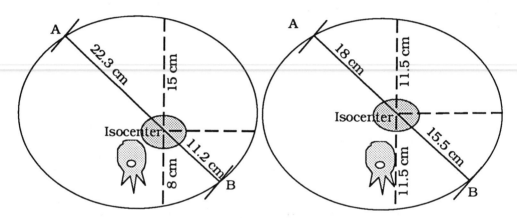

Fig. 7.13. In both of these situations, the isocenter was set at the center of the target in the anterior and the lateral view, and the gantry was then angled until the spinal cord was out of the field. The depths of the isocenter were 22.3 and 11.2 cm, respectively, in the setup on the left and 18 and 15.5 cm, respectively, in the setup on the right; a considerable difference in both cases.

Residual disease within a large region may be treated through lateral fields, or a treatment plan consisting of multiple fields may be used. In complex multiple-field plans, it is sometimes necessary to deliver additional dose to the spinal cord, and it would therefore be advantageous to discontinue the large anterior and posterior fields before spinal-cord tolerance is reached.

Design of treatment fields for lung tumors and for other sites near the diaphragm should be done under flouroscopy to permit observation of the motion of the target during respiration and to allow adequate margins around the target. Detailed field arrangements for treatment of lung tumors are described in *Treatment Planning and Dose Calculations in Radiation Oncology.*

ESOPHAGUS

Treatment techniques for treatment of carcinoma of the esophagus are described in *Treatment Planning and Dose Calculation in Radiation Oncology*. As with other malignancies in the thorax, the standard technique consists of opposed anterior and posterior fields until spinal-cord tolerance is reached, followed by boost fields using cord-sparing techniques. Because of the pattern of spread along the mucosa of the esophagus, generous margins in the cephalad and caudal direction are always necessary. Intraluminal brachytherapy can also be used in treating small obstructing lesions in the esophagus to maintain an open lumen (page 315, Chapter 9).

BREAST

Techniques to treat patients with carcinoma of the breast are very complex. The problem of matching multiple fields on a very irregular surface without causing over- or underdosage at the junctions is quite difficult. Most techniques described in the literature address only the ideal normal patient. Because of the many variations in a) the patient's size, b) the breast size and shape, c) the presence or absence of the breast, d) the patient's ability to elevate the arm, e) the size and location of an incision or drain site, and e) the thickness of the patient's chest wall, a technique developed for one patient may not be useful when treating another. Other factors that must be considered include, for example, whether the internal mammary nodes or the axillary nodes need treatment and whether the patient has had previous irradiation to the other breast or the lung, or to the thoracic segment of the spinal cord. Breast-treatment techniques that offer flexibility must be developed in order to accommodate these situations.

The most important factor in successful field reproducibility is patient positioning and immobilization. The conventional position is supine with the arm on the involved side raised above the head to allow tangential fields across the chest to clear the arm. The head is usually turned away from the irradiated side. The use of an Alpha Cradle®* with an arm support and a handle greatly improves the ability to reposition the patient precisely from treatment to treatment. Patient comfort, which is paramount to the ability to maintain the position for the duration of the treatment, is also improved by the use of these positioning devices (Bentel 1990). Prior to the daily treatment, the patient must be repositioned with the alignment lasers in the treatment room (Fig. 7.14) to insure that this complex treatment setup is reproduced (Bentel 1984 A).

---

*Smithers Medical Products, Inc., 391 Geneva Avenue, Tallmadge, Ohio 44278

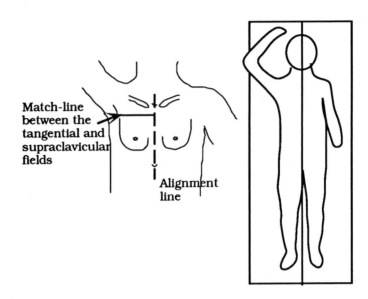

Fig. 7.14. For successful repositioning of the patient, alignment with the laser light system is vital. While the couch angle is on 0°, the patient is aligned on the couch (right) and a realignment line is marked on the patient for future setup.

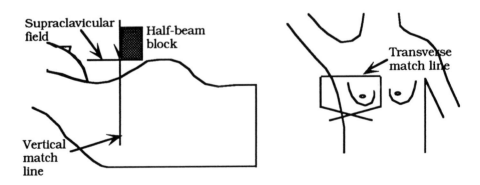

Fig. 7.15. Vertical and transverse match lines are created by using a half-beam block on the anterior supraclavicular field (left) and by turning the couch on the tangential fields to prevent beam divergence into the supraclavicular field. The deep margins of the tangential fields are shaped by customized blocks to create a straight line on the skin surface.

The breast treatment technique developed and used at Duke University Medical Center since 1978 offers the simplicity and flexibility necessary to treat patients in many, but not all, situations. This technique, described elsewhere (Bentel 1982, 1984 B, 1989) uses two custom-shaped tangential fields directed across the chest. (See Fig. 7.74 in *Treatment Planning and Dose Calculation in Radiation Oncology*.) The fields are shaped so that the deep margins of the fields are curved to match the patient's midline on the anterior skin surface or the edge of an internal mammary field. The deep margin basically follows the curvature of the lung as seen in the beam's-eye view in Figure 7.24. The couch is turned to cause the cephalad margin of the two fields to match the supraclavicular field in both transverse and vertical directions (Fig. 7.15). The central axis of the supraclavicular field is placed on the cephalad margin of the tangential fields and the inferior half of this field is then blocked. This half-beam block-technique causes the match line to be vertical without divergence, thus matching the cephalad border of the tangential fields.

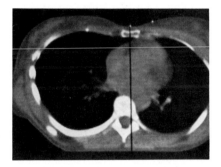 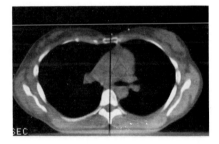

Fig. 7.16. A small rotation of the patient's upper torso is sometimes noted when one arm is elevated and the head turned to the side. Therefore, the patient's spine and sternum often do not superimpose in the anterior view. See vertical line (left). Placement of the internal mammary-node field should be made with respect to the sternum and not the spinal column. Elevation of both arms and keeping the head straight eliminate the rotation in many patients (right).

The conventional position tends to rotate the patient's upper torso causing the sternum and the spine to be misaligned in the vertical plane (Fig. 7.16 left). An alternate method is to position the patient with the head straight and with the chin extended then have the patient raise both arms above the head (Fig. 7.16 right). Such a symmetric position is more reproducible and does not cause the difficulties with field matching otherwise encountered in patients who later return for treatment of metastatic disease in the spine. Alignment of the patient's body under fluoroscopy, while using the spinal axis to determine when the patient is straight, is a good practice. However, setting the anterior internal mammary field with respect to the spinal axis could cause great errors because of the patient rotation previously mentioned.

In patients in whom the breast is situated high on the chest, the vertical match line in the cephalad margin is at an angle rather than transversely across the chest so that breast tissue is included while the axilla is excluded (Fig. 7.17). This is accomplished by using a couch angle that produces a match line at the desired angle across the patient's chest (Fig. 7.18). This angle is referred to as the "neutral" angle. The supraclavicular field is treated with the couch in the neutral angle and the couch is then turned in opposite directions for the two tangential fields to make the cephalad field edges coincide. In other techniques, this problem is solved by the addition of an angled insert on top of the treatment couch which causes the patient's chest to be elevated, thus lowering the breast by gravity (Fig. 7.19). This technique is simple, but in patients who are also treated through a supraclavicular field, it will cause more lung volume to lie within the field.

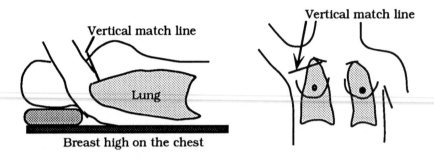

Fig. 7.17. The breast in some patients is situated very high on the chest, and including the breast tissue while avoiding the axilla is very difficult. The cephalad margin of the tangential fields can be placed at an angle across the chest.

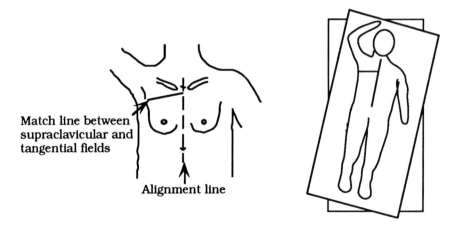

Fig. 7.18. The patient must be be positioned straight on the couch (right). The cephalad margin of the tangential fields is placed at an angle across the chest by turning the couch until the desired direction of the margin is reached.

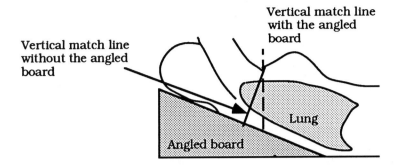

Fig. 7.19. An angled board, placed under the patient's chest to make the breast tissue fall caudal by gravity, will cause more lung tissue to be within the anterior supraclavicular field.

In some cases, particularly in elderly or obese patients, the breast tends to fall laterally, thus making it difficult to include the entire breast without also including a large volume of lung tissue. Stockinette around the patient can help hold the breast up and away from the lateral aspect of the chest. In extremely obese patients, the stockinette may not be strong enough. Keeping the patient's brassiere on while treating may be an option but it is not possible to make use of skin marks under the brassiere. One cup from the patient's brassiere may be strapped around the chest to hold the breast in the desired position. Use of tape and other strapping material is frequently unsatisfactory.

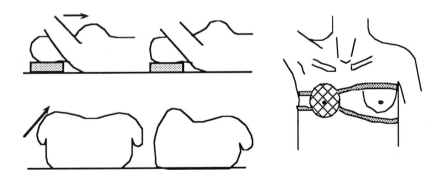

Fig. 7.20. A breast which is very high on the chest is difficult to treat (upper), particularly in patients who have difficulty raising the arm. A breast which falls laterally (lower) is also difficult to treat without including a significant volume of lung. A breast strap can be used to hold the breast in the desired place during treatment (right).

A device consisting of a double, adjustable ring with a thin, stretchable mesh (fish net) clamped between the rings, can be placed around the breast and held in place by adjustable straps stretched around the patient's chest (Fig. 7.20). The mesh can then be tightened to flatten the breast and reduce the height, thus allowing smaller fields to be used, a real advantage because of the field-size limitation often encountered when using wedges.

If everything fails and the entire breast cannot be satisfactorily included in the tangential fields, the field borders may have to be compromised and the sections of the breast which lie outside the tangential fields be treated using electron fields. In patients in whom the breast is situated high on the chest, for example, and all breast tissue cannot be included in the tangential fields, it can be treated through the supraclavicular field using alternating photon and electron beams to reduce the dose to the underlying lung tissue.

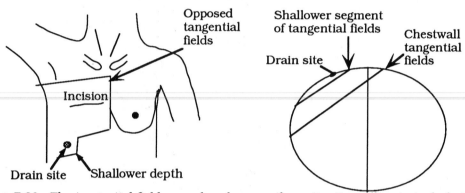

Fig. 7.21. The tangential fields are placed across the patient's midline to include the incision and the internal mammary nodes. A drain site just below the standard tangential fields can be included in the same tangential fields by extending them caudal and using the beam-shaping blocks to reduce their depth.

Including incisions and drain sites may not always be necessary, but when it is, this can cause a problem, particularly in patients in whom the surgeon placed these outside the areas normally included in routine breast treatment fields (Fig. 7.21). A drain site, placed caudal to the normal margin of the tangential fields, can be included by making the tangential fields slightly longer (Fig. 7.21). Customized beam-shaping blocks can also be designed to include such a drain site. A lead marker should be placed on the site during the simulation procedure so that the blocks can be designed appropriately. If the drain site is located outside either the medial or the lateral tangential field margins, the depth will have to be greater at this particular point (Fig. 7.22). In a similar fashion, customized beam shaping can be made to include an incision which otherwise would be outside the tangential fields. Breast treatment techniques which allow customized beam shaping are superior because they provide the option of tailoring the design of the fields. Figure 7.23 illustrates a patient presenting with a difficult problem which was solved by using customized beam shaping and non-opposed tangential fields.

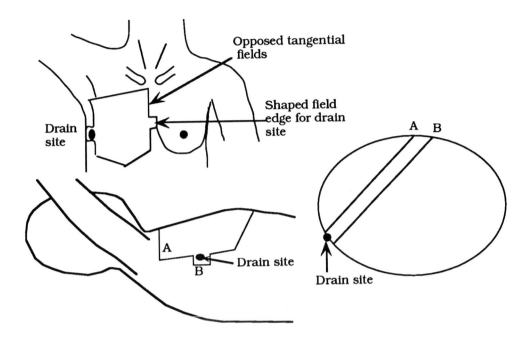

Fig. 7.22. A drain site (or any other site that needs to be treated) just outside the standard tangential fields can be included by extending the tangential fields. Customized blocks are then used to minimize the depth of the tangential fields at other points along the deep margin. (A) in this illustration represent the normal tangential fields while (B) represents the depth of these fields at the drain site.

Wedges are used in an attempt to improve the dose uniformity within the tangential fields. Such wedges will partially compensate for the curvature of the patient's chest and/or breast in the transverse plane. Dose variations within the tangential fields must also be considered in the sagittal plane when evaluating the dose distribution. An axial contour through the central axes of the beams will be useful in selecting the wedge angle (page 72, Chapter 3) that will give the most uniform dose distribution in that plane. Dose distributions calculated on axial contours near the cephalad and caudal margins of the tangential fields, where the shape of the contour can be quite different, will show whether the selected wedge angle is acceptable on these contours also. In patients who have had a mastectomy, the axial chest-wall contour usually has a steep curvature; therefore, 45° wedges are usually needed to produce an acceptable dose distribution, while in patients with a moderately large breast, 30° wedges are usually satisfactory. As a rule, a patient with a large breast requires less wedge angle; thus, in a patient with a very large breast, no wedge at all may result in the best dose uniformity.

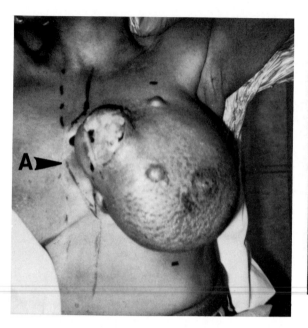
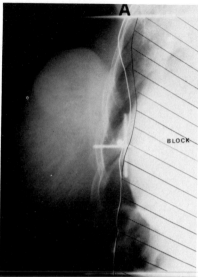

Fig. 7.23. A patient with advanced disease in the breast creates very difficult geometric problems (upper left), but the volume of irradiated lung can be minimized by using customized beam shaping (upper right). This tumor extended across the patient's midline on the skin surface. A CT study was used to determine beam angles and field shape. The fields were not opposed but were angled so that the large node near the sternum could be included in both tangential fields without including more lung volume than absolutely necessary. A lead wire (A on the radiograph) was placed on the skin marks (A on the photograph) indicating palpable disease. The deep field margins, shaped by customized blocks, were extended to allow more margin around the disease.

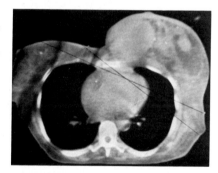

Due to the slope of the patient's chest in the beam's-eye view, the beam near the cephalad margin passes through a thinner part of the wedge, causing the dose at this level to be higher than in the central-axis level (Fig. 7.24). In large patients, where the slope of the chest in the beam's-eye view is greater, the dose is further increased because the beam passes through an even thinner part of the wedge. This dose inhomogeneity is more pronounced with larger wedge angles, and wedges of small angle usually produce the best dose uniformity in both contours.

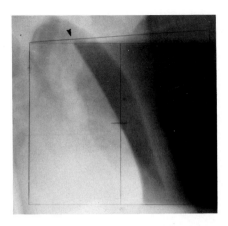
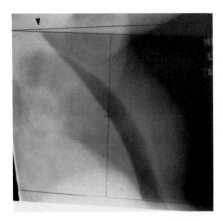

Fig. 7.24. The curvature of the patient's chest wall in the beam's-eye view causes variation in the thickness of wedge material which the beam will pass through in the cephalad margin (arrow left). The dose is usually highest at this point unless compensators are used. In the patient on the right, the field extended farther into the thin segment of the wedge (arrow); therefore the dose is higher than in the patient on the left.

Use of electron beams to treat the chest wall requires very careful determination of the chest wall thickness at all levels. The electron energy is selected when one has ascertained the maximum depth within the treatment field. Areas with shallower depth must be covered by an adequate thickness of tissue-equivalent material (bolus) to prevent high doses in the underlying lung tissue.

Multiple electron fields should be avoided when possible because of the difficulties associated with matching. Electron-arc techniques result in uniform dose and eliminate these matching problems. Compensating material must be placed on the chest wall to provide a uniform depth. Shielding of the surrounding area must be placed directly on the patient or very near the patient's skin.

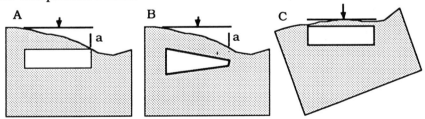

Fig. 7.25. When an electron arc is used to treat the chest wall, the dose will be higher where the radius is smaller (a); however, it may be offset by the increased SSD at this level (A). Shaping the field so that it is narrower where the radius is smaller will improve dose uniformity (B). Elevation of the chest until the chest wall is horizontal will eliminate both the problem of shaping the field and also of longer SSD (C).

The dose near the cephalad margin of the field may be higher because of the smaller radius of the chest at this level (Fig. 7.25A). This higher dose may, however, be balanced out by the increased SSD where the radius is smaller. Careful dose measurements must be made to determine if the field needs to be shaped so that it is narrower where the radius is smaller (Fig. 7.25B). Because the chest wall often has a quite irregular shape, the task of delivering uniform dose in an electron arc is monumental and approximations must be made. Elevating the upper torso until the chest wall becomes horizontal will eliminate both the problem of increased SSD and the necessity of field shaping (Fig. 7.25C).

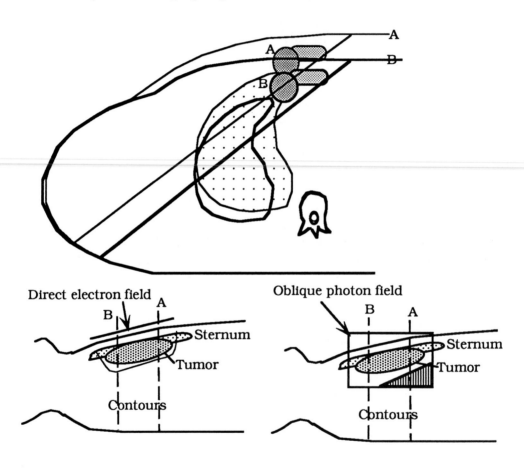

Fig. 7.26. The greatest depth of the tumor used in selecting the electron energy should be measured off each image, when an anteriorly located lesion is considered for electron therapy. The electron cones should then be placed perpendicular to the skin surface in an effort to eliminate air gaps. If oblique photon fields are contemplated, the target must be outlined by "stacking" the images in the usual fashion. The field is set to include the target in all levels, and normal tissues within this field can then be shielded.

Patients with parasternal tumors present a special problem because they are difficult to treat without also including a large volume of underlying lung tissue. When the parasternal mass is small, a direct electron field may be adequate. However, in patients with tumors that are large or are contiguous with the breast tissue, it is necessary to treat both the parasternal mass and the breast in contiguous fields. When an electron field is contemplated, the maximum depth of the tumor mass must be measured from the skin surface of each CT or MRI image rather then by "stacking" the images as described for oblique photon fields in *Treatment Planning and Dose Calculation in Radiation Oncology* (Figs. 4.26 and 4.27).

Figure 7.26 shows two contours superimposed (A and B) with the tumor mass as it appears in each image. If tangential fields are contemplated, the deepest field margin must be deep enough to include the deepest segment of the target in the beam's-eye view (Fig. 7.26, lower right). The fields can then be shaped, as previously described, to reduce the volume of normal tissue. When an electron field is used, the maximum tumor depth must be determined on each individual image and the most appropriate electron energy selected. The electron beam should enter the patient perpendicular to the surface to minimize the air gap and thus improve dose uniformity at a specified depth (Fig. 7.26 lower left).

HEAD AND NECK

Most tumor sites in the head and neck region are treated by applying parallel opposed lateral fields to the primary lesion and bilateral cervical lymph node groups, together with an anterior field to include the lower neck and supraclavicular nodes. Such standard treatment techniques are described in more detail in *Treatment Planning and Dose Calculation in Radiation Oncology,* and only special problems will be discussed here.

Treatment of head and neck malignancies requires precise repositioning and immobilization of the patient. The proximity of the lens of the eye, the optic chiasm, the spinal cord, and the brain requires very precise reproducibility of the setup, particularly when the prescribed dose to the target area exceeds the tolerance of these neighboring organs. Devices and techniques used in the position and immobilization of these patients have been described in *Treatment Planning and Dose Calculation in Radiation Oncology.* A few additional paragraphs are included here to enhance that section, however.

POSITIONING AND IMMOBILIZATION

As in all sites, the two most important factors in reproducing and maintaining the patient's position during head and neck treatment, are comfort and immobilization. A pillow or other support under the patient's head needs to be comfortable yet it needs to support the patient's head in the desired position. The height of the support will vary with the patient's size and also with the desired degree of head tilt (Fig. 7.27A). In a large patient, the head support needs to be higher off the couch surface if the patient is to be comfortable, simply because the axis of the patient's body is higher (Fig. 7.27B). The patient must rest comfortably in the head support to eliminate straining (Fig. 7.28A). When the head is so far extended that only the patient's neck and not the head is resting on the support, the patient is not comfortable and the position can be reproduced only with great difficulty (Fig. 7.28B). Adding a piece of styrofoam under the patient's chest will elevate the chest, put less strain on the neck, and tilt the head back farther (Fig. 7.28C). The curvature of the patient's cervical spine can also be altered by changing the head tilt or the support under the head (Fig.7.29).

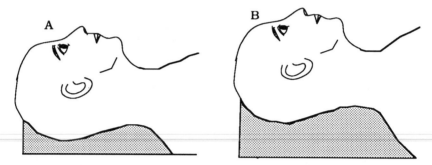

Fig. 7.27. A patient's head must rest comfortably on the appropriate size support (A). For a larger patient, whose shoulders elevate the head off the couch more, a larger head support may be needed (B).

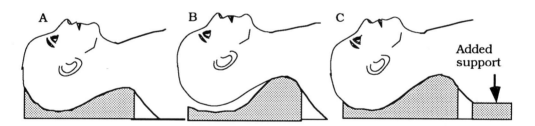

Fig. 7.28. It is sometimes necessary to tilt the patient's head back. In (A) the head is not back far enough. In (B) the head is tilted, but the patient is uncomfortable and the head no longer rest in the support. In (C) the chest is also elevated on a styrofoam support. This helps tilt the head back without patient discomfort.

In the treatment of pituitary lesions through a three-field or arc technique, the head is often tilted forward with the chin tucked down on the chest to allow an anterior field to enter behind the eyes (Fig. 7.30A). Such a forward tilt tends to cause the patient to slip down on the treatment couch. A board fastened to the treatment couch below the feet, on which the patients can brace themselves, helps prevent the patient from slipping down (Fig. 7.30C).

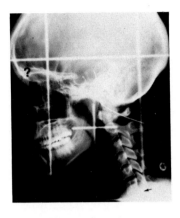 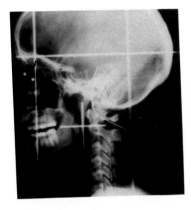

Fig. 7.29. Changing the support under the patient's head also changes the curvature of the spine. The radiograph on the left was taken with a larger support and the corner of the beam is in the spinal canal, making any subsequent field matching practically impossible. The radiograph on the right was taken with a smaller head support. Here the spine is straight and well inside the field. Note also the absence of lead markers at the eyes (left).

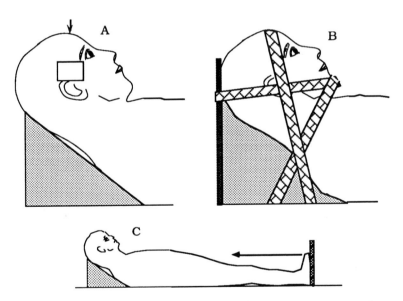

Fig. 7.30. For pituitary treatment, the head is built up on a customized support that fits the curvature of the head and shoulders. Straps around the head fastens the head to the treatment couch. To prevent downward slippage, a foot board can be added on which the patient can brace himself.

A comfortable head support helps the patient maintain position without excessive straining. Standard head supports are sometimes insufficient because of an unconventional head position, but a customized head support can be made by using a set of foaming agents* that swell up and form a mold around the patient's head and shoulders in the desired position (Fig. 7.30B). The patient's head is immobilized in this position using strips of radiolucent material fastened to a baseplate or to the treatment couch.

The angle at which the radiation beam impinges on the patient's surface is defined either by the angles of the machine or by the position of the patient. For example, a true anterior field implies that the beam axis is parallel with the patient's sagittal plane. If the patient's body is rotated 10°, the gantry of the machine must also be rotated 10° in order to achieve a true anterior field (Fig. 7.31). In the head and neck area, this becomes more of a problem than in any other site because it may be difficult to position the patient's head precisely straight. When lateral fields are used to treat tumors near the lens, it is particularly important to position the head so that the lenses of the eyes are on a horizontal plane. In patients where the tumor has caused proptosis, horizontal alignment of the lenses is almost impossible. Therefore, it may be necessary to turn the patient's head until the two lenses lie on a horizontal line or to angle the gantry until the two lenses are parallel with the beam direction (Fig. 7.31).

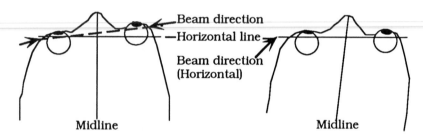

Fig. 7.31. If a patient has proptosis in one eye, the lenses will not be aligned even when the head is straight. The beam can then be angled until the lenses are out of both opposing fields. If the patient's head is not straight, the beam can also be angled until the lenses of both eyes are out of the beam.

TREATMENT TECHNIQUES

In the treatment of practically all head and neck tumors, it is necessary to treat the regional lymphatics. This is routinely achieved via lateral fields that include a segment of the cervical spinal cord. Following the delivery of a dose lower than the spinal-cord tolerance, the fields are reduced off the spinal cord, and the anterior neck along with the primary tumor is treated to a higher dose. If this is accomplished without moving the central axis of the beam but rather through customized blocks almost one half of the field is shielded (half-beam block). In this way as much as possible of the cervical

---

*Smithers Medical Products, Inc., 391 Geneva Avenue, Tallmadge, Ohio 44278

lymphatic area is included without beam divergence into the spinal cord. Field reduction also allows improved matching of an electron field in those patients where the posterior cervical lymphatics overlying the spinal cord need to be treated to a higher dose. A second field reduction is often made to boost to the primary tumor site to high doses, often in the range of 6000 to 6500 cGy.

Since treatment-field reduction usually begins 5 to 6 weeks following the initial simulation, there is a small risk that marks initially made on the patient have migrated as they are refreshed during the course of treatment. The patient's weight may also change during this time period, causing the overlying skin to shift with respect to the underlying tumor. Head and neck tumors that are accessible through the mouth should be marked with a gold seed so that inclusion of the tumor can be verified on simulation and port films. These seed markers may migrate during the course of treatment. Because of these considerations and because the boost fields usually are designed with very small margins around the target, it is a good practice to resimulate and to verify the position of the marking seed prior to treating the boost fields.

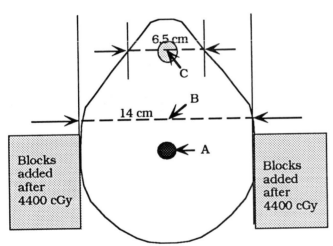

Point (A) receives 4400 to 4500 cGy depending on the off-axis factor

Point (B) receives 4400 + 1600 cGy following spinal-cord shielding

Point (C) receives 6600 to 6900 cGy depending on the off-axis factor + a boost of 1000 to 1500 cGy

Fig. 7.32. In head and neck treatment, the dose can unintentionally be quite high when the central axis is moved for the boost and the prescribed dose is calculated at the central axis of each set of fields. This patient received 4400 cGy at the central axis of the large neck fields plus 1600 cGy following spinal-cord shielding for a total of 6000 cGy. A boost, consisting of 1500 cGy calculated at the isocenter of the small boost fields, was then given. The two central-axis doses were added together and the intended 7500 cGy was recorded in the chart. However, because the patient's neck was thinner in the anterior aspect (larynx), the dose at (C) was approximately 6600 cGy before the boost was given, resulting in a total dose in the larynx of 8000 cGy.

As in many other areas treated via opposed fields, the dose prescription is routinely made on the central axis at the midplane of the patient. Unless compensators are used, the dose inhomogeneity within lateral head and neck fields can be significant. For example, lateral opposed fields used to treat a larynx tumor would also include the cervical lymph nodes. The central axis of such a field would usually be where the lateral diameter is about 12 to 14 cm and the prescribed dose would be calculated at mid-depth (6 to 7 cm). Because the neck is thinner in the anterior aspect where the larynx is situated, the dose at this point will be higher than the prescribed central-axis dose. The overflattening of most beams from linear accelerators also causes the dose at this point to be higher than at the central axis. In some patients the dose increase can be on the order of 10% to 15%. When the fields are reduced and the central axis is moved to the larynx, the dose is calculated at mid-depth, (usually on the order of 3-4 cm) at this level.

A patient who receives 4400 cGy at the central axis of the large opposed fields and then an additional 1600 cGy with shielding of the spinal cord, could receive as much as 6600 to 6900 cGy in the larynx, while only 6000 cGy is delivered at the central axis of the field. An additional 1000 to 1500 cGy to the larynx through small boost fields would result in a total laryngeal dose of well over 8000 cGy rather than the intended 7000 to 7500 cGy (Fig. 7.32).

The lower neck and supraclavicular lymph nodes are routinely treated via an adjacent anterior field. The cephalad field margin and the caudal margin of the lateral fields must be carefully matched in such areas. A small block over the spinal cord in either the lateral fields or in the anterior field should be inserted regardless of what field-matching technique is used because small errors in field setup, patient motion, etc., could cause an overlap in the spinal cord.

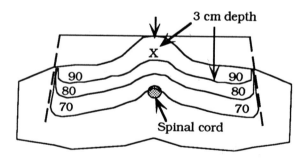

Fig. 7.33. The dose in an anterior bilateral supraclavicular field is often prescribed at 3 cm depth along the central axis. In this patient, because of the curvature of the patient's contour, the longer distance to the supraclavicular nodes, and the value of the off-axis ratio, the dose at 3 cm depth in the supraclavicular nodes is 90% while at 3 cm depth along the central axis it is 95%.

Since the anterior field is usually not opposed, it is treated via an SSD technique and the dose is often prescribed at a small depth or at D_{max} on the central axis. When bilateral lower-neck and supraclavicular lymph nodes are treated, the central axis is in the patient's midline. The prescription point, therefore, does not represent the location of either of the treated lymph node groups and is often shielded by an anterior spinal-cord block. The stated dose to these lymph node groups is thus different from the dose actually delivered (Fig. 7.33).

The risk of tumor recurrence at the site of a tracheostomy is relatively high in patients with larynx cancer. A midline spinal-cord block in the anterior supraclavicular field would also shield the stoma and must therefore be omitted. Bolus material, placed on the edges surrounding the stoma, will reduce the skin sparing and increase the dose to the tissues that are at risk for recurrence. This bolus can be doughnut-shaped to allow air exchange through the tracheostomy site during the treatment. Consideration should be given to the possibility of an increased dose in the spinal cord as a result of the lack of tissue and the creation of an air column in front of the spinal cord in patients with a tracheostomy (Fig. 7.34). If an electron beam is used to boost the stoma dose, the added air space in front of the spinal cord may be of less concern as the bone in the vertebral body attenuates much of the electron beam. The effect on the electron beam of the tissue between each vertebral body is more complex. In most patients, the cervical spine is curved, thus, the anterior beam is rarely perpendicular to the vertebral bodies but passes through any given vertebral body at an angle (Fig. 7.34). The beam must therefore pass through some thickness of bone at all levels before reaching the spinal cord.

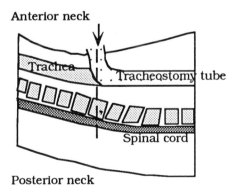

Fig. 7.34. An air column caused by a tracheostomy can result in increased dose in the spinal cord.

NASOPHARYNX

Delivering high doses to tumors in the nasopharynx presents a difficult problem because of the proximity of the brain stem, spinal cord, and brain tissue.

The primary tumor and the regional lymphatics are treated using beam energies of 4 to 6 MV. When doses in excess of 5500 to 6000 cGy are necessary in the primary tumor, higher beam energy might be considered in order to achieve some sparing of the temporomandibular joints. Cervical lymph nodes may be treated using electron beams.

A boost to the primary tumor may be delivered via an intracavitary implant using cesium-137 sources (page 286, Chapter 9).

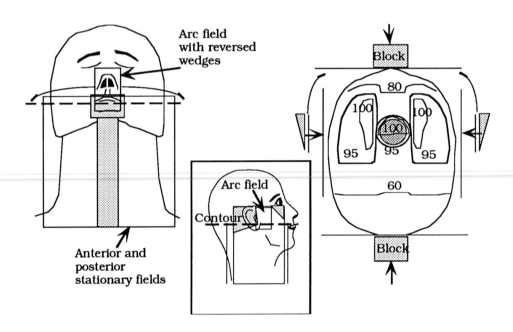

Fig. 7.35. A nasopharynx boost can be delivered via arc fields. Anterior and posterior fields to treat the cervical lymph nodes often extend higher than the arc fields. A midline block must therefore be used in the anterior and posterior fields to shield the high-dose area created by the arc fields.

Another boost technique consists of an arc using a small field with a high-energy photon beam. The patient's head is tilted back so that the beam enters below the eyes. An 180° arc with wedges that are reversed midway through the arc will deliver a cylinder-shaped, uniform high-dose volume with rapid dose fall-off in the surrounding tissue. If the cervical lymph nodes also require a boost dose, anterior and posterior opposed fields can be used. Since these fields frequently must cover the neck more cephalad than the lower border of the arc field, an overlap will occur. A midline block must therefore be used to shield the high-dose area created by the arc (Fig. 7.35). The width of this shielding block must be carefully calculated to prevent high-dose areas within the overlap region.

CENTRAL NERVOUS SYSTEM

WHOLE BRAIN

Whole brain irradiation in the management of brain metastasis is often initiated without simulation of the treatment fields. The treatment fields are set up so that the beam flashes over the entire head in three directions and only the caudal margin is defined by the collimator of the treatment machine. A line is routinely drawn from the eyebrow through the auditory canal to the posterior processes of the skull (Fig. 7.36). Whole brain treatment fields, often used to treat metastatic brain tumors, must be lower in order to include the whole brain as indicated by the sagittal and coronal MRI images in Fig. 7.37.

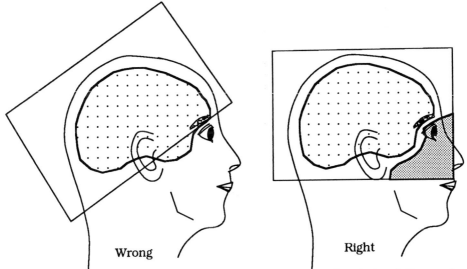

Fig. 7.36. Whole brain treatment fields are often set up without simulation and as a result the inferior margin is often too high, leaving part of the brain untreated (left).

Divergence of the beam into the eye on the opposite side is always a problem if the entire cranial contents are to be treated. The proximity of the eyes is demonstrated in Figure 7.38. Centering the beam very near the eye minimizes beam divergence but will require very large fields (Fig. 7.39). As in any other patient being treated near the eye, a marker should be placed on the lateral canthus (page 164, Chapter 6) of each eye to document radiographically where the eyes are with respect to the beam (Fig. 7.40). This helps guide the physician in shaping the treatment field and it also helps document the exclusion of the eye from the radiation beam. An explanation of precisely what the marker on the radiograph represents should be written on the radiograph, that is, whether it represents the lateral canthus, the lateral aspect of the bony orbit, or anything else. Labelling on radiographs is also discussed in Chapter 6 (page 155).

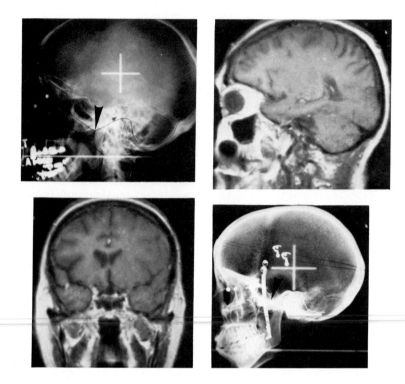

Fig. 7.37. A lateral radiograph (upper left) demonstrating the lower margin of the brain as traced from the sagittal MRI image through the eye (upper right). The coronal image (lower left) shows the caudal margins of the temporal lobes and the lateral radiograph (lower right) shows lead markers placed in the cranium indicating the lower aspect of the brain.

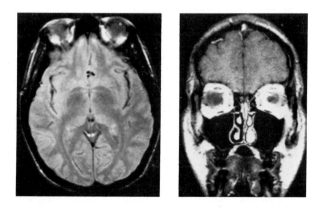

Fig. 7.38. Axial and coronal MRI images of the brain show the proximity of the eyes. Inclusion of the entire contents of the brain in lateral fields while excluding the eyes requires very close margins.

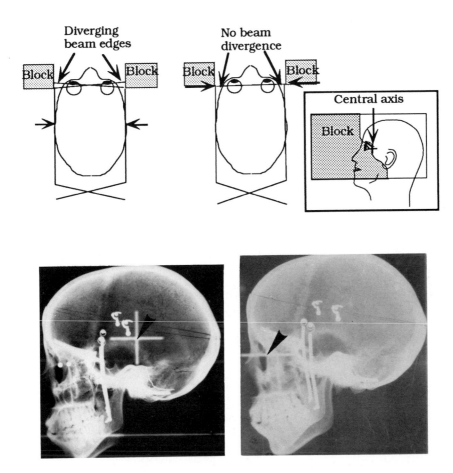

Fig. 7.39. A lateral radiograph of a cranium (lower left) and a diagram (upper left) showing the appearance of the lateral bony ridge of the eye when the beam is centered on the skull (cross hair and arrow). An eye shield placed at the lead marker on the entrance side, will not shield the opposite eye because of beam divergence. To minimize opposing-beam divergence into the eyes, the central axis of the fields can be placed behind the lens (cross hair and arrow) and the anterior half of the field is shielded (right radiograph and center diagram). Such half-beam blocked fields can be very large (upper right insert).

LIMITED VOLUME

As a result of the great progress made in recent years with the help of CT and MRI, in diagnosing and ascertaining the extent of brain tumors, it is possible to treat many of these tumors adequately with small fields. Improved immobilization methods, beam-shaping capabilities, and three-dimensional treatment planning have also contributed to the precision with which brain tumors can be irradiated. In retreatment of already irradiated brain tumors, dose limitation in normal brain tissue is paramount;

therefore, a very high degree of precision is needed. Such tumors are sometimes considered for interstitial implants (discussed on page 304, Chapter 9). Because some brain tumors, especially craniopharyngioma, are very slow growing, patients with recurrent tumors may return many years following initial irradiation. In these cases, a thorough review of the patient's previous irradiation is necessary. This is often difficult because there is poor documentation of precisely where the treatment fields were on the patient, dose delivery is poorly reported, machine data are unavailable, treatment records have been lost, or some combination of these difficulties exists.

Tumors not requiring irradiation of the entire brain (astrocytoma, craniopharyngioma, brain stem tumors, boost fields, etc.) can be treated via a variety of multiple-field techniques. Dose-limiting tissues in this region are the optic chiasm, the lens of the eye, and normal brain tissue. The direction of the beams and the position of the patient must be such that the dose in these organs is minimized. Deep-seated tumors should be treated using high-energy photon beams to limit the dose to peripheral brain tissue. Anterior and posterior fields may be used in addition to lateral opposed fields depending on the location of the tumor and the patient's ability to either extend the chin up or tuck it down on the chest, so that irradiation of the eyes can be avoided. Such a four-field technique would deliver less than 50% of the target dose to the non-target tissue within the entrance and exit region of the beams.

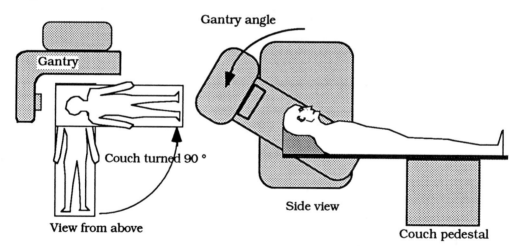

Fig. 7.40. A vertex field can be treated by turning the treatment couch 90° and then rotating the gantry until the desired beam angle has been achieved.

A three-field technique, using lateral opposed wedged fields and a vertex field, as described for treatment of pituitary lesions in *Treatment Planning and Dose Calculation in Radiation Oncology*, can be used if the patient's position permits. Wedges are necessary in the lateral fields to prevent a hot spot near the intersection of the vertex field. The vertex field is treated either by having the patient's head tilted forward or by turning the couch 90° so that the patient's sagittal plane is parallel with the gantry rotation. The gantry is then turned until the beam enters the patient's head at the desired angle (Fig. 7.40). When the lateral fields are treated, the collimator must be angled until the wedge direction becomes parallel with the central axis of the vertex field (Fig. 7.41). The disadvantage of this technique is that the vertex field, depending on the size and the angle at which it is directed, often exits in the thyroid or the mouth, or else follows the axis of the spinal cord. Another disadvantage is inability to obtain verification radiographs of the field position.

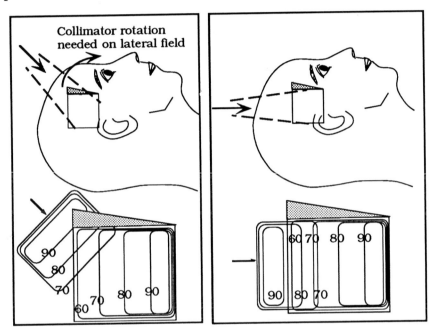

Fig. 7.41. The wedge orientation must always be such that the isodose tilt is parallel with the direction of the vertex field. The wedge orientation in the left diagram requires a collimator rotation to make the tilt of the isodose curves parallel with the intersection of the vertex field. The arrangement in the right-hand diagram is correct.

Small brain tumors are also well suited for treatment via rotation and arc techniques. Such techniques are described in *Treatment Planning and Dose Calculation in Radiation Oncology* and will therefore be described only briefly here. Using a small field and a high-energy photon beam will reduce dose in the periphery of the brain. A full rotation (360°) usually means that the beam must traverse head-support arrangements and sometimes a segment of the treatment couch. Uncertainties in the dose distribution and in the calculation of the beam attenuation are then introduced. These problems can be eliminated by an anterior arc limited to 180° or 270°. A wedge would be needed in such an arc to avoid a higher dose anterior to the axis of rotation. The wedge must be reversed midway through the rotation so that the thick part of the wedge is always directed anteriorly. (See Figs. 6.16,

6.17, 6.18, 7.88, and 7.131 in *Treatment Planning and Dose Calculation in Radiation Oncology.*)

Reirradiating patients with recurrent brain tumors sometimes presents a problem, particularly in patients treated many years ago when orthovoltage beams were often used to treat deep-seated tumors. Because of the increased dose in the entrance/exit region resulting from parallel opposed low-energy beams, sparing of these areas becomes paramount when reirradiation is necessary. Techniques that avoid or minimize the dose to these previously irradiated areas must be used. For example, recurrent brain tumors, previously treated through parallel opposed lateral fields, can be treated through anterior and posterior opposed fields, either alone or in combination with a sagittal arc technique which will minimize dose in the lateral aspect of the brain (Fig. 7.42).

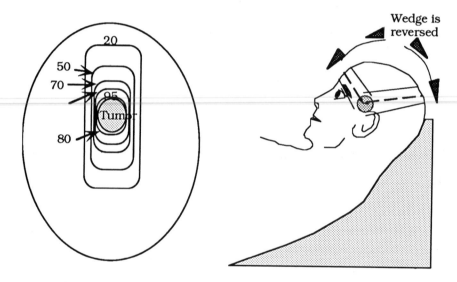

Fig. 7.42. A sagittal arc can be used when the lateral aspect of the brain already has been treated to tolerance doses.

CRANIO-SPINAL IRRADIATION

In many patients it is necessary to treat the entire central nervous system (CNS). This type of treatment is described in great detail in *Treatment Planning and Dose Calculation in Radiation Oncology,* therefore, only some of the problems will be discussed here. This treatment is complicated by the fact that several adjacent fields must be used. Typically, the brain is treated through lateral opposed fields while the spinal axis is treated via one or two posterior fields. Field matching between the two posterior spinal fields is usually accomplished by calculating the separation between the two fields on the skin surface. Matching the margins of the lateral fields with the margin of the most cephalad posterior field is more complicated. It can be accomplished by turning the collimator on the lateral fields until the caudal margin is parallel with the diverging field edge of the posterior field. The number of degrees by which the collimator is turned depends on the length of the posterior spinal field and on the SSD at which the field size is defined. The caudal field margins of the two lateral fields diverge into the posterior spinal field and cause an overlap. This can be avoided by turning the couch so that the two caudal field margins become parallel and cross the patient's neck in a straight line, that is, perpendicular to the sagittal axis of the patient. The number of degrees by which the couch must be turned depends on the field size and the distance at which that field size is defined. The locations of these field junctions are usually moved two or three times during a course of treatment to minimize the chances of over- or underdosage in the spinal cord. The field junction is often shifted by increasing and decreasing the field sizes of the two fields on either side of the junction (Bentel 1990).

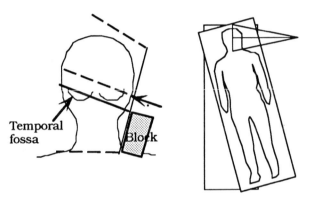

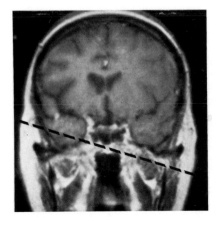

Fig. 7.43. A couch angle on the lateral brain fields can cause the temporal lobe on the opposite side to be missed. The sagittal MRI (right) shows the position of the temporal fossa. The line across the image indicates the blocked edge in the diagram (above left).

While the practice of turning the couch for the lateral fields solves the field-matching problem, it creates a problem of beam divergence away from the most inferior aspect of the temporal fossa (Fig. 7.43).

It is difficult to treat the entire brain without having divergence into the eye on the opposite side. The solution previously described, was to set the central axis of the beam at the lateral canthus of the eye to avoid beam divergence into the opposite eye. While the practice of fixing the central axis of the field at the lateral canthus eliminates eye irradiation, it sometimes causes a problem with matching of the posterior spinal field. It is not always possible to make the cephalad field edge flash over the top of the head in one direction and at the same time have the caudal edge match the cephalad margin of the posterior spinal field in the other direction (Fig. 7.44A). When the caudal margin overlaps into the posterior spinal field, the match line with the diverging posterior spine field must be defined using secondary blocking (Fig. 7.44B). Field matching at the junction by secondary blocking is possible, but it requires new blocks each time the junction is shifted and it also requires that the block be cut precisely parallel with and to the exact location of the diverging posterior field margin. If the treatment machine has independently moving collimator leaves, as many modern machines do, this problem can easily be solved by setting the field margins asymmetrically.

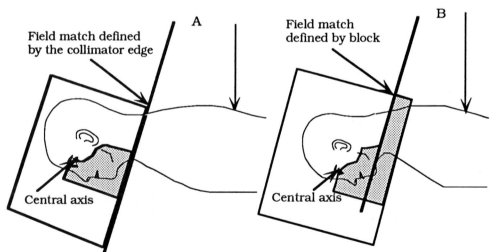

Fig. 7.44. When the patient's chin is extended and the field is centered at the orbit, the field-matching border with the posterior field can be defined by the collimator. However, if the chin is tucked down, the distance from the central axis to the field-matching point is decreased and the margin must be defined by customized blocks.

The precise depth of the spinal cord along its axis is sometimes difficult to determine. Lateral radiographs with the patient in treatment position and a lead wire along the posterior surface is probably the most reliable method. It is, however, sometimes very difficult to see the vertebral column on a lateral radiograph, particularly at the level of the shoulders.

The practice of prescribing the dose at an average depth of the spinal cord can result in quite unexpected doses. For example, in the patient in Fig. 7.45 (upper), taking the depth at four points along the spinal axis (cervical, thoracic, central axis, and lumbar) would result in an average depth of 6.5 cm. A prescription of 150 cGy calculated at 6.5 cm depth would result in delivery of 192 cGy at D_{max} on the central axis (%DD is 78% for a 4 MV photon beam). However, the depth of the spinal cord at the central axis is only 5.5 cm, so the dose in the spinal cord here is really 161 cGy (%DD is 84) which is 7% higher than the prescribed dose. At points where the spinal cord in fact is at 6.5 cm depth, the dose will often be higher than calculated because of the off-axis ratio and also because the SSD at this point may be different from that at the central axis of the beam. If we calculate the dose in the upper thoracic spine (at A in Fig. 7.45), where the spinal cord is at 6.5 cm depth and the SSD is the same as in the central axis, we find that the dose is 157 cGy rather than the prescribed 150 cGy (150 cGy x 1.05 [OAR]), a 5% increase.

If the prescribed dose was calculated at the depth of the spinal cord on the central axis (5.5 cm depth), the dose at D_{max} would be 179 cGy (%DD 84). Now, if we calculate the dose at the upper thoracic spinal cord at 6.5 cm depth, the dose would be 147 cGy (179 [dose at D_{max}] x 0.78 [%DD] x 1.05 [OAR]) which is 2% lower than the prescribed dose. Other dose variations will of course be observed because of the curvature of the spinal cord (Fig.7.45).

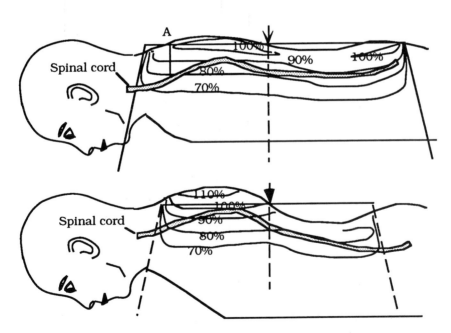

Fig. 7.45. Isodose distributions in the sagittal plane in a patient with a horizontal skin surface (upper) and in a patient where the posterior surface is not horizontal (lower).

Some patients are unable to lie prone without propping the chest up on the arms. If no attempt is made to make the posterior surface horizontal, the result would be similar to that shown in Fig. 7.45 (lower). Although the depth of the spinal cord is practically unchanged, the thoracic segment of the chest, where the dose is already highest, is now raised, causing the SSD to be shorter and thus increasing the dose further.

Calculation of the isodose distribution in the sagittal plane of the posterior field provides information with regard to the dose along the entire spinal axis. The sagittal contour of the patients in Fig. 7.45 was obtained by reducing the outline of the patient's contour from a lateral radiograph to actual size. The isodose distribution was then calculated on the life-size contour. Because of the curvature of the patient's posterior surface and variations in the depth of the spinal cord along its axis, the dose in the patient with a horizontal contour varies from 70% to approximately 92% in the thoracic spine. Figure 7.45 also shows the dose distribution along the spinal canal in a patient where the posterior surface is not horizontal. In this case, the dose varies from a minimum of approximately 75% in the lumbar spine and a segment of the upper thoracic spine to a maximum of 100 % in the thoracic spine.

In summary, an attempt should be made to keep the patient's posterior surface horizontal, an isodose calculation should be made on the sagittal contour, and the dose gradient within the spinal canal should be considered in the prescription. Problems associated with matching of adjacent fields in the spinal cord are discussed in Chapter 6 (pages 157-163).

HODGKIN'S DISEASE

The progress made in the treatment of Hodgkin's disease in recent years constitutes one of the major accomplishments of cancer therapy. The success of the treatment can be attributed to improved radiation therapy techniques as well as many new chemotherapeutic regimens. The prognosis for patients with Hodgkin's disease is largely determined by the initial management. Therefore, special attention must be given to the precision of the treatment in these often young and curable patients.

Improvements in radiation techniques include the ability to treat many lymph node groups in large contiguous fields, thus eliminating the risks associated with field matching. Also, the ability of utilizing custom-designed shielding blocks to tailor the treatment fields to suit each particular patient's needs has contributed to the accuracy with which the treatment can be delivered. Another more recent development is the improved ability to delineate the target volume by using CT and MRI imaging. Modern linear accelerators allow large fields to be treated at normal distances. This makes it possible to treat both anterior and posterior mantle fields and the anterior and posterior para-aortic fields with the patient in the same position, thus minimizing the risks of over- or underdosage in the match region between these areas. Last, positioning and immobilization devices, along with laser alignment systems, greatly improve the ability to reproduce the patient's position from treatment to treatment (Bentel 1991).

Elevation of the patient's arms above the head moves the axillary nodes away from the lateral chest wall, allowing shielding of the lung parenchyma without also shielding the axillary nodes (Fig. 7.46). The design of the mantle and para-aortic fields requires knowledge of both the tumor location and the patient's normal anatomy. In patients who have palpable lymph nodes, marking with lead wire or lead shot during the simulation procedure is helpful when the treatment fields are designed. It is also good practice to palpate these lymph nodes during the first setup to ensure that they actually are included in the treatment field with acceptable margins.

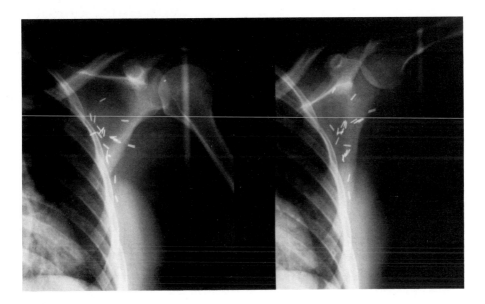

Fig. 7.46. Elevating the patient's arm pulls the axillary nodes out away from the chest wall, allowing larger margins around the nodes while sparing the lung parenchyma. (Reproduced with permission from Bentel, G.C.: Positioning and immobilization of patients undergoing radiation therapy for Hodgkin's disease, *Medical Dosimetry*, 16, 111 (1991). Courtesy Pergamon Press, Inc., Elmsford, NY.

Marking the splenic pedicle with metallic clips during the removal of the spleen will facilitate the design of the para-aortic and splenic-pedicle treatment fields (Fig. 7.47). In patients without metallic clips, other means of localizing the splenic pedicle, such as ultrasound, must be used. The information gained from the localization procedure must be used very carefully because the projection of the diverging radiation beam can cause the spleen to be missed (Fig. 7.48). As in any other site, only the tissues in the patient's mid-depth will be projected in the same fashion on anterior and posterior parallel opposed radiographs.

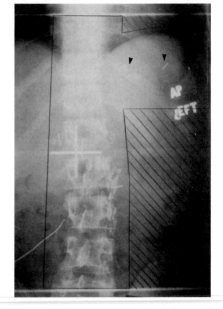

Fig. 7.47. Metallic clips marking the site of the spleen.

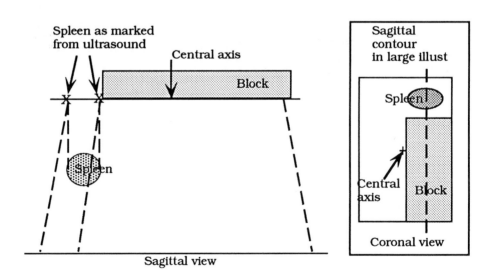

Fig. 7.48. The skin marks made during ultrasonic localization of the spleen must be used with caution. Only when the beam is centered on this volume will it be included in both the anterior and the posterior fields. The spleen and the para-aortic lymph nodes are usually treated in the same fields, causing the central axis to be at some distance from the spleen. Because of the beam divergence, the margins around the spleen should be very generous or the spleen could be partially missed.

The gap between the mantle and para-aortic/splenic fields must be very carefully calculated and measured because the patient's sloping chest can cause a significant error in the field separation (Keys 1990). Tattoos made on the patient's skin surface to indicate the margins of previously treated fields must not be totally relied on, because changes such as weight loss or gain, swelling, and growth (in the case of children) can alter the relationship between tattoos and the underlying anatomy.

REFERENCES

Bentel, G.C., Laser repositioning in radiation oncology, <u>Applied Radiology</u> 13, July/August (1984 A).

Bentel, G.C., A reproducible field matching technique for treatment of breast carcinoma, (Abstract) <u>Int. J. Radiat. Oncol. Biol. Phys.</u> 10, Supp. 2, 177 (1984 B).

Bentel, G.C., Nelson, C.E., Noell, K.T., <u>Treatment Planning and Dose Calculation in Radiation Oncology</u>, Pergamon Press, Inc., Elmsford, NY, 1989.

Bentel, G.C., Positioning and immobilization device for patients receiving radiation therapy for carcinoma of the breast, <u>Medical Dosimetry</u> 15, 3 (1990).

Bentel, G.C. , Halperin, E.C. , High dose areas are unintentionally created as a result of gap shifts when the prescribed doses in the two adjacent areas are different, <u>Medical Dosimetry</u> 15, 179 (1990).

Bentel, G.C., Positioning and immobilization of patients undergoing radiation therapy for Hodgkin's disease, <u>Medical Dosimetry</u> 16, 111 (1991).

Johns, H. E., Epp, E. R., Cormack, D. V., Fedoruck, S. O., Depth dose data and diaphragm design for the Saskatchewan 1000 curie cobalt unit, <u>Br. J. Radiol.</u> 25, 302 (1952).

Kalend, A.M., Park, T.L., Kalnicki, S., Meek, A.G., Bloomer, W.D., Solowsky, E.L., Clinical use of a wing field with transmission block for the treatment of the pelvis including the inguinal nodes, <u>Int. J. Radiat. Oncol. Biol. Phys.</u> 19, 153 (1990).

Khan, F. M., Moore, V. C., Levitt, S. H., Effect of various atomic number absorbers on skin dose for 10 MeV x-rays, <u>Radiology</u> 109, 209 (1973).

Keys, R., Grigsby, P. W., Gapping fields on sloping surfaces, <u>Int. J. Radiat. Oncol. Biol. Phys.</u> 18, 1183 (1990).

Richardson, J.E., Kerman, H.D., Brucer, M., Skin dose from cobalt 60 teletherapy unit, <u>Radiology</u> 63, 25 (1954).

Rosenthal, D.I., Sailer, S.L., Varia, M., Sherouse, G.W., Tepper, J.E., Optimizing peritoneal surface and renal dose distribution in whole abdominal radiation therapy (Abstract), <u>Int. J. Radiat. Oncol. Biol. Phys.</u> 19, Supp. 1, 256 (1990).

Shanahan, T.G., Mehta, M.P., Bertelrud, K.L., Buchler, D.A., Frank, L.E., Gehring, M.A., Kubsad, S.S., Utrie, P.C., Kinsella, T.J., Minimization of small bowel volume within treatment fields utilizing customized "Belly Boards," Int. J. Radiat. Oncol. Biol. Phys. 19, 469 (1990).

Willett, C.G., Linggood, R.M., Stracher, M.A., Goitein, M., Doppke, K., Kushner, D.C., Morris, T., Pardy, J., Carroll, R. , The effect of the respiratory cycle on mediastinal and lung dimensions in Hodgkin's disease, Cancer 60, 1232 (1987).

PROBLEMS

1. A belly board

   a) promotes small bowel movement
   b) helps to keep all the flabby skin folds out of the treatment field
   c) helps to keep the small bowel out of the pelvis

2. A patient with rectal carcinoma is best treated

   a) in supine position via a posterior and opposed lateral fields that are flashing over the posterior surface
   b) in prone position via only lateral fields that are flashing over the posterior surface
   c) in prone position via a posterior and opposed lateral fields that are flashing over the posterior surface

3. Partial kidney shielding is best accomplished by means of

   a) 5 HVT blocks in both the anterior and posterior fields, throughout the course of treatment
   b) partial shielding of the kidneys during the first week of treatment only
   c) partial shielding of the kidneys in the anterior and posterior fields until kidney tolerance is reached, followed by total removal of the blocks
   d) partial shielding of the kidneys in both the anterior and the posterior field until kidney tolerance has been reached, followed by total shielding of the kidneys

4. The volume of lung within an anterior supraclavicular field can be reduced when treating a patient with breast carcinoma by

   a) elevating the arm higher
   b) treating the supraclavicular field every other day only
   c) trying to move the breast lower on the chest wall by placing an angled board under the chest
   d) moving the breast down on the chest wall and making the match line between the tangential fields and the supraclavicular field as high on the chest as possible

5. To make patients more comfortable during treatment it is a good idea to

   a) make them lie prone
   b) provide supports under the head, knees, and arms
   c) place a soft pillow under the back

6. To minimize beam divergence into the eye on the opposite side, when treating a brain through opposed lateral fields

    a) the collimator can be angled so there is no divergence
    b) the beam is centered just behind the eye
    c) the patient's head is turned when each field is treated so that the beam exits behind the eyes
    d) the gantry can be angled so that the beam exits behind the eyes

7. A vertex field is difficult to treat because

    a) the gantry and the collimator must be turned
    b) the couch and the gantry must be turned
    c) the couch and the gantry must be turned, and sometimes the collimator also
    d) there is no reliable way of obtaining a port film, because the beam exits along the patient's torso

8. When the entire spinal axis must be treated, the patient's posterior surface should be as flat as possible

    a) to make field matching easier
    b) to make the dose more uniform
    c) so the position and matching of adjacent fields can be reproduced

9. Lateral brain fields and a posterior spinal field are best matched by

    a) turning the collimator when treating the lateral fields and turning the couch when treating the posterior spinal field
    b) turning the couch when treating the lateral fields and turning the collimator when treating the posterior spinal field
    c) turning the collimator and the couch when treating the lateral fields
    d) turning the couch and the collimator when treating the posterior spinal field

10. When treating the para-aortic lymph nodes and the splenic pedicle through parallel opposed isocentric fields, clips marking the splenic pedicle will always appear on port filmsat the same position with respect to the central axis of the beam

    a) if the central axis is on the clips
    b) if the clips are at the same depth in the patient as the isocenter
    c) a and b are correct
    d) a and b are wrong

SOLUTIONS

1.	c	6.	b
2.	c	7.	c
3.	d	8.	b
4.	d	9.	b
5.	b	10.	c

CHAPTER 8

DOSE CALCULATIONS IN BRACHYTHERAPY

Almost immediately following the discovery of radium by Marie and Pierre Curie in 1898, it was used to treat cancer by placing it in direct contact with the tumor. The placement of sealed radioactive sources into or immediately adjacent to tumors is referred to as brachytherapy. Brachy, meaning short, is used here in the context of therapy at a short distance (see footnote on page 31). The advantage of this method is that very high doses can be delivered locally to the tumor in a matter of hours while very low doses are delivered in the surrounding normal tissue.

Isotopes used in brachytherapy can be embedded in surface applicators which are placed directly on the tumor, or can be inserted into specially designed apparatus which are placed into body cavities (intracavitary), various tubular organs (intraluminal), or directly through the tumor (interstitially). In each of these methods, the radioactive material is sealed inside a shell which prevents escape of radioactivity into the tissues. The technical aspects of such brachytherapy applications are described in Chapter 9.

EMITTED RADIATION

Various types of radiation are produced by radioactive isotopes, including alpha, beta, and gamma rays. Emitted alpha particles are useless in the treatment of malignant disease because they lack penetrating power. Beta particles, which are somewhat more penetrating (the range is typically 3 mm or less), may be useful for treatment of very superficial lesions, especially those of the eye. Gamma rays can have very high penetrating power and are commonly used.

Filters, consisting of platinum or a platinum/iridium alloy, are often built into the walls surrounding an isotope to prevent non-useful low-energy radiation from penetrating. The size and shape of a radioactive source depends on how it is to be used and can be either in the shape of a needle, seed, tube, plaque, or in solution.

ACTIVITY

Much of the early work with radioactivity and dose determination was carried out using radium. The very slow decay of radium makes it an excellent standard from which to determine the radioactivity of other isotopes.

The activity of an isotope is defined as the number of disintegrations per time unit such as seconds, minutes, or hours. Because it is such an important concept, a special SI* unit for activity, the becquerel (Bq), has been defined. One becquerel equals one disintegration per second. Another unit of activity, which has been used for many years, is the curie (Ci). Early experiments with radium indicated that 1 gram of radium underwent 3.7×10^{10} disintegrations per second, and this disintegration rate (or activity) was later chosen as the unit for the activity of all nuclides. A sample decaying at this rate of 3.7×10^{10} disintegrations/sec was said to have an activity defined as 1 curie. Thus, 1 gram of radium has an activity of 1 curie, and 1 milligram of radium has an activity of 1/1000th curie or 1 millicurie. The becquerel and the curie are both named after famous physicists who did much of the early work on radioactivity and radium (Chapter 1).

DECAY

Radium decays to form daughter substances that are themselves unstable. Decay of successive daughters eventually results in a stable substance that does not decay any further. The rate at which these decays occur is characteristic of the internal nuclear structures of the various daughters. The time required for a radioactive isotope to lose half of its original activity is the half-life or $T_{1/2}$. The rate of decay of radium is very slow and the half-life is about 1600 years. The half-lives for some of the radioactive isotopes frequently used in radiation oncology are listed in Table 8.1. Isotopes decay with half-lives ranging from microseconds to millions of years. When the half-life and the present activity are known, it is possible to calculate the activity of a given isotopic sample at any future or past time.

---

* Système Internationale (International System)

TABLE 8.1

PHYSICAL CHARACTERISTICS OF SOME ISOTOPES USED IN RADIATION
ONCOLOGY

Isotope	Exposure rate constant (R/hr/mCi at 1 cm)	Half-life	Energy of gamma ray (MeV)	Half-value layer (cm Pb)
Radium-226	8.25	1600 years	avg. 1.2	1.3
Cesium-137	3.1	30 years	0.66	0.65
Cobalt-60	12.9	5.26 years	1.2	1.2
Strontium-90	-	28 years	Beta emitter	-
Iridium-192	4.61	74.3 days	avg. 0.380	0.3
Gold-198	2.34	2.7 days	0.412-1.09	0.33
Iodine-125	1.66	59.6 days	0.035	0.003
Iodine-131	2.3	8 days	Many	0.31
Phosphorus-32	-	14.3 days	Beta emitter	-

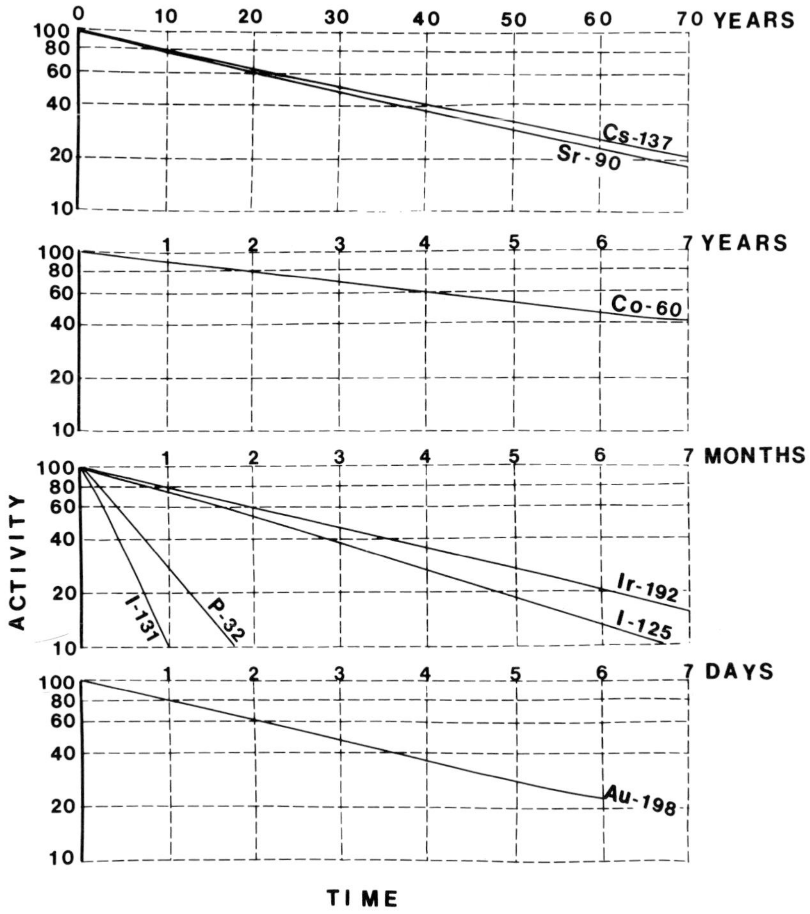

Fig. 8.1. Decay of some commonly used isotopes plotted on semilogarithmic paper.

Figure 8.1 shows the decay of a number of commonly used isotopes in radiation oncology. A straight line is drawn on semilogarithmic paper from the point, on day 0, when the activity is 100% through a point one half-life later when the activity is 50% or half of its original value. Intermediate values can then be easily determined. Similar graphs are useful in a clinic where many isotopes are used and where it is frequently necessary to quickly find the current activity of a given isotope.

RADIUM

Radium-226, the earliest and once the most commonly used isotope in brachytherapy, has largely been replaced by artificially produced isotopes. This change is in part due to the hazards associated with radium. Radium disintegrates very slowly to form radon (Rn-222), which is a hazardous radioactive gas. Despite double encapsulation of the activity, the risk of radium escaping from a broken or damaged source represents a serious hazard. This risk, combined with the increased availability of reactor-produced isotopes, has led to a gradual decline in the use of radium for brachytherapy.

ARTIFICIALLY PRODUCED ISOTOPES

Many radioactive isotopes are used in the diagnosis and treatment of disease. This section is limited to a description of the ones most commonly used in radiation oncology.

CESIUM-137

Cesium-137 (Cs-137), with a half-life of 30 years, is recovered from fission products made in a nuclear reactor. Cesium-137 has largely replaced radium in the treatment of gynecologic malignancies because it has no gaseous decay products and is therefore much safer in clinical use than radium. The gamma ray energy of Cs-137 is 0.662 MeV.

COBALT-60

Cobalt-60 (Co-60) has a half-life of 5.26 years and produces in each disintegration 2 gamma rays (1.17 and 1.33 MeV) with an average energy of 1.2 MeV. The relatively high penetrating power of Co-60 makes it an excellent isotope for use in teletherapy. The first Co-60 source for medical use was produced in 1951 in Canada and was used by Johns and co-workers in the first Co-60 teletherapy machine for external beam therapy in 1952 (page 31, Chapter 2). More recently, Co-60 has been used in ophthalmic plaques for the treatment of ocular melanomas.

STRONTIUM-90

Strontium-90 (Sr-90) became available in 1952 as a beta-ray applicator frequently used for the treatment of pterygium, a benign condition of the cornea. Strontium-90, a pure beta-emitter, decays with a half-life of 28 years. The maximum beta ray energy from Sr-90 is 0.54 MeV, while the daughter product, yttrium-90 (Yt-90), produces a penetrating beta particle with a maximum energy of 2.27 MeV. The Sr-90, foil-bonded in silver, is covered with a polythene plastic of about 0.5 mm thickness. The low-energy beta particles from the strontium are stopped by the silver and are thus prevented from exiting the source itself. The beta particles from Yt-90 are ideal for the treatment of superficial lesions of the eye. The dose falls very rapidly away from the applicator and is approximately 20% at 2 mm depth in tissue. The dose rate on the surface of such an applicator is in the range of 100 cGy/sec, and thus each treatment is delivered in seconds.

IRIDIUM-192

Iridium-192 (Ir-192) has become increasingly popular in brachytherapy. Iridium has a half-life of 74.3 days and emits beta particles with a maximum energy of 0.670 MeV, which are largely eliminated by the stainless steel capsule, as well as 11 gamma rays with energies ranging from 0.136 to 0.613 MeV. The effective gamma energy is approximately 0.380 MeV and the half-value thickness (HVT) is approximately 3 mm lead (Pb). Iridium-192, a reactor-produced isotope, is usually manufactured in the shape of seeds approximately 3 mm long and 0.5 mm in diameter. Nylon ribbons, containing iridium seeds, can be purchased to specification as to seed spacing, ribbon length, and seed activity. The ribbons are placed inside hollow plastic tubing which is first inserted into the tumor (page 288, Chapter 9).

All of the isotopes mentioned above for brachytherapy are left in place in the patient for a limited period of time until the desired dose is delivered, after which they are removed and stored or disposed of. There are, however, several short-lived radioactive isotopes which are used for permanent implantation. Such implants are used in treatment of deep-seated tumors where removal is not possible.

GOLD -198

Gold (Au-198) has a half-life of 64.7 hours and emits primarily gamma rays, most of which have an energy of 0.412 MeV. In the form of seeds or grains, the material is suitable for permanent implants because of the relatively short half-life. After complete decay the small inert masses cause no adverse affects and can remain in the tissues permanently. Gold seeds have largely replaced Rn-222 seeds for permanent implantation. Because gold emits only 3 gamma rays (maximum energy is 0.412 MeV), in contrast to the complex penetrating spectrum of radium, protection problems are much more easily solved, and exposure to personnel is minimized. Another advantage of gold over radon is that, although the major gamma activity of both isotopes disappears after about 1 month, some minor gamma activity from radon daughters persists for many years.

IODINE-125

Iodine-125 (I-125), which is also available in seed form, (commonly 4.5 mm long and 0.8 mm in diameter) is used in permanent implants but can also be used in removable implants. Iodine-125 has a half-life of 59.6 days and in addition to some very non-penetrating radiations that are absorbed by the 0.05 mm titanium wall of the seed, emits 0.274 and 0.355 MeV photons. Some I-125 seeds are made with two to five resin spheres containing absorbed I-125 and an x-ray marker. The titanium end welds, sometimes seen on radiographs, will cause an asymmetric dose distribution around the seed. This anisotropy should be taken into account in the dose calculation (Ling 1976, 1979, 1983, Krishnaswamy 1978). Another type of I-125 seeds are made with a silver rod, serving both as an x-ray marker and as a carrier for the I-125 (Fig. 8.2). The distribution of the activity within this type of seed may be sufficiently non-uniform to cause significant dose variations along the seed. Various gun-type applicators have been developed to insert these permanent seeds directly into accessible yet non-resectable tumors (pages 309-314, Chapter 9).

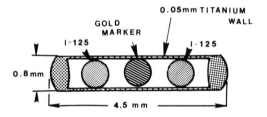

Fig. 8.2. Two types of I-125 seeds; two resin spheres with I-125 and a gold x-ray marker in the center (upper); a silver rod with I-125 (lower).

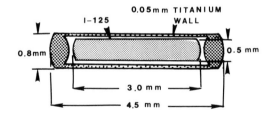

PHOSPHORUS-32 AND IODINE-131

Phosphorus-32 (P-32) and Iodine-131 (I-131) are other artificially produced isotopes that are used for therapeutic purposes. Phosphorus-32 decays by beta-minus emission with a maximum energy of 1.71 MeV and a half-life of 14.3 days. Chromic phosphate (P-32) in suspension is used in attempts to treat diffuse microscopic disease in the intraperitoneal space or thoracic cavity by direct deposition into the cavity; a colloidal form of gold-198 is sometimes used in a similar fashion.

Iodine-131 in the form of sodium iodide is given orally for the treatment of thyroid carcinoma and also for benign thyroid conditions. It decays by beta and gamma emission with a half-life of 8 days. The maximum gamma energy is 0.723 MeV. Caution must be used due to the undesired gamma radiation from I-131. These uses of P-32 and I-131 in liquid (unsealed) form are not discussed further in this book.

THE EXPOSURE RATE CONSTANT

The rate at which radiation arrives at a point near a radioactive source is related to the activity and to the energy and the number of photons emitted in each decay. It is called the exposure rate at the point and it can be expressed in terms of roentgens per hour or R/hr: the exposure concept is explained and the unit R is defined on page 19 in *Treatment Planning and Dose Calculation in Radiation Oncology* (Bentel 1989) and in radiation physics text.

The exposure rate at 1 cm away from a 1 mCi point source is called the exposure rate constant for the source material. Since the exposure rate at 1 cm from a 1 mCi point source of radium-226 filtered by 0.5 mm of platinum (Pt) is 8.25 R/hr, we can say that the exposure rate constant for radium is 8.25. The values for some other sources are given in Table 8.1. If we know the constant and the number of mCi of the isotope in question we can easily calculate the exposure at any distance, bearing in mind that the rate falls off as the inverse square of the distance. Thus at 3 cm from a 4.2 mCi (or mg) radium source the exposure rate is

$$\frac{4.2 \times 8.25}{(3)^2} = 3.85 \, \text{R/hr}$$

It is often convenient to express the activity of other isotopes in terms of milligram radium equivalent (mg Ra eq). When the activity of another isotope is expressed in terms of mg Ra eq, we mean that it produces the same exposure rate at a specified distance as a radium source of a specified activity. A Cs-137 source containing 1 mg Ra eq thus delivers the same dose rate at the treatment distance as 1 mg of Ra-226 filtered by 0.5 mm Pt.

The exposure rate constant for Ir-192 from Table 8.1 is 4.61. If we wanted to deliver 8.25 R/hr at 1 cm (the same as 1 mCi of radium-226), it would be necessary to use

$$\frac{8.25}{4.61} = 1.79 \, \text{mCi of Ir-192}$$

Thus, 1 mg Ra eq of Ir-192 contains 1.79 mCi of iridium.

In the rare event that we would need to find the number of mg Ra-226 needed to deliver the same dose as 1 mCi of another isotope, the equation is inverted. To deliver 4.61 R/hr (the exposure rate of 1 mCi of Ir-192) the amount of Ra-226 is

$$\frac{4.61}{8.25} = 0.56 \, \text{mg}$$

One mCi of Ir-192 is thus equivalent to 0.56 mg Ra.

SPECIFICATION OF SOURCES

Radioactive sources are specified by their physical length, active length, activity or strength, and by their filtration. The active length is obviously always smaller than the physical length because of the encapsulating material which surrounds the radioactivity. The walls of each source consist of a platinum alloy and, in some sources, also of ordinary iridium (non-radioactive), which strengthens the walls. A 0.5 mm thick sheath of platinum surrounding the radium is sufficient to filter out all alpha and most beta particles emitted by the radium and its daughter products. Only the gamma rays (average energy 1.2 MeV) escape. The encapsulating material also prevents escape of radioactive material into body tissues and fluids.

THE PHYSICAL FORM OF BRACHYTHERAPY SOURCES

TUBES

Tubes are the standard capsules for radioactive sources used in the treatment of gynecologic disease. These tubes contain either Ra-226, Co-60, or more recently, Cs-137. The usual range of activity is 5 to 25 mg Ra eq.

Radioactive tubes are inserted into devices designed to fit into the uterine canal, cervix, and vagina. These devices require that the exterior size and shape of the tubes be standardized. The standard physical dimensions of cesium tubes are 20 mm in length and approximately 3 mm in diameter. The length of the radioactive segment is obviously less, usually 14 mm. (See Chapter 2, page 14 in *Treatment Planning and Dose Calculation in Radiation Oncology*.) Smaller "microsources," which fit only into specially designed apparatus, have more recently been introduced.

NEEDLES

Radium-226 used for interstitial treatment is usually encapsulated in a shield shaped like a needle. These needles are longer than tubes but have a smaller diameter to allow easy insertion into tissue. An eyelet in one end is necessary for attaching the thread used to suture the needle in place and also to withdraw it. The other end of the needle is sharp. The physical length of each radium needle is usually 2.5 to 5.5 cm, while the active length is shorter. The outer diameter is less than 2 mm. The activity is less than in tubes, usually 0.33 or 0.66 mg Ra eq/cm of active length. Since the active lengths are 1.5 to 4.5 cm the total activity therefore ranges from 0.5 to 3 mg Ra eq/needle.

The activity of a radium source is always specified in milligrams or millicuries of radium. This activity is usually uniformly distributed within the active segment of the tube or needle. Needles with uniform linear activity may be "full-strength" or "half-strength." A full-strength needle has 0.66 mg radium per cm and a half-strength needle has 0.33 mg/cm. Needles with higher activity in one end are referred to as "Indian club" needles because of the shape of the resulting dose distribution. A needle with higher activity in both ends is similarly referred to as a "dumbbell" needle.

SEEDS

Radioactive seeds placed interstitially, such as Rn-222, have been used for many years. These seeds are left in place permanently since their half-life is short. Short-lived I-125 and Au-198 seeds are also left in place permanently while Ir-192 seeds are removed after a few days when the desired dose has been delivered; the longer half-life of Ir-192 prevents safe permanent implantation. The beta component of the radiation is filtered out by 0.1 mm of Pt. The activity per seed is usually less than 1 mg Ra eq but can be higher when ordered for special situations.

FLUIDS

The most frequently used radionuclides administered as a fluid are I-131 and P-32. Gold-198 and I-131 are often used for treatment of thyroid carcinoma, and P-32 is usually deposited in the peritoneal or pleural space for treatment of diffuse microscopic disease. Phosphorus-32, a beta-emitter, has a range in tissue of millimeters, and its distribution within the cavity is uncertain. Gravitational effects are believed to cause increased concentration in the lower segments of the cavity, which change with the patient's position. Removal of radioactive fluids is impossible, and short-lived isotopes must therefore be used.

OPHTHALMIC APPLICATORS

Some conditions of the conjunctiva, primarily pterygium, are effectively treated with a Sr-90 source which has a half-life of 28 years. Beta particles from the daughter product Yt-90 are used. This source is encapsulated in a small, circular applicator placed directly on the conjunctiva. The dose rate at the surface of the applicator is very high, about 100 cGy/sec. Penetration is very poor, so the dose falls off very rapidly with depth. The dose at 1 mm depth is only 50% of the dose at the surface and at 4 mm depth, it is only 5%; thus, the dose to the lens is very low. A typical Sr-90 applicator is shown in Fig. 8.3.

Other applicators in the form of plaques are used for treatment of ocular melanomas (Fig. 8.4). The plaques are usually circular and have a concave surface to provide a snug fit over the curved surface of the eye. Several eyelets are provided for suturing the plaques onto the sclera, because they are usually left in place several days. Cobalt-60 plaques with diameters of 10 to 15 mm are available commercially, but other isotopes with shorter half-life and less penetration such as I-125 or Ir-192 can be used in customized plaques. In Co-60 plaques, the radioactivity, which is not removable, is distributed in a circular pattern over the inner (concave) surface of the plaque.

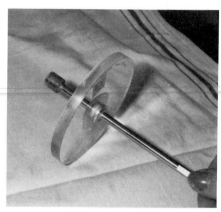

Fig. 8.3. A Sr-90 applicator, frequently used to treat pterygium.

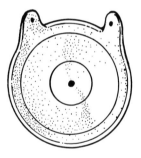 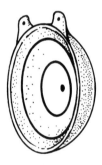

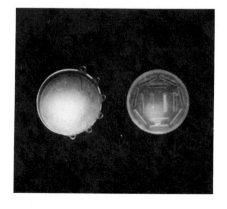

Fig. 8.4. Diagram of a Co-60 plaque used for treatment of ocular melanomas (above). The radioactivity is distributed in a circular pattern. There are two eyelets for suturing the plaque in place. A photograph (right) of an I-125 seed ophthalmic plaque with several suture holes and a seed carrier, which remains inside the metal plaque during the treatment. Also, see Chapter 9, Fig. 9.40.

The most popular ophthalmic plaque in the U.S. consists of two components: an outer metal shield and a seed carrier insert (Fig. 8.4). The plaques are available in various diameters and can thus be selected to best cover the tumor. The metal shield, which consists of a gold alloy, is a spherical shell segment with a "lip" that is at right angles to the back of the plaque. The height of the lip depends on the thickness of the insert and the diameter of the plaque, and is designed to bring the lip to the outer scleral surface. Attached to the lip are several tabs with suture holes. The seed carrier insert, made of silicone rubber, is designed to fit snugly into the concave surface of the metal shield. Molded into the outer surface are seed "troughs" into which I-125 seeds will fit. The pattern of these seed troughs is designed to provide a uniform dose distribution. The seed carriers are discarded after each use, while the metal plaques are reusable.

Cobalt-60 plaques have a total activity of approximately 2 to 3 mCi (not mg Ra eq), while the activity in customized plaques varies depending on the isotope used and the size of the lesion to be treated.

DOSE CALCULATION

Dose determinations from radium, made by the pioneers in the early 1900s, can be applied to other isotopes also and are therefore presented following the description of modern, artificially produced isotopes.

Calculation of the dose or exposure from sources used for intracavitary or interstitial applications requires knowledge of the dose per hour at some distance from a source when a known number of curies or millicuries of activity is present. Since most sources are encapsulated in some material, the exposure will also be affected by the amount of filtration such capsules provide. The exposure rate constant (Γ) provides the link between activity (in curies) and exposure (in roentgens). The exposure rate (X_r) is found by taking the exposure rate constant, multiplying by the activity (A), and dividing by the square of the distance (r) to include the inverse square factor.

$$X_r = \frac{\Gamma \times A}{(r)^2} \qquad (8.1)$$

The exposure rate constant for radium is 8.25 R/hr at 1 cm from 1 mCi (Table 8.1). Using equation 8.1, the exposure rate 50 cm from a 20 mCi point source of radium filtered by 0.5 mm of platinum is

$$\frac{8.25 \text{ R cm}^2 \text{ hr}}{\text{hr mCi}} \times \frac{20 \text{ mCi}}{(50 \text{ cm})^2} = 0.066 \text{ R/hr}$$

A roentgen to cGy factor (f_{tis}) must be applied to convert exposure in air to absorbed dose in muscle. The recommended f_{tis} value is 0.963 (Johns 1983). All tables in this chapter have been converted to cGy.

Another popular method often used to describe a treatment with radium and radon is mg hr (or mCi hr). Milligram hour is the number of mg (or mCi) of radium or radium equivalent inserted multiplied by the number of hours the source was left in place. For example, 15 mg Ra eq left in place for 10 hours represents 150 mg hr. Milligram hours do not tell the dose delivered at a specific point unless the arrangement of the sources is also known. For example, a 10 mg Ra eq source left in place for 1 hour (10 mg hr) delivers 79.5 cGy (10 x 8.25 x 0.963) at 1 cm from the source. However, 10 mg Ra eq in four sources arranged in a linear fashion and left in place for 1 hour also represent 10 mg hr, but the dose at 1 cm from the center of each source (19.86 cGy) can not be added because this dose is delivered at four different points. In most implants, several sources are used and they are often arranged to produce a dose distribution which conforms to the target. It is therefore very unlikely that the sources are arranged so that all of them are at the same distance from a common dose calculation point.

Ovoids of various diameters and with a central canal for the source are often used in gynecologic implants. Here, the dose on the ovoid surface will vary depending on the size of the ovoid if the mg hr remain unchanged. In this situation, the mg hr must be increased in order to maintain the same dose on the ovoid surface (mucosa) as the ovoid size increases.

SIEVERT INTEGRAL

A difficulty with the concept described via equation 8.1 is that it allows the calculation of exposure only from point sources. While some non-point sources may be considered as approximate point sources at large distances, the rationale for brachytherapy involves the concept of treating at short distances away from non-point sources. For example, the treatment of gynecologic malignancies with radium or cesium involves the calculation of the dose at positions only 2 or 3 cm away from tubes that are 2 or 3 cm long. This involves calculating the dose via the evaluation of an integral, the Sievert integral (Sievert 1921, 1930, Johns 1983), a process too complicated to do routinely by hand.

The dose from a linear source can be found by considering the source to be divided into many small segments and applying an inverse square law calculation and a filtration correction factor to each segment. Adding together or "integrating" the doses contributed at the calculation point by each segment gives the dose rate from the entire source. Figure 8.5, for example, illustrates that the distance from segment a to the dose calculation point (P) is longer than from segment c to P. Furthermore, the thickness of filtration which the radiation from segment a traverses (a to b) is greater than that which the radiation from segment c traverses (c to d). The dose contributed at P by segment a is thus lower than that contributed by segment c because of the longer distance and also because of the increased attenuation by the greater thickness of filtration through which it travels. When very large numbers of segments are considered, the mathematical expression used to add all of the segment doses together is called the Sievert integral.

Dose rates are similarly calculated around a source, and by joining points of equal dose, dose-rate distributions are displayed. These calculations are very tedious to do by hand, but computer methods are routinely applied in clinical brachytherapy.

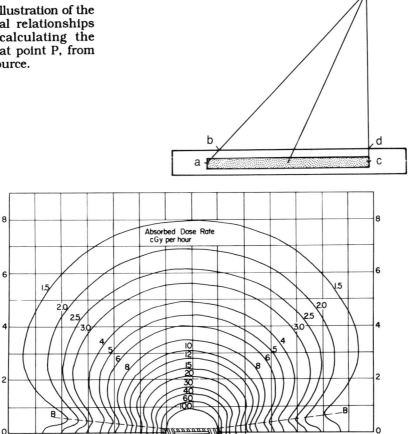

Fig. 8.5. Illustration of the geometrical relationships used in calculating the exposure at point P, from a linear source.

Fig. 8.6. Dose-rate distribution around a 13.3 mg radium tube filtered by 1.0 mm platinum. Note the small cone of more intense dose at 0 cm away from the source, that is, at the axis of the source. (Reproduced with permission from Johns, H.E. and Cunningham, J.R.: *The Physics of Radiology.* Courtesy Charles C. Thomas, Springfield, IL, 1983.)

Figure 8.6 illustrates a computer-calculated dose-rate distribution around a 13.3 mg radium source. The dose rate along the axis of the tube is less than it is at right angles to the tube because of the increased effect of oblique filtration. Maximum oblique filtration occurs at the corners of the tube, while along the exact axis of the source, part of the attenuating encapsulation is replaced by the less attenuating radioactive material itself. As a result, there is a small cone of more intense radiation at the axis of the source.

Fig. 8.7. A point source (left) and a linear source (right) delivering the same dose (100 cGy/hr) at a given distance from the source (X). However, at a longer distance, the linear source delivers a higher dose (Y). The inverse square law does not apply to linear sources.

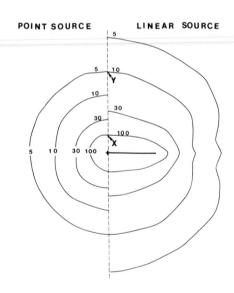

For linear sources, the dose rate is lower than that calculated by the inverse square law, particularly at points close to the source. This is expected since the photons travelling from the extremes of the source have a longer distance and also must traverse oblique filtration. As the distance from the source increases, the effect diminishes and the dose rates approach that of point sources (Fig. 8.7).

DOSAGE SYSTEMS

Several systems of dosimetric planning for brachytherapy have been devised over the past 50 years. The Paris system (Regaud 1929, Dutreix 1982,

1987), the Paterson-Parker or Manchester system (Paterson 1938, 1979), and the Quimby system (Quimby 1944, Glasser 1961) are the most widely used. The three systems differ in the rules of implantation, definition of dose uniformity, and the method used in reference-dose specification (Dutreix 1988). While the Paterson-Parker system was designed to distribute the radium in a non-uniform fashion to achieve a reasonably uniform dose distribution, the Paris and Quimby systems were designed to distribute the radium itself in a uniform fashion which provides a non-uniform dose distribution. Figure 8.8 shows a comparison of the dose-rate distributions from the Quimby and the Manchester systems.

Both the Manchester and the Quimby systems provide tables giving the mg hr necessary to deliver 1000 cGy for implants of various sizes and shapes. The original tables have been converted from roentgens to cGy but have not been corrected for the attenuation and scattering of radiation in the surrounding tissue, which are assumed to compensate for each other. This approximation is valid to within a few percentage points.

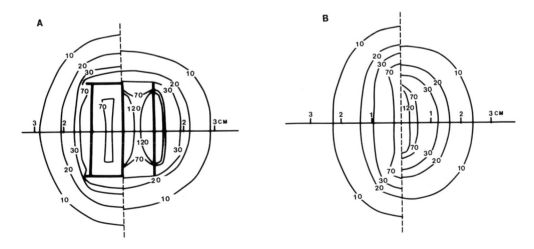

Fig. 8.8. Comparison of a Paterson-Parker-type and a Quimby-type implant. Only one-half of each implant (Paterson-Parker on the left and Quimby on the right) is shown side-by-side. A plane along the needles is shown in (A) and a plane across the needles is shown in (B).

The Quimby System

Quimby calculated and tabulated dose distributions for linear radium sources with different active lengths and wall thicknesses. The tabulated data give the cGy/hr at locations "along" as well as "away" from the axis of a 1 mg radium source. Tables 8.2 and 8.3 take account of the f-factor (roentgen to cGy conversion factor) and the oblique filtration through the radium salt and the source capsule.

The example below illustrates the use of Quimby's tables for linear sources in a typical gynecologic implant consisting of a tandem containing three sources and a pair of ovoids, each containing one source (Fig. 8.9).

Calculating the dose at X from sources A, B, C, D, and E using Table 8.2:

Source A

(2 cm away, 3 cm along)
0.57 cGy/mg hr x 15 mg = 8.55 cGy/hr

Source B

(2 cm away, 1 cm along)
1.56 cGy/mg hr x 10 mg = 15.6 cGy/hr

Source C

(2 cm away, 1 cm along)
1.56 cGy/mg hr x 10 mg = 15.6 cGy/hr

Source D

(4.5 cm away, 0 cm along)
0.4 cGy/mg hr x 15 mg = 6.0 cGy/hr

Source E

(2 cm away, 0 cm along)
1.89 cGy/mg hr x 15 mg = 28.35 cGy/hr

Total dose in cGy/hr at X = 74.1.

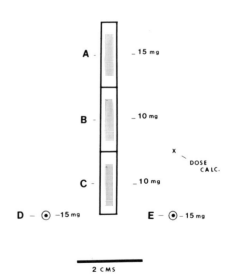

Fig. 8.9. Diagram illustrating point calculation from linear sources.

TABLE 8.2

CGY/MG HR DELIVERED TO LOCATIONS ALONG AND AWAY
BY LINEAR RADIUM SOURCE
(1.5 CM ACTIVE LENGTH) FILTERED BY 0.5 MM PT(IR)*

Distance Away From Source (cm)	Distance Along Source (cm)										
	0	0.5	1.0	1.5	2.0	2.5	3.0	3.5	4.0	4.5	5.0
0.5	20.4	16.9	8.06	3.25	1.62	0.90	0.56	0.37	0.24	0.15	0.10
0.75	10.9	9.30	5.64	2.92	1.62	0.99	0.66	0.44	0.32	0.24	0.17
1.0	6.69	5.95	4.11	2.48	1.54	0.99	0.68	0.48	0.35	0.26	0.21
1.5	3.27	3.03	2.41	1.75	1.23	0.88	0.64	0.48	0.36	0.29	0.23
2.0	1.89	1.79	1.56	1.25	0.97	0.74	0.57	0.45	0.36	0.28	0.23
2.5	1.23	1.18	1.07	0.92	0.75	0.62	0.50	0.40	0.33	0.27	0.23
3.0	0.86	0.84	0.77	0.70	0.60	0.51	0.42	0.36	0.29	0.25	0.22
4.0	0.49	0.48	0.46	0.43	0.39	0.35	0.31	0.28	0.24	0.21	0.19
5.0	0.31	0.31	0.30	0.29	0.27	0.25	0.22	0.21	0.19	0.17	0.15

*Modified from data of Greenfield et al. (Greenfield 1959).

Reproduced with permission from Hendee, W.R.: *Radiation Therapy Physics*. Courtesy Year Book Medical Publishers, Inc., Chicago, IL, 1981.

TABLE 8.3

CGY/MG HR DELIVERED TO LOCATIONS ALONG AND AWAY
BY LINEAR RADIUM SOURCE
(1.5 CM ACTIVE LENGTH) FILTERED BY 1.0 MM PT(IR)*

Distance Away From Source (cm)	Distance Along Source (cm)										
	0	0.5	1.0	1.5	2.0	2.5	3.0	3.5	4.0	4.5	5.0
0.5	18.0	14.9	7.28	2.49	1.10	0.58	0.32	0.20	0.11	0.08	0.05
0.75	9.68	8.24	4.86	2.41	1.24	0.70	0.43	0.28	0.21	0.13	0.09
1.0	6.02	5.28	3.56	2.11	1.24	0.76	0.50	0.33	0.24	0.17	0.13
1.5	2.93	2.69	2.12	1.54	1.03	0.74	0.52	0.38	0.28	0.21	0.16
2.0	1.70	1.61	1.38	1.09	0.84	0.64	0.48	0.38	0.28	0.23	0.17
2.5	1.11	1.06	0.95	0.81	0.67	0.54	0.43	0.34	0.27	0.23	0.18
3.0	0.77	0.75	0.70	0.62	0.53	0.44	0.37	0.31	0.25	0.22	0.18
4.0	0.44	0.43	0.41	0.39	0.35	0.31	0.27	0.24	0.21	0.18	0.16
5.0	0.28	0.28	0.27	0.26	0.24	0.23	0.20	0.19	0.17	0.15	0.13

*Modified from data of Greenfield et al. (Greenfield 1959).

Reproduced with permission from Hendee, W.R.: *Radiation Therapy Physics*. Courtesy Year Book Publishers, Inc., Chicago, IL, 1981.

Quimby's system of uniform distribution of radioactivity within a one- or multiple-plane implant gives a non-uniform dose distribution within the implanted volume. The center of the volume receives substantially higher dose than the periphery (Fig. 8.8).

The following example of dose calculation illustrates the use of Quimby's tables giving the mg hr necessary to deliver 1000 cGy at different distances from a surface applicator. Using Quimby's approach, a surface mold is to be constructed to treat a 4 x 6 cm lesion. A dose of 3000 cGy is to be delivered in 48 hours at the center of the lesion which is 1 cm below the plane of the radium sources (filtration 0.5 mm Pt[Ir]).

Here we use Table 8.4, modified from Quimby's data, providing the product of the amount of radium and exposure time in hours, that is, the mg hr required to deliver 1000 cGy at various distances along a line perpendicular to the center of the implant plane. From Table 8.4, 453 mg hr are required for 1000 cGy. The number of mg hr required for 3000 cGy is

$$\frac{453 \text{ mg hr} \times 3000 \text{ cGy}}{1000 \text{ cGy}} = 1359 \text{ mg hr}$$

To deliver the treatment in 48 hours, the required mg of radium is

$$\frac{1359 \text{ mg hr}}{48 \text{ hr}} = 28.3 \text{ mg}$$

The radioactivity must be uniformly distributed over the mold.

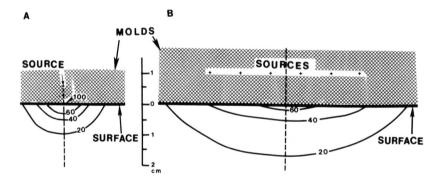

Fig. 8.10. A very small surface mold (A) with a radioactive source embedded 0.5 cm above the surface delivers 40 cGy/hr at 0.5 cm depth in tissue. A larger surface mold (B) with several radioactive sources but containing the same total activity as in (A) embedded 1.0 cm above the surface also delivers 40 cGy/hr at 0.5 cm depth in tissue. The maximum tissue dose in (A) is 100 cGy while in (B) it is 63 cGy/hr; a considerable improvement in %DD in (B).

TABLE 8.4

MILLIGRAM HOURS REQUIRED FOR ABSORBED DOSE OF 1000 CGY AT
LOCATIONS ALONG A LINE PERPENDICULAR TO CENTER OF
APPLICATOR OR IMPLANT PLANE*+

Circular Applicators
(Diameter in cm)

Distance (cm)	1	2	3	4	5	6
0.5	47	80	110	181	234	319
1.0	145	187	234	319	394	482
1.5	301	345	426	506	598	725
2.0	528	577	646	745	846	977
2.5	782	846	920	1016	1229	1346
3.0	1160	1224	1298	1404	1522	1665

Square Applicators
(Length of side in cm)

Distance (cm)	1	2	3	4	5	6
0.5	49	85	122	210	266	372
1.0	150	200	253	348	431	544
1.5	314	367	442	544	638	782
2.0	532	606	686	795	910	1064
2.5	777	846	952	1075	1213	1458
3.0	1160	1224	1351	1479	1617	1777

Rectangular Applicators
(Dimensions in cm)

Distance (cm)	1 x 1.5	2 x 3	3 x 4	4 x 6	6 x 9	8 x 12
0.5	54	110	152	305	606	1016
1.0	157	228	291	453	772	1181
1.5	317	394	496	664	1005	1442
2.0	538	628	761	930	1319	1777
2.5	767	894	1053	1213	1617	2128
3.0	1181	1266	1420	1617	2054	2660

*Modified from data of Quimby et al. (Goodwin 1970).
+The radium sources are distributed uniformly across the plane and filtered by 0.5 mm Pt(Ir).

Reproduced with permission from Hendee, W.R.: *Radiation Therapy Physics*. Courtesy Year Book Medical Publishers, Inc., Chicago, IL, 1981.

In small surface applicators, the radioactive sources must be placed closer to the tumor than in larger applicators (Fig. 8.10). In Fig. 8.10 (A), the source is placed 0.5 cm from the surface and the dose rate is 40 cGy/hr at 0.5 cm depth in tissue. In Fig. 8.10 (B) six sources are placed 1.0 cm from the surface. The dose rate at 0.5 cm depth in tissue is also 40 cGy/hr; however, the surface dose is approximately 63 cGy/hr in (B) and 100 cGy/hr in (A). (See inverse square law for point sources vs. linear sources, Fig. 8.7).

If all dimensions (length, width, and height) of an implant are approximately the same, tables for volume implants must be used. As an example, a cylindrical volume 3 cm in diameter and 4 cm long is implanted and 3000 cGy is desired in 72 hours. (See the Manchester system for a similar case.)

Here we use Table 8.5, which is modified from Quimby's data, providing the mg hr required to deliver 1000 cGy in a volume implant designed according to the Quimby system. We find that for a volume of 28 cm³, 554 mg hr (interpolated value) are required to deliver 1000 cGy.

The number of mg hr required to deliver 3000 cGy is

$$\frac{554 \text{ mg hr} \times 3000 \text{ cGy}}{1000 \text{ cGy}} = 1662 \text{ mg hr}$$

TABLE 8.5

MILLIGRAM HOURS REQUIRED FOR MINIMUM ABSORBED
DOSE OF 1000 CGY IN VOLUME IMPLANT*

Volume (cm³)	Mg hr for 1000 cGy	Diameter of Sphere (cm)	Mg hr for 1000 cGy
5	213	1.0	43
10	340	1.5	106
15	415	2.0	192
20	468	2.5	298
30	575	3.0	415
40	660	3.5	505
60	798	4.0	612
80	926	4.5	718
100	1064	5.0	841
125	1192	6.0	1138
150	1330	7.0	1490
175	1479		
200	1596		
250	1788		
300	1915		

---

*Modified from data of Quimby et al. (Goodwin 1970). The radium sources are distributed uniformly and filtered by 0.5 mm Pt(Ir).

Reproduced with permission from Hendee, W.R.: *Radiation Therapy Physics.* Courtesy Year Book Medical Publishers, Inc., Chicago, IL, 1981.

To obtain 1662 mg hr in 72 hr, we need

$$\frac{1662 \text{ mg hr}}{72 \text{ hr}} = 23 \text{ mg ra}$$

Caution must be used when tables of dose rates or mg hr are consulted. For example, using Quimby's tables with a Paterson-Parker system implant would be erroneous, and vice versa.

The Paterson-Parker System

The Paterson-Parker system was devised to deliver a reasonably uniform dose to a plane or a volume. Elaborate rules for distribution of the radioactivity within the volume were developed along with tables, which give the mg hr necessary to deliver 1000 cGy at various treatment distances from the implant. In Quimby's approach, the number of mg hr required to deliver 1000 cGy is higher than in the Manchester system because with Quimby's approach the *minimum* dose is 1000 cGy. In the Manchester system the absorbed dose is approximately 1000 cGy *throughout the volume*.

An exposure rate constant correction from 8.4 R per hour at one cm from 1 mg of radium to the current value of 8.25 must be made when using older Paterson-Parker tables. A roentgen to cGy factor (f_{tis}) of 0.963 should be applied to convert exposure in air to absorbed dose in muscle.

The distribution rules for surface applicators and planar implants are:

(1) On a single plane, a fraction of the radium should be arranged uniformly around the periphery, while the remainder should be spread as evenly as possible over the area itself. The fraction of the radium used in the periphery should be as follows:

Area:	<25 cm^2	25 - 100 cm^2	> 100 cm^2
Peripheral Fraction:	2/3	1/2	1/3

(2) A common arrangement is a row of parallel needles with active ends crossed by means of needles at right angles to the first part of the implant (Fig. 8.11). In many anatomical situations, it is impossible to cross one or both ends of the implant. When only one end is crossed, the area that is treated should be considered as 90% of the length of the implant and when neither end is crossed the treated area should be considered as 80%, that is, for each uncrossed end, the treated area should be taken as 10% less than the nominal area. Use of Indian club needles, previously described, eliminates the need for a crossing needle at the end of uniformly implanted needles. Dumbbell needles, also previously described, have greater activity at both ends and do not require crossing needles at either end.

(3) Needles arranged as such a series of parallel lines should not be more than 1 cm from each other or from the crossing ends.

Similarly, the spacing of seeds should not exceed 1 cm from each other.

(4) In two-plane implants, the radium on each plane should be arranged as in rules 1), 2), and 3), and the planes should be parallel to each other.

(5) If two planes differ in area, the area to be used for table-reading purposes is the average of the two, and the total amount of radium is prorated to each plane.

When the radium is distributed on two planes, the mg hr found from the table has to be increased by a factor depending on the distance between the planes, except for planes separated by 1 cm. These factors are

Separation (cm):	1.5	2.0	2.5
Factor:	1.25	1.4	1.5

It must be recognized that with larger separation between the planes the dose between the planes is decreased.

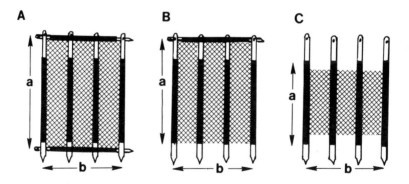

Fig. 8.11. Diagrams of different arrangements of radioactive needles for planar implants. The shaded areas indicate the areas used for calculating the dose. To calculate the number of cubic cm (cm³) of the treated slice of tissue one would use a x b x 2h, where h is the treatment distance in the third dimension and 2h is the thickness of the slice of tissue treated. If the treatment distance (h) is 0.5 cm the slice thickness (2h) is 1 cm.

Special cases

(1) A single plane of needles or seeds can satisfactorily treat a slice of tissue 1.0 to 1.25 cm thick in which the radium plane is the center. When a thicker slice of tissue must be treated, two planes will be necessary. A two-plane implant can satisfactorily treat a block of tissue 2.5 cm thick. From Fig. 8.12 and Table 8.6, it is obvious that the dose between the planes is decreased if the separation of the planes is increased.

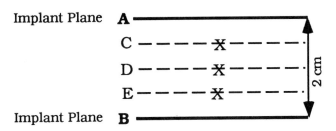

Fig. 8.12. Two implant planes separated by 2 cm. The dose at (X) on plane D is the same from both implant planes while the dose at (X) on planes C and E is higher. Point (X) on plane C receives higher dose from implant plane A than from B.

TABLE 8.6

DOSE CALCULATION FOR A TWO-PLANE IMPLANT

Distance	Plane C 0.5 cm	Plane D 1 cm	Plane E 1.5 cm
Mg hr/1000 cGy	618	967	1392
Dose for 600 mg hr in plane A	971 cGy	620 cGy	431 cGy
Dose for 600 mg hr in plane B	431 cGy	620 cGy	971 cGy
Dose for 1200 mg hr in planes A and B	1402 cGy	1240 cGy	1402 cGy

In this example, the area of each plane is 38 cm² and the planes are separated by 2 cm. The dose is calculated using Table 8.7. The dose from implant plane A (600 mg hr) along plane C (0.5 cm away) is 971 cGy. From Table 8.7 we find that 618 mg hr deliver 1000 cGy at 0.5 cm distance, so 600 mg hr deliver

$$\frac{600 \text{ mg hr} \times 1000 \text{ cGy}}{618 \text{ mg hr}} = 971 \text{ cGy}$$

TABLE 8.7

SURFACE APPLICATORS AND PLANAR IMPLANTS

The table gives R_A, the number of mg hr required to deliver 1000 cGy to muscle tissue for different areas and treatment distances. Filtration 0.5 mm Pt. The table may be used for planar implants by using a treatment distance of 0.5 cm.

Area (cm²)	\ Treatment Distance (cm)									
	0.5	1.0	1.5	2.0	2.5	3.0	3.5	4.0	4.5	5.0
0	32	127	285	506	792	1139	1551	2026	2566	3166
1	72	182	343	571	856	1204	1625	2100	2636	3295
2	103	227	399	632	920	1274	1697	2172	2708	3349
3	128	263	448	689	978	1331	1760	2241	2772	3383
4	150	296	492	743	1032	1388	1823	2307	2835	3450
5	170	326	531	787	1083	1436	1881	2369	2896	3513
6	188	354	570	832	1134	1495	1938	2432	2956	3575
7	204	382	603	870	1182	1547	1993	2490	3011	3634
8	219	409	637	910	1229	1596	2047	2548	3067	3694
9	235	434	667	946	1272	1645	2099	2605	3123	3752
10	250	461	697	982	1314	1692	2149	2660	3178	3809
12	278	511	755	1053	1396	1780	2247	2769	3284	3917
14	306	557	813	1120	1475	1865	2341	2870	3389	4027
16	335	602	866	1184	1553	1947	2429	2968	3490	4131
18	364	644	918	1245	1622	2027	2514	3063	3585	4240
20	392	682	968	1303	1690	2106	2601	3155	3682	4341
22	418	717	1021	1362	1755	2180	2683	3242	3777	4441
24	444	752	1072	1420	1821	2252	2764	3326	3872	4540
26	470	784	1122	1477	1881	2328	2841	3405	3962	4634
28	496	816	1170	1530	1943	2398	2917	3484	4047	4730
30	521	846	1215	1582	2000	2468	2997	3562	4131	4824
32	546	876	1261	1635	2060	2532	3073	3639	4220	4915
34	571	909	1305	1688	2119	2598	3145	3713	4306	5000
36	594	935	1349	1743	2179	2662	3215	3787	4389	5089
38	618	967	1392	1793	2234	2726	3285	3859	4466	5174
40	642	994	1432	1843	2290	2787	3351	3931	4546	5258
42	664	1024	1472	1894	2344	2848	3421	4003	4626	5341
44	685	1053	1511	1942	2399	2908	3484	4071	4706	5422
46	708	1080	1550	1990	2452	2966	3548	4139	4781	5505
48	729	1110	1585	2037	2504	3025	3612	4207	4857	5586
50	750	1141	1619	2083	2556	3082	3676	4275	4929	5668
60	851	1283	1790	2319	2815	3362	3974	4605	5288	6054
70	947	1426	1944	2532	3059	3628	4257	4913	5632	6419
80	1044	1567	2092	2726	3301	3891	4532	5213	5958	6756

Filtration (mm Pt)	0.3	0.5	0.6	0.8	1.0	1.5
Correction to mg hr	-4%	0	+2%	+6%	+10%	+20%

This table was prepared from the original by Meredith (Meredith 1967) by multiplying his values by C = 1.064.

Reproduced with permission from Johns, H.E. and Cunningham, J.R.: *The Physics of Radiology.* Courtesy Charles C. Thomas, Springfield, IL, 1983.

The dose on plane D will be the same from the two implant planes, that is, 620 cGy each. The dose on planes C and E will be the same, but C will receive a higher dose from implant plane A than from implant plane B because of the shorter distance. As the implant planes are separated farther, the dose on plane D will decrease.

Figure 8.13 shows three radioactive sources indicating the 10 cGy/hr line from each source. The combined dose along lines B and C is the same, but it is higher than along lines A and D because they are closer to the center of the implant. The doses along lines E and G are the same, but are lower than along line F which crosses the implant at the center. The intersection of lines B and F, for example, lies within all three 10 cGy/hr lines, while the intersection of lines A and E lies within only one 10 cGy/hr line. This illustrates the higher dose at the center of an implant when the activity is uniformly distributed.

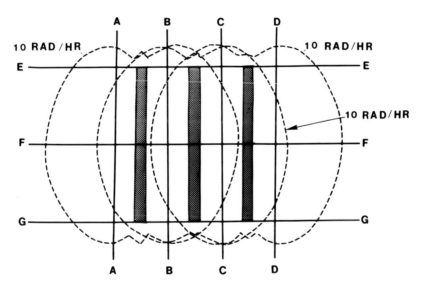

Fig. 8.13. Three sources (shaded) and the 10 cGy/hr line from each source. The sum of these dose-rate lines shows lower dose toward the ends of the sources and also in the periphery. The dose is highest in the center.

Example #1
In this example, we will calculate the amount of radium required to deliver 3000 cGy in 48 hr at 1 cm from the center of a 4 x 6 cm (24 cm²) planar implant. From Table 8.7, which gives the number of mg hr required to deliver 1000 cGy at various distances from surface applicators and planar implants, 752 mg hr are required for a uniform dose (±10%) of 1000 cGy over the entire treated area. The original values of required mg hr to deliver 1000 R given by Meredith (Meredith 1967) have been multiplied by 1.064 to

describe the required number of mg hr to deliver 1000 cGy in tissue rather than 1000 R in air.

The number of mg hr required for 3000 cGy is

$$\frac{752 \text{ mg hr} \times 3000 \text{ cGy}}{1000 \text{ cGy}} = 2256 \text{ mg hr}$$

The number of mg radium required is

$$\frac{2256 \text{ mg hr}}{48 \text{ hr}} = 47 \text{ mg}$$

Example #2
    Using Table 8.7, calculate the amount of radium required to deliver 2000 cGy 0.5 cm from the center of a 6 x 6 cm implant in 40 hr. From Table 8.7, 594 mg hr is required to deliver 1000 cGy at 0.5 cm from the center of the implant. The number of mg hr required for 2000 cGy is therefore

$$\frac{594 \text{ mg hr} \times 2000 \text{ cGy}}{1000 \text{ cGy}} = 1188 \text{ mg hr}$$

Since 40 hr are available, the number of mg radium required is

$$\frac{1188 \text{ mg hr}}{40 \text{ hr}} = 29.7 \text{ mg}$$

(2) Elongated rectangular implants result in lower dose rates requiring increased mg hr. The reasons for this lower dose is somewhat similar to the elongation effect in rectangular external fields described in Chapter 5 (page 121). The elongation rules given by Paterson and Parker are:

        length/width = 2; increase mg hr by 5%
        length/width = 3; increase mg hr by 9%
        length/width = 4; increase mg hr by 12%

For example, an implant which is 10 x 5 cm has a length/width ratio (elongation factor) of 2 (10/5) so the mg hr should be increased by 5%.

Volume implants are used when the three dimensions, length, width, and height, are approximately the same. The original distribution rules by Paterson and Parker for volume implants were limited to geometric forms such as cylinder, sphere, or cuboid (brick) forms (Fig. 8.14). The spherical form can really only be obtained using seeds. The cuboid shape is obtained using multiplanar implant rules rather than by using volume rules.

Distribution rules for volume implants and the number of mg hr necessary to deliver 1000 cGy to the volume are given in Table 8.8.

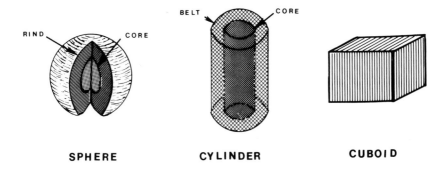

SPHERE   CYLINDER   CUBOID

Fig. 8.14. Diagrams illustrating different geometric shapes of implants.

TABLE 8.8

VOLUME IMPLANT

R_V - mg hr to give 1000 cGy to volume implant:
Radium equivalent for filtration of 0.5 mm Pt.

Volume (cm³)	R_V mg hr	Distribution Rules:
5	106	Volume should be considered
10	168	as a surface with 75%
15	220	activity and core with 25%
20	267	
30	350	Rules for cylinders:
40	425	Belt - 50% activity with minimum 8 needles
50	493	Ends - 12.5% of activity on each end
60	556	Core - 25% with minimum of 4 needles
80	673	For each uncrossed end, reduce volume by
100	782	7.5%
140	979	
180	1156	

Length/ Diameter:	1.5	2.0	2.5	3.0
Increase mg hr:	3%	6%	10%	15%

Volume (cm³)	R_V mg hr
220	1322
260	1479
300	1627
340	1768
380	1902

This table was prepared from the original by Meredith (Meredith 1967) by multiplying his values by C = 1.064.

In this example, we will calculate the number of mg hr required to deliver 2000 cGy in 48 hr in a 3 x 5 x 6 cm implant (90 cm³). From Table 8.8, 728 mg hr is required to deliver 1000 cGy. The number of mg hr required to deliver 2000 cGy is therefore

$$\frac{728 \text{ mg hr} \times 2000 \text{ cGy}}{1000 \text{ cGy}} = 1456 \text{ mg hr}$$

Since 48 hr are available, the number of mg Ra required is

$$\frac{1456 \text{ mg hr}}{48 \text{ hr}} = 30.3 \text{ mg Ra}$$

distributed according to the volume implant rules in Table 8.8.

Here we will use Table 8.8 to calculate the dose rate from a 6 x 5 x 3 cm (90 cm³) volume implant. The implant is designed according to the rules in Table 8.8 and contains 30 mg radium. From Table 8.8, we find that 728 mg hr deliver 1000 cGy. The dose rate is

$$\frac{1000 \text{ cGy} \times 30 \text{ mg}}{728 \text{ mg hr}} = 41.2 \text{ cGy/hr}$$

The number of hours required to deliver 2000 cGy is therefore

$$\frac{2000 \text{ cGy}}{41.2 \text{ cGy/hr}} = 48.5$$

The Paris System

Like the Quimby system, the Paris system, developed in the 1920s (Regaud 1929), utilizes uniform distribution of the radioactivity and the rules can be applied to volumes of any shape. The spacing of the sources ranges from 5 to 10 mm for small volumes to 15 to 22 mm for large volumes. The longer the sources are, the higher the dose will be around each source, thus allowing greater spacing. The tolerance of the irradiated tissues must also be considered in choosing the spacing. The high-dose volume in the immediate neighborhood of the radioactive source should never exceed 1 cm in diameter.

The uniform spacing of sources in the Paris as in the Quimby system causes the dose to be higher in the center of the implant than in the periphery. This increased central dose is greater with larger implants. While in the Manchester system the treated volume is decreased by 10% when uncrossed ends are used, in the Paris system, 15% of the length is considered untreated at each end of the radioactive length. The radioactivity should therefore extend 15% beyond the target volume in each direction. When the target volume involves the skin or the mucosa, the use of loops or "hairpins" is recommended. The loop and the transverse section of the hairpin act as a substitute for a crossed end.

In the Paris system, the reference dose, as represented by the isodose line corresponding with the treated volume (minimum tumor dose), is 85% of what is called the basal dose. The basal dose is determined by finding the average dose at several low-dose points inside the perimeter formed by the most exterior sources of an implant (Fig. 8.15). The high-dose volume in the immediate neighborhood of each radioactive source is the volume enclosed by an isodose surface along which the dose is twice the reference value.

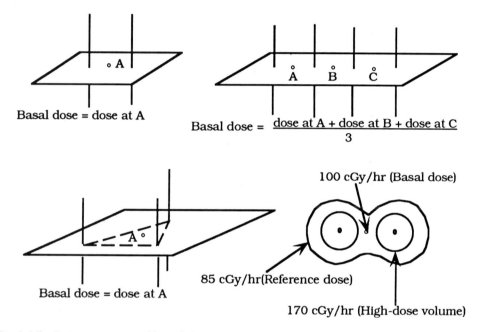

Fig 8.15. Determination of basal dose in the Paris system above. Diagram illustrating basal dose, reference dose, and high-dose volume in a two-ribbon implant (lower right).

PERMANENT IMPLANTS

The calculations described thus far have assumed that the implant is temporary and that the radioactive material is eventually removed from the patient, usually after several days. Implants with short-lived isotopes wherein the sources are left in place can be permanent. When the activity eventually decays, small seeds of inert metal are left behind with no adverse effects.

The determination of the number of millicurie hours required for a permanent implant involves the concept of the average life of a radionuclide. The average life (T_{avg}) of a radionuclide is the time that would be required for the complete decay of the activity assuming that it continued to decay at its initial rate; in fact the rate of decay (that is, the activity) gets less as time goes on, but if it continued at its original rate, the isotope would "last" at its original activity for a time T_{avg} and would then stop emitting. It can be shown that the average life is related to the half-life as follows:

$$T_{avg} = 1.44\, T_{1/2} \tag{8.2}$$

Note that the average life is lower than the half-life.

To calculate the number of millicurie hours required for a permanent implant, the number of milligram hours of radium required to treat the lesion is determined as in the case of temporary implants. This number is multiplied by the ratio of the exposure rate constants (previously explained) of radium and the nuclide to be used and yields the number of millicurie hours required. This number is divided by the average life to yield the number of millicuries of a radionuclide required to deliver the dose desired. The example below illustrates this procedure:

Example: Determine the number of millicuries of I-125 required for a single-plane implant 3 x 3 cm in area, if the dose in a plane at 0.5 cm is to be 4000 cGy.

From Table 8.7, 235 mg hr of radium per 1000 cGy is required for this implant, so to deliver 4000 cGy, if we used radium, we would need

$$\frac{235 \text{ mg hr} \times 4000 \text{ cGy}}{1000 \text{ cGy}} = 940 \text{ mg hr}$$

Iodine-125, however, gives only 1.66 R/hr at 1 cm from 1 mCi and when inserted can be considered to last for a time equal to the average life of I-125. The average life is 1.44 times the half-life, that is, for I-125 the half-life is 59.6 days, and so

$$T_{avg} = 1.44 \times 59.6 \text{ days} \times 24 \text{ hr} = 2060 \text{ hr}$$

$$T_{avg} = 2060 \text{ hr}$$

Each mCi of I-125 permanently implanted is therefore equivalent to

$$\frac{1.66}{8.25} \times 2060 \text{ mg hr} = 414.5 \text{ mg hr}$$

Therefore the number of mCi of I-125 needed to give the required 940 mg hr that we found from Table 8.7, as above is

$$\frac{940}{414.5} = 2.27 \text{ mCi}$$

SOURCE LOCALIZATION

Despite careful planning of the source distribution, the radioactivity can never be arranged precisely as planned, so determination of the actual distribution achieved during the insertion is necessary (Fig. 8.16). This can be accomplished by taking orthogonal radiographs (that is, at right angles to each other) of the implant. The central axes of the two x-ray views cross at or near the center of the implant. Two such radiographs (conveniently made by using the isocentric capabilities of a simulator, which can be rotated through 90° between exposures while centered on the implant) provide sufficient information for a computer to reconstruct, in three dimensions, the geometry of the implant. Placement of metal clips to mark tumor margins is recommended to allow the relationship between the dose distribution and the tumor to be evaluated.

The orthogonal radiographs, of which examples are shown in Fig. 8.16, are enlarged views of the implant as well as of the patient, as described in Chapter 4 of *Treatment Planning and Dose Calculation in Radiation Oncology*. A magnification ring with known dimensions can be placed at the same distance in the beam as the implant to facilitate calculation of the true size, or one can set a known field size (conveniently 10 x 10 cm) at the isocenter when a simulator is used. If we know the distance to the isocenter, the magnification can be calculated. For example, if the distance to the isocenter is 100 cm and the field size is 10 x 10 cm, then the appearance of a 14 x 14 cm field on the radiograph means that the magnification is 1.4 (140/100 = 1.4).

An anterior and a lateral radiograph are usually taken but the films do not always have to be horizontal and vertical. Provided they are orthogonal (at 90° to each other) they can be taken at *any* angles separated by 90°. In entering the three-dimensional source locations into treatment planning computers a coordinate system must be used. The conventional system is with the x axis from the patient's left to right, the y axis from cephalad to caudal, and the z axis from anterior to posterior (see Chapter 4 of *Treatment Planning and Dose Calculation in Radiation Oncology*). An anterior film would therefore represent the source position along the x and y axes, while the lateral film would represent the seed position in the z and y axes. The origin of the coordinate system, which of course must be the same point on both radiographs, is chosen to be a point which can be identified on both films and should be near the center of the implant. Using an isocentrically mounted simulator unit, where the central axis is indicated by a cross hair, this point would ideally be the origin.

Identification of the sources is made easier if the magnification is the same on both radiographs. Since the y axis is common to both films, the distance from the origin can be compared for each point when sources are identified. For example, the source with the largest y coordinate on one x-ray will also have the largest y coordinate on the other. After all sources have been identified, the coordinates of each seed (or each end of each linear source) on each film is sequentially entered into a treatment planning computer with a digitizer. All source coordinates are corrected for magnification by the computer and are stored as x, y, and z coordinates for use in the dose calculation. Errors in source location are discovered by the computer through inconsistencies of the y coordinates.

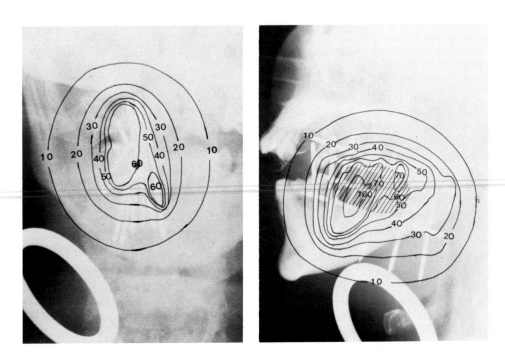

Fig. 8.16. Radium needles implanted in a carcinoma of the tongue. The radioactivity is not always arranged precisely as planned. A magnification ring is used to facilitate calculation of actual dimensions.

Identification of each source on each image is tedious, but keeping in mind how each source should appear on each view is helpful. For example, sources positioned at an angle with respect to the beam will appear foreshortened, while sources positioned perpendicular to the beam will appear enlarged. Figure 8.17 illustrates the appearance of two needles of equal length (A - B and C - D) on orthogonal images. Source C - D appears foreshortened in both images while source A - B appears enlarged in the lateral view and as a point source in the anterior view. From this we know that the source, which appear shorter, is inserted at an angle with respect to the radiographic images, while the other source, which appear as a point source on the anterior view, is inserted parallel with the anterior image and perpendicular to the lateral.

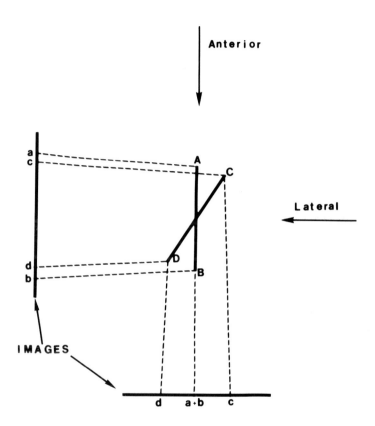

Fig. 8.17. Two sources of equal length appear different on an anterior and a lateral image. Source C - D is foreshortened (appears shorter than the real length) in both images. Source A - B appears as a point source on the anterior image and is actually enlarged on the lateral view.

A more complex method of determining source location, which does not involve orthogonal radiographs, is the stereo-shift technique in which the patient or the x-ray tube is shifted horizontally a certain distance between the exposures (Fig. 8.18). The x and y coordinates can be found on either of the two images and the z coordinate can be derived from the known geometry of the two radiographs (Khan 1984). This method is useful in implants where sources can not be identified by orthogonal films, for example, when a large number of seeds are used or when some sources are obscured by bone or lead shielding (Anderson 1975, Sharma 1982).

COMPUTER DOSE CALCULATION

Dose calculations using tables give a very good guide to the required amount of radioactivity and the number of hours the implant must be left in place to deliver the treatment. For information about the dose distribution surrounding an implant, however, computer calculations in multiple planes are necessary.

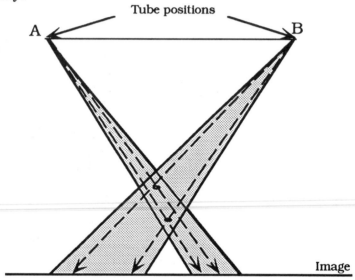

Fig. 8.18. Diagram illustrating a stereoshift technique for source localization where the tube is shifted from position A to position B.

Computer calculation of dose distributions consists of summing the dose contributed by each source at grid points arranged in a three-dimensional lattice pattern and by connecting points receiving the same dose rate (cGy/hr). The dose-rate distributions can then be viewed in any plane within the implant. To perform the dose summing, it is necessary to input the source position in three dimensions. This is usually accomplished from orthogonal x-rays, using a digitizer as described above.

In a uniformly implanted volume, dose-rate distributions calculated on three planes (between the implant planes, across and along the implanted needles or rows of seeds) is often sufficient for evaluation of the dose distribution (Fig. 8.19), while in a non-uniform implant additional planes may be necessary.

The dose-rate distributions calculated in planes parallel to the films can be enlarged and superimposed on the radiographs. Caution should be used in interpreting the dose distribution with respect to the tumor volume. The dose distribution in any one plane represents a very narrow segment of the implant, and the distribution can be quite different at a slightly different plane.

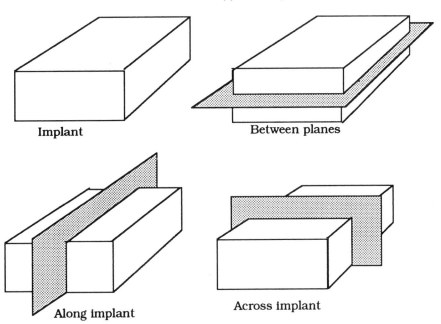

Fig. 8.19. Dose-rate distributions are usually calculated along, across and between two planes in a rectangular implant.

DOSE SPECIFICATION

One of the shortcomings of most computer programs is the failure to allow the user to outline the target volume or the anatomical structures within or near the implant. Dose specification in brachytherapy is therefore, in most cases, complicated by the inability to localize the target volume precisely with respect to the dose distribution. The very steep dose gradient near the implant and the very hot spots near each source also complicate the dose specification. Most physicians prescribe the treatment to the dose-rate line that adequately encompasses the target volume as viewed in multiple planes. There are obviously areas of significantly higher dose within that volume.

The significance of the rate at which brachytherapy treatment (which is continuous rather than fractional, as in teletherapy) is delivered has been discussed in the literature by several authors (Hall 1964, Pierquin 1973, 1976). Experience of delivering continuous irradiation at dose rates on the order of 25 to 100 cGy/hr to a total dose of 6000 to 7000 cGy in a large number of patients has been described by Pierquin (Pierquin 1973, 1976). More recently, remote afterloading apparatus, described in Chapter 9 (page 317), has been used to deliver brachytherapy treatments at very high dose rates (on the order of several hundred cGy per hour). The biological effect of such high-dose rates, on tumors and normal tissues, are not fully known (Fu 1990). Inconsistencies in dose specification, dose determination, and treatment techniques among treatment centers using high-dose-rate methods makes the interpretation of results very difficult.

REFERENCES

Anderson, L.L., Dosimetry of interstitial radiation therapy, Handbook of Interstitial Brachytherapy, Hilaris, B.S. (ed.), Publishing Sciences Group, Acton, MA 1975.

Bentel, G.C., Nelson, C.E., Noell, K.T., Treatment Planning and Dose Calculation in Radiation Oncology, Pergamon Press, Inc. Elmsford, NY, 1989.

Dutreix, A., Marinello, G., Wambersie, A., Dosimetric du system de Paris, Dosimétrie en Curiethérapie, Masson, Paris, France, 1982.

Dutreix, A., Marinello, G., The Paris System, Modern Brachytherapy, Pierquin, B., Wilson, J. F., Chassagne, D. (eds.), Masson, New York, NY, 1987.

Dutreix, A., Can we compare systems for interstitial therapy? Radiotherapy and Oncology 13, 127 (1988).

Fu, K.K., Phillips, T.L., High-dose-rate versus low-dose-rate intracavitary brachytherapy for carcinoma of the cervix, Int. J. Radiat. Oncol. Biol. Phys. 19, 791 (1990).

Glasser, O., Quimby, E.H., Taylor, L.S., Weatherwax, J.L., Morgan, R.H., Physical Foundations of Radiology (3rd ed.), Harper & Row, New York, NY, 1961.

Goodwin, P.N., Quimby, E.H., Morgan, R.H., Physical Foundations of Radiology, (4th ed.), Harper & Row, New York, NY, 1970.

Greenfield, M., Fichman, M., Norman, A., Dosage tables for linear radium sources filtered by 0.5 and 1.0 mm of platinum, Radiology 73, 418 (1959).

Hall, E.J., Bedford, J.S., Dose rate: Its effect on the survival of He La cells irradiated with gamma rays, Radiat. Res. 22, 305 (1964).

Hendee, W.R., Radiation Therapy Physics, Year Book Medical Publishers, Inc., Chicago, IL, 1981.

Johns, H.E., Cunningham, J.R., The Physics of Radiology, Charles C. Thomas, Springfield, IL, 1983.

Khan, F.M., The Physics of Radiation Therapy, Williams & Wilkins, Baltimore, MD, 1984.

Krishnaswamy, V., Dose distribution around an I-125 seed source in tissue, Radiology 126, 489 (1978).

Ling, C.C., Interstitial implant of I-125 seeds - absolute activity calibration and angular distribution measurement with an Si (Li) detector (Abstract), 4th Int. Conf. Med. Phys., Ottawa, Canada 1976, Special Issue, Phys. Can. 32, 16, 9 (1976).

Ling, C.C., Anderson, L.L., Shipley, W.U., Dose inhomogeneity in interstitial implants using I-125 seeds, Int. J. Radiat. Oncol. Biol. Phys. 5, 419 (1979).

Ling, C.C., Yorke, E.D., Spiro, I.J., Kubiatowicz, D., Bennett, D., Physical dosimetry of I-125 seeds of a new design for interstitial implant, Int. J. Radiat. Oncol. Biol. Phys. 9, 1747 (1983).

Meredith, W.J. (ed.), Radium Dosage: The Manchester System (2nd ed.), Livingston, Ltd., Edinburg and London, UK, 1967.

Paterson, R., Parker, H.M., A dosage system for interstitial radium therapy, Brit. J. Radiol. 11, 252 (1938).

Paterson, R., Parker, H.M., Radium Dosage - The Manchester System, Meredith, W.J. (ed.), The Williams & Wilkins Company, Baltimore, MD, 1949.

Pierquin, B., Chassagne, D., Baillet, F., Paine, C.H., Clinical observations on the time factor in interstitial radiotherapy using iridium-192, Clin. Radiol. 24, 506 (1973).

Pierquin, B., The destiny of brachytherapy in oncology, Am. J. Roentgenol. 127, 495 (1976).

Quimby, E.H., Dosage tables for linear radium sources, Radiology 43, 572 (1944).

Regaud, C., Radium therapy for cancer at the radium institute, Am. J. Roentgenol. 21, 1 (1929).

Sharma, S.C., Willamson, J.F., Cytacki, E., Dosimetric analysis of stereo and orthogonal reconstruction of interstitial implants, Int. J. Radiat. Oncol. Biol. Phys. 8, 1803 (1982).

Sievert, R.M., Die Intensitätsverteilung der primären Gamma-Strahlung in der Nähe medizinischer Radiumpräparate, Acta. Radiol. 1, 89 (1921).

Sievert, R.M., Die Gamma-Strahlungsintensität an der Oberfläche und in der nächsten Umgebung von Radiumnadeln, Acta. Radiol. 11, 249 (1930).

PROBLEMS

1. The half-life of an isotope is

   a) the thickness of a given material necessary to reduce the intensity by half of the original value
   b) the time required for a nuclide to divide in half
   c) the time required for a nuclide to lose half of its original activity

2. Match the nuclides in the left-hand column with the half-lives in the right-hand column

Isotope		Half-lives
___	cobalt-60	a) 30 years
___	gold-198	b) 28 years
___	iridium-192	c) 74 days
___	cesium-137	d) 59.6 days
___	iodine-125	e) 2.7 days
___	strontium-90	f) 5.26 years

3. The exposure-rate constant for radium is defined as

   a) the exposure rate at a point 1 cm away from 1 mCi of unfiltered radium
   b) the exposure rate at a point 1 cm away from 1 mg of radium filtered by 0.5 mm of platinum
   c) the exposure rate at a point 1 cm away from 1 Curie of radium filtered by 0.5 mm of platinum

4. A half-strength radium needle has a linear activity of

   a)   0.66 mg Ra/cm
   b)   0.33 mg Ra/cm
   c)   0.1 mg Ra/cm

5. The Manchester and the Quimby dosage systems

   a)   use the same distribution rules for the radioactivity but differ in the prescription point
   b)   use the same dosage tables but differ in the distribution rules for the radioactivity
   c)   use different tables and different distribution rules for the radioactivity

6. Calculate the time necessary to deliver 2000 cGy at 0.5 cm from a surface mold which is constructed to treat a 2 x 3 cm area. The mold contains a total of 20 mg Ra eq of iridium-192 which is uniformly distributed. (Use Table 8.4.)

7. Calculate the mg Ra eq required to deliver 3000 cGy in 48 hrs in a 2 x 2.5 x 3 cm volume implant. (Use Table 8.5.)

8. Calculate the mg Ra eq needed to deliver 3000 cGy in 42 hrs at 0.5 cm from a 6 x 6 cm single-plane implant where the radioactivity is distributed according to the Manchester system. (Use Table 8.7.)

9. Calculate the time needed to deliver 2000 cGy in a 4 x 4 x 5 cm volume implant containing 20 mg Ra eq distributed according to the Manchester system. (Use Table 8.8.)

10. In the Paris system

    a) the reference dose is 85% of the high-dose volume

    b) the reference dose is determined by finding the average dose rate at several points inside the implant

    c) the reference dose is 85% of the basal dose

11. Calculate the number of mCi of I-125 needed to deliver 2000 cGy at 0.5 cm in a 4 x 4 cm single-plane permanent implant.

SOLUTIONS

1. c

2. cobalt-60   f

    gold-198   e

    iridium-192   c

    cesium-137   a

    iodine-125   d

    strontium-90   b

3. b

4. b

5. c

6. 11 hrs

7. 35.9 mg Ra eq

8. 42.4 mg

9. 67.3 hr

10. c

11. 1.62 mCi

CHAPTER 9

PRACTICAL APPLICATION OF BRACHYTHERAPY
TECHNIQUES

The development of artificial isotopes, afterloading techniques, and automatic devices with remote control has stimulated renewed interest in brachytherapy and has also brought about the almost complete replacement of interstitial radium needles which therefore will not be discussed further in this text. Brachytherapy can be carried out using either external surface molds, intracavitary, interstitial, or intraluminal techniques, or in some situations, a combination of these methods.

AFTERLOADING

Insertion into the tumor or cavities adjacent to the tumor of hollow applicators that later are loaded with the radioactive sources is referred to as an afterloading technique. This technique, originally developed for the purpose of reducing exposure to personnel (Grigsby 1991), has also made it possible 1) to plan an implant and prepare needed apparatus in advance and 2) to plan the optimal loading of an implant after the apparatus is inserted but before the radioactivity is actually loaded.

Tumors of unusual shape or that are located adjacent to radiosensitive tissue benefit particularly for advance planning. Tumor size and shape, as well as outlines of anatomical structures, are established by use of CT, MRI, and orthogonal radiographs. The optimal source strength and distribution of the radioactivity are then calculated with the aid of a treatment-planning computer. Some computer software has optimization capabilities in which the computer can calculate these variables once the tumor volume is entered and dose constraints (minimum, maximum dose, etc.) have been set by the user. Many of the implants described in this chapter were planned in advance and then an appliance (mold or template) was built to hold the radioactivity in place.

Idealized plans can be calculated in advance but often cannot be implemented in practice. However, in a short time computers can calculate dose-rate distributions in three dimensions around the actual implant before the loading of the radioactivity takes place. The activity and spacing of sources are calculated from localization films taken with the apparatus in place. In gynecologic implants using cesium-137 or other isotopes in the shape of tubes, the dose distribution can be altered by changing the spacing and the activity of the sources within the already inserted apparatus. Sources can also be removed early in the case of a hot spot, but this practice is not recommended except in extreme situations. In many situations, however, adding a tube or source is not possible. In the case of seed ribbons, which are usually purchased in advance with fixed seed activity, spacing, and length, optimization is limited by the availability of seeds at the time of the loading. However, the dose deposited by the seeds in a ribbon can be modified by leaving the ribbon in place for a different length of time.

PREPARATION OF SURFACE MOLDS AND CUSTOMIZED APPLICATORS

Surface molds, which have been briefly mentioned previously, are used when well-circumscribed surface lesions must be treated to high doses. Surface molds can be prepared to fit snugly over the surface of the lesion and the adjacent region. Pathways for radioactive ribbons are embedded in the mold at a distance from the lesion and spaced so that a uniform dose is delivered in the lesion when the implant is loaded. Lead shielding can be added in the mold to reduce total body dose to the patient and to personnel. Straps and hooks can also be built into the mold for anchoring the mold to the patient. Surface and intracavitary applicators, which conform to body surfaces or cavities and which contain built-in pathways for afterloaded radioactive ribbons, can be constructed to fit practically any shape.

The procedure for making afterloadable surface applicators is very similar to that used for making the custom-designed intracavitary applicators described later in this chapter. Before a suitable applicator can be fabricated, a detailed replica of the surface anatomy or cavity must be made. A model of the cavity alone is sufficient for lesions lying entirely within a cavity and distal to the exterior surface (Fig. 9.1). In those situations where the lesion extends to the margins of the cavity, it is appropriate to include a generous area of the exterior surface to which the applicator can be attached. The model should always encompass an area which is larger than that requiring treatment.

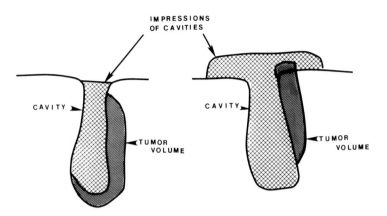

Fig. 9.1. An impression of the cavity alone is sufficient when the lesion lies entirely within the cavity (left). When the lesion extends outside the cavity, the impression must also include a generous area of the exterior surface.

Details of the anatomy must be precisely mirrored in the replica for a snug and comfortable fit of the applicator (Fig. 9.2). Irregular surfaces and recesses also increase stability and adhesiveness while the applicator is in place. Precise details of the tumor are helpful in the assessment of the area to be treated and for determination of necessary margins around the tumor.

An impression of the area or cavity under consideration is made with dental impression alginate.* The alginate consists of a powder which when mixed with water becomes a creamy mixture and sets in 2 minutes to an elastic rubbery compound. Unfortunately, this material shrinks and deteriorates quite rapidly and is therefore not itself suitable for use as final mold material. Impressions made of the entire face require that provision be made for breathing. A syringe barrel with at least 1 cm diameter provides an excellent airway when placed in the patient's mouth (Fig. 9.3).

The negative impression is filled with plaster or dental stone to form a replica (Figs. 9.2 and 9.3). The dental stone consists of a powder which is mixed with water until it becomes creamy. This mixture sets and becomes rock-hard in about 2 to 3 hours. When possible, the tumor should be marked on the patient before the impression material is poured onto the surface. This allows tumor markings to be transferred onto the impression material and subsequently onto the replica of the patient. The impression material gives a very detailed surface, including that of a raised tumor. Tumor dimensions and position with respect to the subsequently constructed

---

* Jeltrate ®, Registered trade name of the L.D. Caulk Co.

applicator are determined either via the transposed marks, the raised replica of the tumor, or in the case of a body cavity, via radiographic examination with the applicator in place (Fig. 9.4). The source distribution and activity necessary to deliver the desired treatment can be planned from this information. The plastic tubes, which will provide pathways for the afterloaded radioactive ribbons, are arranged within the cavity that is obtained when another negative impression of the replica is made. Transparent acrylic is then poured into this cavity leaving the hollow plastic tubes in place.

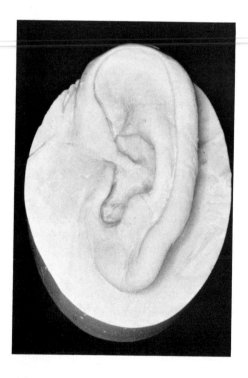

Fig. 9.2. A detailed replica of the anatomy is necessary for a snug, yet comfortable, fit of customized applicators.

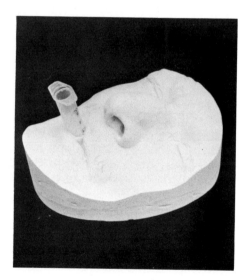

Fig. 9.3. A syringe barrel in the patient's mouth provides adequate airway when impressions of the entire face are necessary. In this replica, the syringe remained as part of the impression of the patient's face.

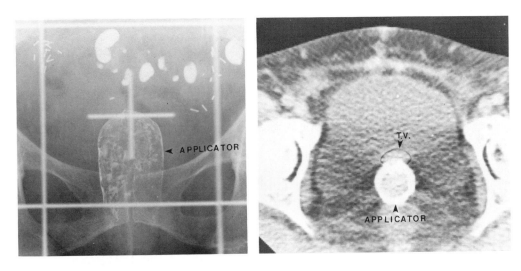

Fig. 9.4. Radiographic examination with a customized vaginal applicator in place.

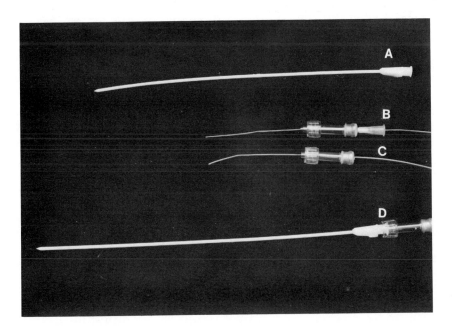

Fig. 9.5. A Luer lock glued onto a plastic needle (A). A hypodermic needle is pushed through the rubber top of a heparin lock to facilitate pushing the radioactive ribbon through to the desired length (B). The needle is then withdrawn leaving the radioactive ribbon secured in the heparin lock (C). The heparin lock is secured in the Luer lock (D). The rubber top of the heparin lock prevents the radioactive ribbon from sliding in or out.

The pathways provided in molds for afterloading radioactive ribbons must obviously have a caliber larger than that of the ribbons. Plastic needles or other plastic tubing can be used. The plastic needles, also referred to as Flexiguides®™†, have the advantage of having a very strong sharp point, making it possible to insert them directly into tissue.

In some customized applicators, pathways are built to facilitate the insertion of the plastic needles beyond the mold and into the adjacent tissue. The pathways must then be large enough to accept the larger caliber of the plastic needles. The radioactive ribbons must be anchored securely inside the plastic needles. To do this, a Luer lock (Fig. 9.5) can be glued onto the open end of the plastic needle (Boyer 1980). The radioactive ribbon is then threaded through a heparin lock to the desired length. The guiding needle is withdrawn and the rubber top prevents the ribbon from sliding out (Fig. 9.5). The radioactive ribbon is then inserted into the plastic needle and the heparin lock is secured onto the Luer lock.

INTRACAVITARY BRACHYTHERAPY OF GYNECOLOGIC MALIGNANCIES

Brachytherapy, as a treatment modality in the management of gynecologic malignancies, has been used since its beneficial effects on tumors were first discovered (Forssell 1912, Béclère 1914). Insertion of radioactive sources into body cavities adjacent to tumors allows delivery of large doses in the tumor while minimizing adverse effects on regional normal tissue. The careless use of brachytherapy can, however, lead to irreversible injury in practically any site.

Intracavitary apparatus used in treatment of gynecologic malignancies is fairly standardized. In instances where the anatomy, sometimes distorted by surgery or tumor, precludes the use of standardized apparatus, individualized applicators, as previously described, can be prepared to conform to the body cavity to be treated. Various types of applicators holding the radioactivity have been used over the years. The inventors or the institutions at which these applicators were first used have often lent their names to such devices. Many of the older types of applicators did not facilitate afterloading techniques.

Some of the first gynecologic applicators were designed to conform to the individual patient's anatomy. The arrangement of the radioactive sources was therefore unpredictable and could result in unacceptable dose distributions. Large bulky tumors, for example, would cause the flexible apparatus to be pushed away from the tumor, resulting in underdosage. Later models of gynecologic applicators have been designed to be rigid and thus, to some extent, make the anatomy conform to the applicator, yet provide some degree of choice of source arrangement within the apparatus.

---

† Registered trade name of Nuclear Associates, Inc.

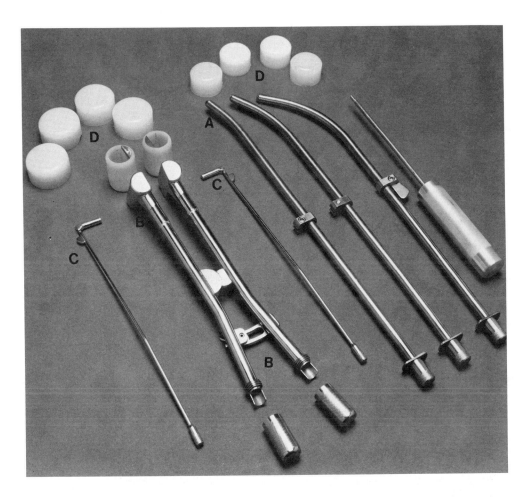

Fig. 9.6. A set of Fletcher-Suit-Delclos intracavitary apparatus. It consists of three tandems with different curvature (A), a colpostat (ovoids) (B) with the inserts for afterloading sources (C), and nylon caps which can be placed over the stainless-steel ovoid to increase the distance from the source to the surface of the ovoid (mucosa) (D). (Courtesy Medical Device Division, 3M Company, St. Paul, MN.)

Afterloading is a technique in which the radioactivity is loaded after the proper placement of the apparatus has been confirmed. Confirmation of placement of the apparatus is usually determined with "dummies" in place. Dummies are radiopaque markers which are identical to the radioactive sources in size and shape but have no radioactivity. Insertion of the apparatus usually takes place in the operating room, while the insertion of the radioactive sources takes place later, ideally in the patient's room, thus reducing unnecessary exposure to personnel, patients, and hospital visitors.

TANDEM AND OVOIDS

Gynecologic malignancies are usually treated using standard apparatus; however, due to unusual tumor volumes or abnormal anatomy, customized apparatus can be used to improve the dose distribution.

A system consisting of a tandem and a pair of ovoids (Fig. 9.6) is the most frequently used afterloading apparatus in the treatment of gynecologic malignancies (Suit 1963, Fletcher 1980). The tandem is a hollow, curved, stainless-steel tube with an internal diameter slightly larger than that of the radioactive sources. (See Chapter 5 in *Treatment Planning and Dose Calculation in Radiation Oncology*, Bentel 1989). The radioactive sources are inserted into plastic tubing which fits inside the tandem and is afterloaded. Tandems are available with different curvatures to best fit each patient. The tandem is inserted into the uterine canal and a keel is placed against the external cervical os to stabilize the position. The radioactive sources are typically loaded into the segment which lies within the uterus only. This usually requires three sources. These sources should extend to the keel but not protrude beyond it. This may require more than three sources or the placement of nylon spacers above or between sources so that the lowest source extends just to the keel. Sources protruding below the keel may deliver excessive doses to the vaginal apex, bladder, and rectum.

A pair of ovoids is placed on each side of the uterine cervix in the vaginal vault with its long axis in an anteroposterior direction. This arrangement causes the ends of each source, where the dose is lower, to be directed toward the bladder and rectum. Each ovoid typically has an exterior diameter of 20 mm and a length of approximately 30 mm. Tungsten shields (Fig. 9.7) are built into the ovoids medially at each end to reduce the dose to the bladder and rectum (Fletcher 1980). The handles of the ovoids protrude from the vagina and are assembled so that pressing the distal part of the handles together separates the ovoids. An insert, containing the source, is afterloaded through the hollow handle down into each ovoid.

Apparatus of this kind is typically inserted in the operating room under general anesthesia. Orthogonal radiographs are obtained, usually in the operating room, to confirm satisfactory geometry and to evaluate the position with respect to the bladder and the rectum. Active sources are customarily not inserted until the patient is in her hospital bed. This reduces exposure to personnel in the operating room, recovery room, and during transfer between these areas.

The activity of the sources to be afterloaded is determined and the time required to deliver the prescribed dose is calculated, usually before the sources are inserted. A pear-shaped dose distribution centered around the cervix is typically desired in treatment of carcinoma of the cervix (Fig. 9.8).

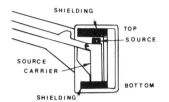

Fig. 9.7. Tungsten shielding is built into the ovoids medially at each end to reduce dose to the bladder and rectum. (Courtesy Medical Device Division, 3M Company, St. Paul, MN.)

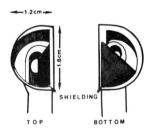

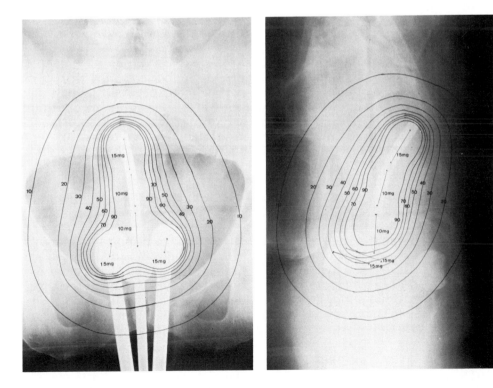

Fig. 9.8. Typical dose-rate distributions from a tandem and ovoid intracavitary application.

The standard source strength used in the tandem is a 15 mg Ra eq cephalad source followed by two 10 mg Ra eq caudal sources. Each ovoid is usually loaded with 15 mg Ra eq. For patients with large vaginal vaults, plastic caps of 2.5 or 3 cm diameter, can be placed over each ovoid. This will increase the distance from the source to the mucosa and thus decrease the dose rate (page 232, Chapter 8). Therefore, the activity in the larger ovoids is often increased to 20 or 25 mg Ra eq. Smaller ovoids, called mini-ovoids, are also available to facilitate placement of sources in the vaginal fornices of patients with a narrow apex.

Selection of source strength in the ovoids depends on the diameter of the ovoid and the separation between them. The separation of the ovoids also has some bearing on source-strength selection for the lowest source within the tandem. Large separation between the ovoids would create a cold area in the cervix between the two ovoids. This can be eliminated by placing a stronger source in the lower aspect of the tandem within the cervical canal. The dose contributed to the bladder and rectum might however limit the strength of this source.

Dose Calculation

Although the crude statement of milligram hours as if it were a measure of dose has, through much accumulated experience, attained some meaning in this site, it can be very misleading and should not be used. Expressing the dose in cGy, however, is associated here with such complex factors that a special dosage system for this type of treatment has been developed.

The difficulties are primarily a result of great variations in shape, size, and type of tumor to be treated. In an attempt to solve the problem of dose prescription, some points, at a distance where the dose is not highly sensitive to small and clinically unimportant alterations in the source position, have been chosen for dose prescription. Such points must be anatomically comparable from patient to patient and should be in such a place as to allow correlation of dose with clinical effects. Thus, points A and B have been designated.

Point A has been selected to represent the paracervical triangle and is defined as a point 2 cm lateral to the center of the cervical canal and 2 cm from the mucous membrane of the lateral fornix in the plane of the uterus (Fig. 9.9). Although point A is defined in relation to important anatomical structures, these cannot be visualized on a radiograph, and it is therefore necessary to establish some convention by which the position of point A can be determined on a radiograph. Experience has shown that, in the average patient, the external cervical os is at the same level as the lateral fornix, so point A can be found by measuring 2 cm up (cephalad) from the external os and 2 cm lateral in a plane perpendicular to the uterine canal (tandem).

Point B is defined as a point 2 cm up (cephalad) from the external cervical os and 5 cm lateral of the patient's midline. In some cases, the uterus may be tilted to one side. In such circumstances, it is assumed that the tissues represented by point A are carried with the uterus, whereas point B, near the

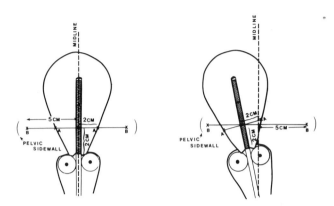

Fig. 9.9. Diagram illustrating the position of points A and B in an ideal situation (left). Frequently, the uterus is tilted toward one side (right). Points A shift with the uterus, while points B, defined with respect to the patient's midline, remain unchanged.

pelvic sidewall, is located in tissues that are not dependent on the position of the uterus and therefore has a fixed position relative to bony structures.

Since many variations of the position of the apparatus are possible, no generalization can be made of the doses delivered to points A and B, and each case must be considered on its own merits. Standardization of the design and loading of applicators which will deliver the same dose rate to point A is another solution to the problem of dose specification.

HEYMAN CAPSULES

Packing the uterine cavity with Cs-137 tubes is occasionally selected for intracavitary treatment of endometrial carcinoma in inoperable patients. The Heyman capsules used for this purpose are stainless-steel cylinders which contain the radioactive tubes (shown in Fig. 5.2 in *Treatment Planning and Dose Calculation in Radiation Oncology*). Each has an eyelet for attaching an instrument used to insert the capsule into the uterine cavity. A long wire is attached to this eyelet. At the end of the wire is a small metal plate which has a number engraved on it. When the capsules are in place in the uterus, these wires protrude out of the vagina and are used to pull out the capsules at the completion of the treatment. The capsules are identified with numbers since they must be pulled out in reverse order from their insertion. Heyman capsules are available with different diameters. Six mm diameter capsules are customarily loaded with 5 mg Ra eq sources. Capsules of greater diameters are loaded with 10 mg Ra eq to produce a dose rate on the exterior surface of the capsule similar to that of the smaller caliber capsule.

VAGINAL CYLINDERS

Cylinders are commonly used for the treatment of vaginal lesions. Burnett cylinders are commercially available, but custom-designed cylinders can quite easily be made in most radiation oncology departments. Burnett cylinders are a set of applicators with different lengths and diameters (Shown in Fig. 5.3 in *Treatment Planning and Dose Calculation in Radiation Oncology*). A blind canal through the cylinder accepts a plastic insert which contains the radioactive tubes. A screw-cap is provided to lock the sources into place inside the cylinder. Sutures are usually placed to maintain the cylinder within the vagina. Afterloading is performed when the positioning of the cylinder has been confirmed. The number of sources and the radioactivity required to deliver the desired dose-rate distributions can be determined before loading takes place.

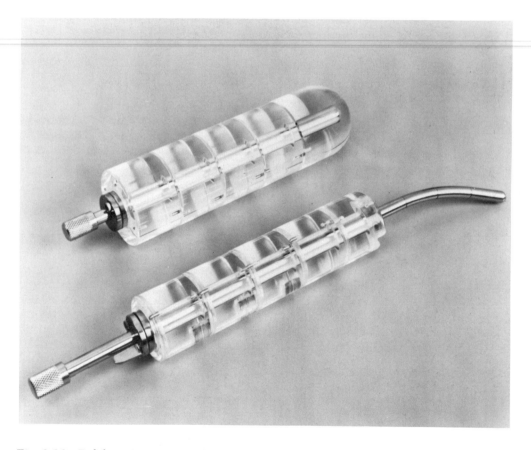

Fig. 9.10. Delclos uterine-vaginal afterloading system. (Courtesy Medical Device Division, 3M Company, St. Paul, MN.)

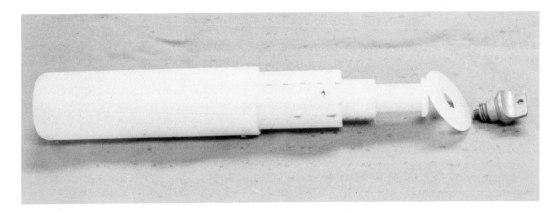

Fig. 9.11. Vaginal cylinder which can hold several cesium-137 tubes and 14 ribbons of Ir-192.

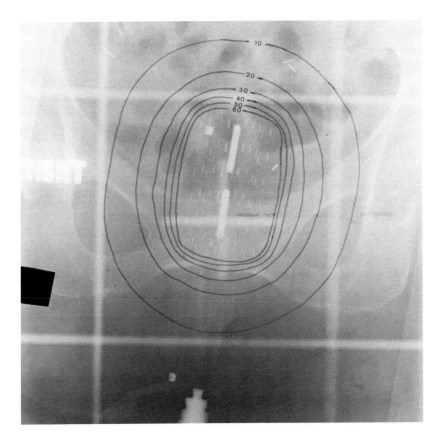

Fig. 9.12. Dose-rate distribution superimposed on the localization film of the vaginal cylinder shown in Fig. 9.11. Two cesium-137 sources were also used in this implant.

The Delclos uterine-vaginal afterloading system is designed for simultaneous treatment of the uterine cavity, cervix, and the vaginal walls. This system consists of a tandem and six sets of segmented plastic cylinders with various diameters ranging from 2 to 4 cm (Fig. 9.10). The uterine tandem fits inside the vaginal cylinder and extends into the uterus. The length of the segment to be loaded and the strength of each source are determined prior to the actual loading of radioactive sources, based on the position of the tumor with respect to the apparatus and the thickness of the tumor. Linear sources are afterloaded via a plastic insert which fits inside the tandem. One disadvantage of this system of linear source arrangement is the increased dose to the bladder and rectum.

Other types of vaginal cylinders are constructed to facilitate simultaneous use of iridium ribbons and cesium tubes (Scott 1966). The pathways that hold the iridium ribbons are distributed lengthwise in two concentric rings with a larger central canal in which cesium tubes can be placed (Fig. 9.11). The length and the pattern into which the sources need to be loaded are determined from orthogonal radiographs. Metal clips marking the lesion are useful in this determination. Figure 9.12 shows a localization film of a patient with such a cylinder in place and with the dose-rate distribution superimposed.

Case presentation

A 63-year-old patient was referred for radiation therapy of recurrent squamous-cell carcinoma of the cervix following a total hysterectomy. She was found to have a very small lesion in the lateral aspect of the superior portion of the left vaginal wall. She was also noted to have a 2 to 3 cm diameter mass in the anterior aspect of the vaginal apex.

She received 4500 cGy to the whole pelvis via external beam irradiation which was followed by an intracavitary application using a vaginal cylinder. The cylinder was loaded with two 4.2 mg Ra eq Cs-137 sources in the apex surrounded by 14 six cm long ribbons of Ir-192 arranged in two cylinder-shaped patterns (Fig. 9.12). The outer circle was 2 mm inside the surface of the apparatus and the inner circle was 1.2 cm from the surface. This delivered 50 cGy/hr at 0.5 cm depth in tissue and remained in place for 30 hours delivering 1500 cGy.

Patients with recurrences in the cervical stump or with bulky tumors in the apex of the vagina often cannot be adequately treated with conventional apparatus (Lichter 1978). The presence of bulky tumor and prior surgery distorts the normal anatomy of the vagina. A customized applicator which will allow adequate source position and which also conforms to the anatomy can then be utilized. Figure 9.13 illustrates some customized applicators.

Case presentation

The vaginal cylinder labelled A in Fig. 9.13 was used for treatment of an elderly lady who, 38 years prior to this illness, had a total hysterectomy followed by whole pelvic irradiation using orthovoltage equipment. She was referred for consideration of radiation therapy for squamous-cell carcinoma in the vaginal apex.

A vaginal applicator, containing 14 iridium ribbons, was custom made for her treatment. The applicator was formed from an impression made of the vagina, and the necessary configuration of the iridium seeds was planned to achieve optimal coverage of the tumor (Fig. 9.14). The applicator was left in place for 50 hours delivering 3000 cGy at 0.5 cm depth in tissue. The procedure was repeated 5 weeks later.

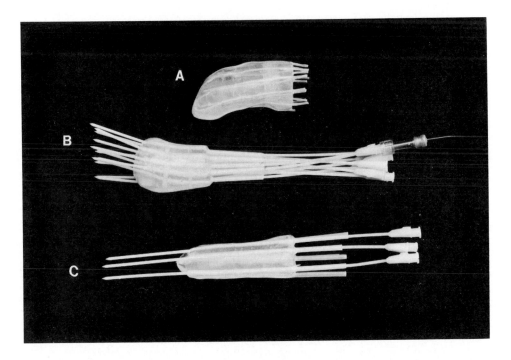

Fig. 9.13. Three customized vaginal applicators. The cylinder labelled (A) was inserted without anesthesia, while (B) and (C), having plastic needles extending beyond the cylinder, were inserted under general anesthesia. Note the heparin lock with a dummy ribbon in place in (B).

Case presentation

This 68-year-old patient had undergone a total hysterectomy for papillary adenocarcinoma of the endometrium approximately 18 months prior to the discovery of a recurrence in the vaginal apex. Surgical resection was not possible due to tumor attachment to the bladder. The patient received 4000 cGy to the whole pelvis via external irradiation followed by a vaginal intracavitary application. A dummy applicator was made from a vaginal impression. The vaginal cylinder labelled B in Fig. 9.13 was constructed to provide a means of having the plastic needles, containing Ir-192 ribbons, extend beyond the mold into the tumor deep to the vaginal vault, thus combining intracavitary and interstitial treatment methods.

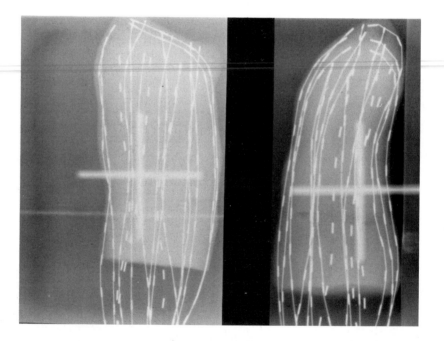

Fig. 9.14. Orthogonal radiographs of the vaginal applicator labelled (A) in Fig. 9.13. Dummy seeds show the built-in source pathways.

During the treatment-planning process, orthogonal radiographs were obtained and a CT examination was carried out with the custom-made dummy applicator in place (Fig. 9.14). The tumor volume was marked with respect to the applicator and following planning of optimal source configuration the final cylinder was made. Eleven open pathways were built in so that the needles could extend beyond the applicator. The tumor extended cephalad of and anterior to the vaginal apex. Some of the pathways were therefore built with a curve to force the plastic needles to continue in an anterior direction beyond the cylinder. This apparatus was inserted under general anesthesia and was afterloaded with eleven ribbons of eight iridium seeds each.

A 12.6 mg Ra eq cesium-137 source was also inserted near the apex via a central blind canal within the applicator. The implant remained in place 29 hours delivering a minimum tumor dose of 2030 cGy.

Case presentation

The vaginal cylinder labelled C in Fig. 9.13 was also constructed to allow the plastic needles to extend beyond the mold into the tissue. It was custom built for a patient with recurrent adenocarcinoma in the apex of the vagina. The vaginal tube was quite narrow and could only facilitate seven pathways. The applicator was inserted under general anesthesia and was afterloaded with seven ribbons containing seven seeds each of Ir-192. The implant remained in place 31 hours delivering 1550 cGy. The patient had received 4500 cGy to the whole pelvis via external beam irradiation prior to the procedure.

Case presentation

Figure 9.15 shows another vaginal applicator used for the treatment of a clear-cell adenocarcinoma of the posterior vaginal wall in a 26-year-old woman. Following resection of the lesion, a vaginal impression was made and a customized vaginal cylinder was fabricated. Preservation of fertility was of concern to the patient and since the lesion was on the posterior wall of the vagina, the anterior half of the mold was filled with a low melting-point alloy to provide shielding. In addition to four pathways for Ir-192 ribbons inside the applicator, a collar with evenly-spaced holes facilitated the insertion of plastic needles into the rectovaginal septum. The applicator was inserted under general anesthesia and five plastic needles were introduced in a semicircular pattern 1 cm posterior to the embedded tubes inside the applicator, thus "sandwiching" the lesion between the planes. Nine Ir-192 ribbons containing six seeds each were afterloaded and remained in place 75 hours delivering 4500 cGy to the posterior vaginal wall.

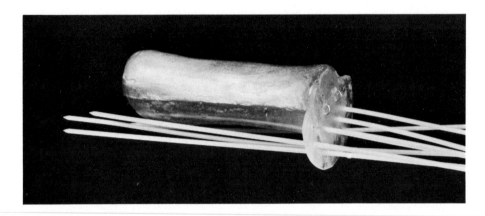

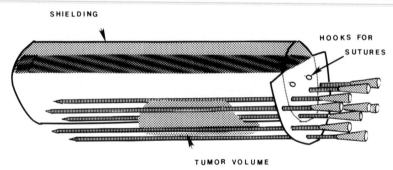

Fig. 9.15. Customized vaginal cylinder used in combination with several interstitial needles "sandwiching" a tumor in the posterior vaginal wall. Lead shielding was added in the anterior half of the applicator.

BLADDER AND RECTUM COMPLICATIONS

Numerous attempts at determining the dose in the bladder and rectum during intracavitary treatments have been made, either with TLDs or an ionization chamber in the rectum or by calculating the dose using orthogonal films (Million 1966, Roswit 1970, Cunningham 1981).

Many authors (Pitts 1930, Gray 1957, Fletcher 1958, Strockbine 1970, Villasanta 1972, Lee 1976, Pourquier 1982, Hamberger 1983, Montana 1983, 1985, 1986, Perez 1984, Orton 1986) have attempted to correlate the dose with the incidence of bladder and rectum injuries.

Contrast in the bladder and the rectum, used in radiographic localization to identify the position of these organs with respect to the implant, probably alters the distance between the radioactive sources and the walls of these organs when the contrast is evacuated and the walls collapse. Due to the very rapid fall-off of dose in brachytherapy very small shifts of the anatomy can result in large differences in dose. When we also consider the changes in the relationship between the sources and the bladder and rectum which occur during a 48 to 72 hour period due to small changes in the patient's position, fecal and gas accumulations, etc., the uncertainties of dose delivered to these organs are further increased. If complication probabilities are to be assessed, it is not appropriate to relate these to the dose at some fixed point in the pelvis, such as point A, or to the number of mg hr used, but rather to the dose actually received at the site of the injury.

Factors other than the dose may affect the complication rate in these organs. Previous surgery, poor nutritional status, anemia, age, and perhaps the dose rate at which the treatment is given are some of these predisposing factors. Technical factors such as the type of apparatus used in the intracavitary treatment, the arrangement of the sources, and the geometry of the application may also have a role in the incidence of complications and must therefore be carefully considered in attempts to reduce the dose delivered to the bladder and rectum.

SURFACE AND INTRACAVITARY BRACHYTHERAPY IN HEAD AND NECK TUMORS

Although less conventional, custom-built applicators holding radioactive ribbons can be used to boost small volumes of persistent or recurrent disease in the head and neck region. The placement of applicators holding radioactive sources directly on the lesion makes invasive procedures unnecessary and because they can be removed and repositioned easily may also, in some patients, be removed overnight to obviate hospitalization. This text will only describe some cases giving a variety of applications. Similar techniques have been described previously (Karolis 1983).

ORAL CAVITY

Interstitial implants in the oral cavity are limited to sites where soft tissue surrounds the lesion. The presence of bone and teeth prevents interstitial implants in sites such as the hard palate and alveolar ridge. Instead, surface applicators can be used to boost the dose to small shallow lesions following external-beam irradiation. Anchoring of surface applicators in the oral cavity is possible with small amounts of denture adhesives, and numerous recesses and ridges can also be utilized to maintain the position of the applicator. A very detailed impression of the entire oral cavity is necessary so that the appliance can be made large enough to include some of the irregular surfaces which will aid repositioning and anchoring.

Case presentation

A 62-year-old female patient with a superficial lesion of the hard palate 2 cm in diameter was referred for radiation therapy. She received 5000 cGy through external-beam irradiation followed by an intraoral surface application.

Figure 9.16 shows a surface applicator fabricated to fit snugly against the hard palate. Tubes, providing pathways for radioactive iridium ribbons, were built into the appliance. Figure 9.17 shows the appliance in place.

Figure 9.18 shows a localization film with the applicator in place carrying 6 ribbons with 47 Ir-192 seeds. The ribbons were separated by 0.5 cm and the seed spacing in the ribbons was also 0.5 cm thus there was one seed in each 0.5 cm^2 of the area. The distribution of the seeds was similar to that for planar implants with one ribbon crossing the proximal end near the lesion. Two metal clips indicated the location of the lesion. The implant remained in place 50 hours delivering 1500 cGy at the 30 cGy/hr line.

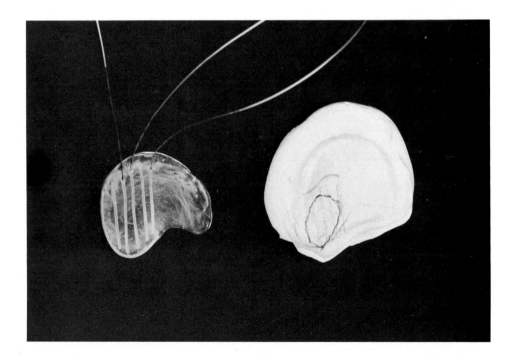

Fig. 9.16. A replica of the hard palate with the tumor marked in black (right). The surface applicator with some dummy ribbons inserted in the pathways (left).

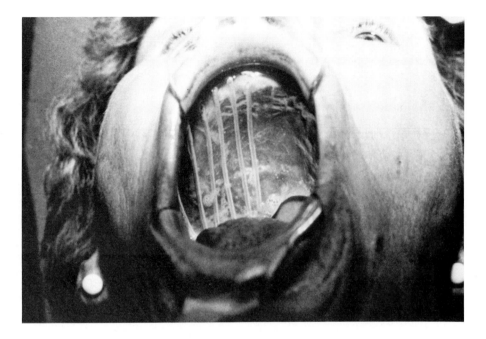

Fig. 9.17. The appliance was held in place against the hard palate by the application of dental adhesive.

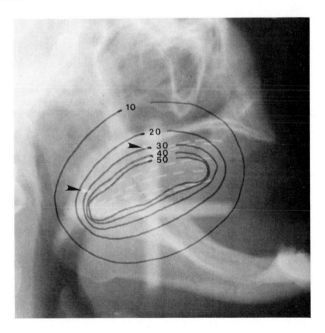

Fig. 9.18. The dose-rate distribution superimposed on the lateral radiograph of the hard palate surface applicator shown in Figs. 9.16 and 9.17. Arrows indicate a seed marking the tumor.

NASAL CAVITY

Surface applicators to boost the dose to small lesions in the nasal cavity, vestibule and the nasal ala are ideal (Ibrahim 1982, Chassagne 1984). Such surface applicators can be removed overnight, and the patient would not require hospitalization. In patients where the lesion is too thick for a surface applicator, a second plane of radioactive ribbons can be implanted interstitially. This would obviously require general anesthesia and hospitalization. A very detailed impression of the nose, particularly the nostrils, is necessary for a snug fit.

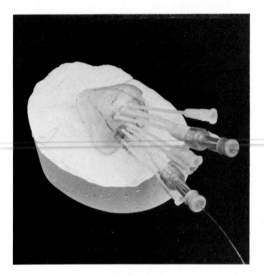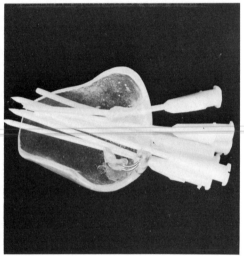

Fig. 9.19. An intracavitary applicator used in an implant in the nasal cavity. Two dummy ribbons are shown inserted in pathways in the applicator. The metal spring was used to clamp the applicator in place.

Case presentation

A 63-year-old male patient was found to have a basal-cell carcinoma of the left nasal cavity. He underwent local resection of the tumor with a skin graft in the nasal septum. The surgical specimen showed tumor cells at the deep margins. The patient then received 3000 cGy via external beam irradiation using a three-field technique with a wax compensator over the nose (shown in Fig. 7.102 in Chapter 7 of *Treatment Planning and Dose Calculation in Radiation Oncology*). This was followed by a treatment using an intracavitary applicator holding Ir-192 seeds. The applicator covered the left ala (Fig. 9.19) and had a cone- shaped segment, holding five ribbons with four iridium seeds each (2 seeds/cm), which fitted snugly into the left nostril. A spring-like wire embedded in the acrylic mold was curved under the septum and into the right nostril where a small soft pad at the end clamped the applicator in place. A small opening in the cone-shaped segment in the left nostril facilitated air flow through the mold making breathing more comfortable. This implant remained in place 25 hours delivering 2500 cGy minimum surface dose to the nasal septum.

Figure 9.20 shows another nasal applicator which was used along with several interstitial plastic needles inserted in the nasal septum, thus combining intracavitary and interstitial techniques.

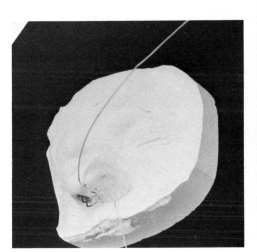 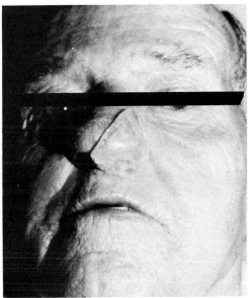

Fig. 9.20. A replica of the patient (left) from which the nasal applicator (above) was made. Several interstitial needles were used.

ORBITAL CAVITY

Tumors recurring subsequent to orbital exenteration can be treated via intracavitary applications. The bony boundaries of the orbit prevents local treatment with interstitial techniques.

Case presentation

A 10-year-old girl had a left orbital exenteration for embryonal-cell rhabdomyosarcoma followed by chemotherapy. Approximately 1 year later she presented with a mass in the upper medial region of the left orbit. The mass was removed and she received 5000 cGy to the left orbit via external beam treatment. She presented again with a recurrence in the same location approximately 6 months later. She received 3000 cGy via external beam treatment which was followed by placement of an intracavitary applicator holding eleven ribbons of Ir-192 seeds in the left orbit (Fig. 9.21).

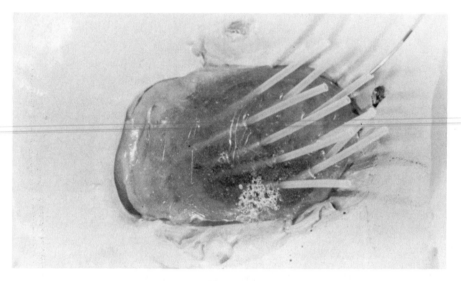

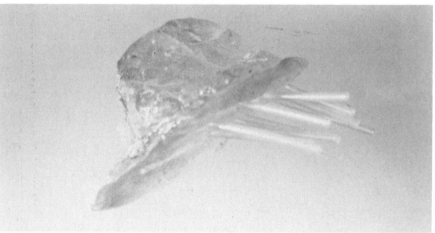

Fig. 9.21. A direct (upper) and a lateral view (lower) of an intraorbital applicator used in the treatment of a recurrent rhabdomyosarcoma.

The applicator was removed intermittently as she wanted to participate in activities with other children in the hospital. It remained in place a total of 60 hours, delivering 3000 cGy. The applicator was made of a tissue-equivalent material consisting of water, gelatin, and glycerin. These ingredients are boiled after the gelatin has been dissolved in the water. The material sets in approximately 2 hours and has a rubbery consistency. It is not as durable as dental acrylic material but it does not deteriorate like the alginate mentioned on page 263. The rubbery mold was comfortable for the patient and could be inserted and removed from the already sore orbit without much manipulation and discomfort.

EXTERNAL AUDITORY CANAL

Although rare, tumors occurring in the external auditory canal can be treated using a customized applicator. The anatomy of the ear provides many structures which increase the stability and fit of the applicator (Fig. 9.22).

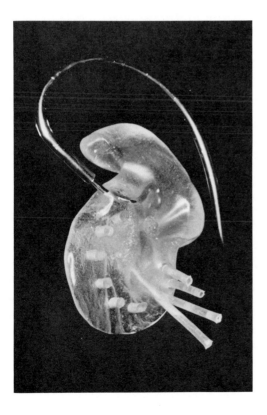

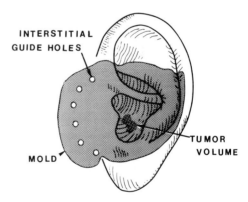

Fig. 9.22. An acrylic applicator used to treat a lesion in the auditory canal (the replica of the ear is shown in Fig. 9.2). The metal loop, which fits around the external ear, was used to stabilize the position. Six holes drilled through the applicator in the preauricular area were used to guide interstitial needles.

<u>Case presentation</u>

A 52-year-old male patient presented with a basal-cell carcinoma of the lower aspect of the external auditory canal. The lesion was resected but the deep margins were positive for tumor. The patient had a history of multiple basal-cell carcinomas treated surgically over several years. An acrylic applicator, containing four tubes for Ir-192 ribbons, was fabricated (Fig. 9.22). The appliance was made to include a semicircle over the preauricular area. Six holes were drilled through this collar 1 cm apart and 1 cm from the segment which was in the auditory canal. Six interstitial needles were planned in this semicircle to achieve a two- plane implant. Planning of four ribbons with four seeds each in the mold and three seeds in each interstitial needle with a seed spacing of 0.5 cm indicated too high a dose in the external auditory canal. It was elected to load only three of the four ribbons in the auditory canal to reduce the hot spot.

The appliance, which was made with an anchoring loop around the ear (similar to those used for eyeglasses), was placed in the ear, and the needles were inserted under local anesthesia only 1 cm deep in the preauricular area. The implant remained in place 48 hours delivering an estimated minimum tumor dose of 1470 cGy. A second procedure included only the four ribbons in the auditory canal. This implant was left in place 96 hours, delivering 4800 cGy, giving a total dose of 6270 cGy.

NASOPHARYNGEAL CAVITY

Treatment of recurrent tumors in the nasopharynx following curative doses of irradiation must be limited to small volumes because of the proximity of vital organs. Consideration must be given to the dose in, for example, the spinal cord, brain, lens of the eye, and the optic chiasm. Interstitial implants are not possible due to the inaccessible location. Intracavitary placement of radioactive sources, usually cesium-137, has been used by several authors (Wang 1966, 1975, Fu 1975, Smith 1979).

A cesium-137 tube secured inside a small (< 2 cm in diameter) Manchester ovoid can be pulled via a nasogastric tube into the nasopharyngeal cavity. The diameter of the ovoid is important in maintaining an adequate distance between the radioactive source and the mucosa. If the source were placed directly on the mucosa, the dose rate would be very high and would fall off very rapidly within the first couple of millimeters. Increasing the distance to the mucosa results in a lower dose rate on the surface, but the fall-off will then be less rapid. The disadvantage with this technique is the necessity of hot loading (with the radioactive sources in place).

An alternative technique is to insert two endotracheal tubes into the nasopharynx through the nostrils (Fig. 9.23). The balloon, near the tip of an endotracheal tube, is filled with contrast. Following radiographic verification, using dummy sources, that the endotracheal tubes are successfully positioned, the tubes are secured to the patient's nose. Plastic tubes, prepared by using the information obtained from the dummy verification, are loaded with the cesium-137 sources and are introduced through each of the endotracheal tubes. Following radiographic verification of the position, the plastic tubes holding the sources are secured to the endotracheal tube. The contrast remains in the bulb during the implant to help in maintaining the distance between the radioactivity and the mucosa. This afterloading technique allows one to verify the position prior to loading and reduces exposure to personnel.

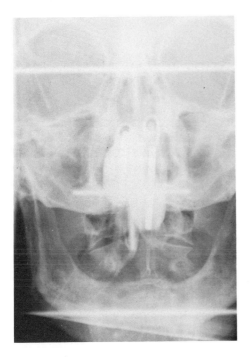 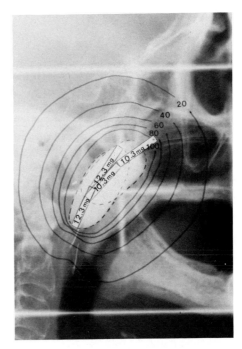

Fig. 9.23. Orthogonal radiographs of an afterloaded nasopharyngeal implant.

Case presentation

An 81-year-old man was referred for consideration of radiation therapy of a recurrent squamous-cell carcinoma in the nasopharynx. Fifteen years prior to the referral he had received 6000 cGy via external beam treatment to the nasopharynx and bilateral cervical nodes. Valium was administered orally 45 minutes prior to the procedure. A 2% cocaine spray was used as a vasoconstrictor in each nostril at the beginning of the procedure.

An endotracheal tube was inserted through each nostril. The position of the endotracheal tubes was confirmed by inserting dummy sources. The bulb of each endotracheal tube was then filled with 5 cc diluted renografin. Two cesium-137 sources were loaded into each tube. Dose calculations showed that higher activity sources were needed in the left tube where the lesion extended to a greater depth. Two 12.3 mg Ra eq sources were inserted on the left side and two 10.3 mg Ra eq sources were inserted on the right side. These sources were left in place 36 hours, delivering 3000 cGy minimal dose to the tumor. The procedure was repeated approximately 5 weeks later, delivering a minimum tumor dose of 6000 cGy.

REMOVABLE INTERSTITIAL IMPLANTS USING OPEN-ENDED PLASTIC TUBING

In anatomic regions where there is no body cavity or orifice to accept radioactive sources, it is necessary to place the radioactivity directly into the tissue. Such removable interstitial implants can only be used in areas that are accessible to direct instrumentation. Insertion of hot needles directly into tumors has largely been replaced by insertion of hollow steel needles or plastic tubing which are threaded through the tumor or tumor bed for subsequent loading of radioactivity (Henschke 1963). There are several different techniques that can be employed, depending on the size and the location of the tumor. Only some of these techniques are summarized in this text.

In soft tissues, hollow stainless-steel needles can be pushed through the tumor at the desired spacing so that both ends are accessible (Fig. 9.24). Plastic tubing with a button at the sealed end is then threaded through each needle. The inside caliber of the tubing can accommodate the radioactive ribbons. The needles are removed over the unbuttoned end, leaving the hollow plastic tubing in place. Another button is pushed onto the tubes close to the skin at the open end to fix the tubes in place. Nylon ribbons containing non-radioactive seeds (dummies) are then inserted into the empty tubing. Orthogonal radiographs are obtained to verify the position and for dose calculation purposes. The dummies are removed and radioactive ribbons, usually Ir-192, are inserted through the open end. Each plastic tube is then sealed by crimping a button or by melting the open end. Although more comfortable for the patient, this flexible system gives rise to a somewhat less uniform dose distribution than the older type of rigid radium needle. This type of implant is particularly useful in treatment of head and neck and breast tumors (Syed 1977), and broader applications are gradually being found.

BREAST IMPLANTS

The conservative management of early carcinoma of the breast with tumor excision (tylectomy) and breast irradiation is becoming increasingly accepted as an alternative to radical mastectomy (Fisher 1977, Prosnitz 1977, Calle 1978, Pierquin 1980). Radiation therapy typically follows the excisional biopsy and usually consists of 4500 to 5000 cGy delivered via external beam irradiation and a boost of 1500 to 2000 cGy to the tumor bed using an electron beam or an Ir-192 interstitial implant (Zwicker 1985). The value of boosting the dose to the tumor bed has been presented by several investigators (Levene 1977, Harris 1981). Typically, the sequence of the radiation therapy is that the interstitial implant follows the external-beam irradiation. However, because the status of the axillary nodes plays an important role in the management of this disease, an axillary dissection is often carried out prior to any radiation therapy. If the axillary nodes are microscopically negative an interstitial implant is sometimes used to boost the tumor area. Since both the axillary node dissection and the interstitial implant require general anesthesia, the two procedures can be carried out at the same operation followed by external beam irradiation.

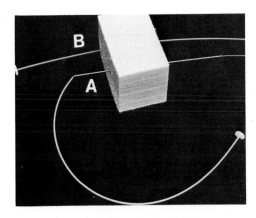

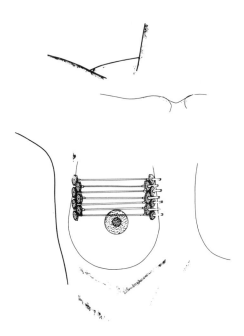

Fig. 9.24. Stainless-steel needles are pushed through the tissues (a block of styrofoam is used in this illustration) until both ends are visible (above). Plastic tubes are pulled through the needles (A) which are then removed leaving the plastic tubes in the tissue (B). Diagram of a breast implant using the open-ended tubing technique (lower right).

An increasingly popular method of interstitial implantation for breast carcinoma is a Quimby-like implant using Ir-192 seeds. The seeds are uniformly distributed throughout the target volume resulting in higher dose in the center of the implant and lower dose in the periphery, with very rapid fall-off outside the implanted volume (Kwan 1983). In the Manchester (Paterson-Parker) system, crossing sources are recommended to achieve dose uniformity within 10% at a distance of 0.5 cm from the implant plane (page 241, Chapter 8). This is not usually possible in breast implants because of the presence of the nipple and areolar region near the implant. In the absence of crossing ribbons, several authors recommend that the source lengths be considerably longer than the target length (Pierquin 1978, 1979, Anderson 1981, 1985, Gillin 1984). The use of extended source length in breast implants, however, is not always possible because it may result in the placement of radioactive seeds in proximity to the skin.

Ideally, the nylon ribbons containing the seeds are spaced 1 cm apart and are parallel with one another. In each ribbon the seeds are spaced 1 cm apart (center to center) and thus there is one seed per cm^3 of tissue. Alternatively, continuous Ir-192 wires, rather than discrete seeds, can be used. These deliver a more uniform dose along the tubes (Marinello 1985). With an activity of 0.33 mg Ra eq per seed, the dose-rate line encompassing the implanted volume is approximately 40 cGy/hr. The dose rate near each seed is considerably higher but falls off very rapidly with distance from the seed. The tubing, into which the nylon ribbons holding the seeds are loaded, creates some distance between the radioactive seed and the tissue, thus reducing the hot spots considerably.

Several afterloading techniques have been described (Boyer 1980, Zwicker 1985), but a typical implant uses the open-ended plastic tubing technique described above. The steel needles are pushed through the breast tissue until each needle exits on the opposite side. When the plastic tubing is pulled through and the rigid steel needles are removed, the flexible plastic tubes tend to follow the curvature of the breast tissue. With dummy seeds in place, the implant is now verified radiographically to facilitate computerized dosimetry. The depth of each tube is measured using dummy ribbons and the radioactive ribbons are cut to appropriate length. The seeds must be well within the breast tissue to prevent very high dose to the skin surface where the plastic tubes enter and exit the breast. The buttons holding the tubes in place are crimped when the loading is completed to prevent the ribbons from shifting during the implant. The loading of the radioactivity can take place in the patient's room or alternatively in the simulation room. The latter permits verification films of the actual sources in place to be taken, but causes a few additional minutes of exposure of the simulator technologist. The transport of the patient to the room also causes additional exposure to personnel, but both can be minimized with good planning and experienced personnel.

Case presentation

A 58-year-old woman noted a lump in the lower outer quadrant of her right breast. A mammogram confirmed the presence of a lesion suspicious for carcinoma. A needle aspirate confirmed the diagnosis of adenocarcinoma and she underwent local excision of a mass 2 cm in diameter. Approximately 1 week later she underwent an axillary dissection and an interstitial implant. Twenty-one lymph nodes removed during the dissection were all negative for malignancy. The implant consisted of two planes with six ribbons in each plane. Ten ribbons had seven seeds each and the remaining two had six seeds each. The dose distribution is shown in Fig. 9.25. The higher dose in the lower aspect of the implant is due to the curvature of the implant causing the calculation plane to be closer to the shallow plane of the implant (Fig. 9.26). The very small areas of high dose rate (80 to 90 cGy/hr) represent points where the calculation plane intersects, or is near, a seed. The implant remained in place 38 hours, delivering 1900 cGy at the 50 cGy/hr line. This was followed by a course of external-beam irradiation consisting of 4600 cGy to the right breast delivered via parallel opposed tangential photon beams.

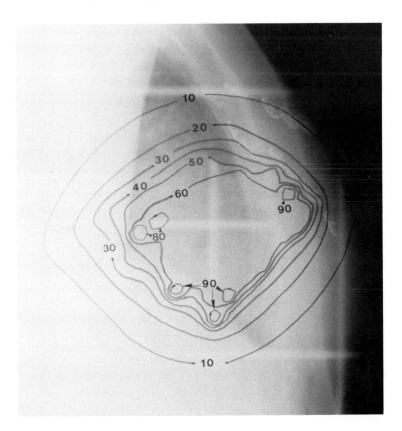

Fig. 9.25. A lateral radiograph of a two-plane breast implant with the resulting dose-rate distribution superimposed.

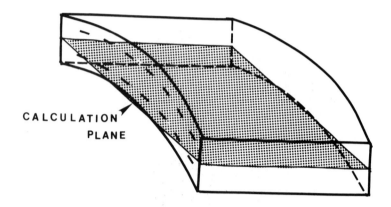

Fig. 9.26. The calculation plane cannot follow a curved implant, so the dose rates are higher where the plane is closer to a row of seeds.

HEAD AND NECK IMPLANTS

The management of head and neck malignancies often includes brachytherapy. Delivering cancerocidal doses of radiation in these sites is often difficult and is limited by the tolerance of adjacent normal tissue. Interstitial implants using radium needles have been used in the management of persistent or recurrent tumors for many years (Fletcher 1980). More recently, nylon ribbons containing Ir-192 seeds have been used. Several techniques, some of which will be described below, have been investigated (Syed 1978, Vora 1983).

Open-ended plastic-tubing techniques, described above for breast implants, are also used in persistent neck nodes or lip tumors.

Case presentation

A 72-year-old male patient with a 2-year history of progressive exophytic growth on the lower lip was referred for radiation therapy when a biopsy revealed well-differentiated squamous-cell carcinoma. Previous biopsies had shown actinic chelitis. On examination, the patient was found to have an exophytic lesion covering the entire lower lip. The lesion infiltrated the entire thickness of the lip but did not extend into the labiogingival sulcus. The oral cavity and the neck were free of disease. The patient received 3000 cGy via external beam followed by an interstitial implant using four ribbons with six Ir-192 seeds each. The technique used was the same as described for the breast treatment. Following insertion of the plastic tubing, dummy seeds were inserted and orthogonal films were obtained for dose calculation. The implant remained in place 50 hours, delivering 3500 cGy at the 70 cGy/hr line (Fig. 9.27).

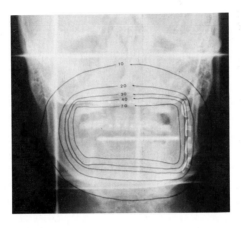

Fig. 9.27. An anterior radiograph of a lower-lip implant with the resulting dose-rate distribution superimposed.

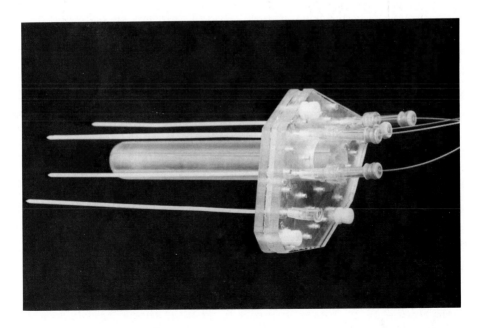

Fig. 9.28. A customized template used for guiding needles in a perineal implant. The pattern of holes drilled for insertion of needles is tailored for treatment of a lesion in the lower pelvis.

TEMPLATE-GUIDED INTERSTITIAL IMPLANTS

BLIND-NEEDLE TECHNIQUES

In anatomical sites where the open-ended plastic tube technique cannot be used, a blind needle (sealed at the pointed end) can be inserted through the tumor and the radioactive ribbons loaded directly into the needles. The spacings and directions of these needles are difficult to control unless some kind of template is used. These difficulties have led to the development of templates which can either be customized or bought commercially. Because template techniques are practically always used with blind needles, the descriptions of these techniques are combined in this text.

TRANSPERINEAL TEMPLATE IMPLANTS

Templates, developed to guide the spacing and parallelism of interstitial needles, are popular in transperineal implants (Ampuero 1983, Feder 1978, Flemming 1980, Martinez 1984, Syed 1977, 1978, 1983). The Syed-Neblett "butterfly" template is probably the most commonly used type. It consists of a removable vaginal obturator and an acrylic perineal plate. Holes drilled through the plate in a predetermined pattern serve as guides for the spacing of the stainless -steel or plastic needles which are inserted in five concentric cylinders around the lateral plane of the vagina. The needles are afterloaded with Ir-192 seeds in nylon ribbons, and a tandem is provided for the placement of intrauterine cesium or radium sources. More recent models are made to facilitate other patterns of needle distribution. The perineal plate in the newer models is made of softer silicone material which is more comfortable for the patient. A removable obturator in the center of the template is inserted into the vagina to stabilize the template. For rectal, prostatic, and urethral lesions, the template is stabilized by threading it over a rectal tube or a catheter in the bladder. Once confirmation of placement is obtained, dose calculations are completed, and radioactive ribbons are inserted into the needles.

Templates can also be customized (Bentel 1990) to suit a particular situation (Fig. 9.28). Such customized templates are superior to standard models because they can be designed with a needle pattern which, when loaded, results in a uniform dose distribution conforming to the shape of the target (Fig. 9.29).

The pattern of guide holes actually used in each implant and the depth to which the radioactivity is inserted can, to a limited degree, be tailored to match the target volume. This, of course, requires very detailed characterization of the target in terms of its size, shape, and location with respect to the obturator or other reference point. For smaller target volumes, smaller templates can be used. Rectal and prostate templates have been developed to treat single sites and provide a much smaller and thus more comfortable template. The combination of an intracavitary tandem containing cesium sources with interstitial iridium seeds in treatment of locally advanced pelvic disease has been described by multiple authors (Feder 1978, Ampuero 1983, Martinez 1984, 1985).

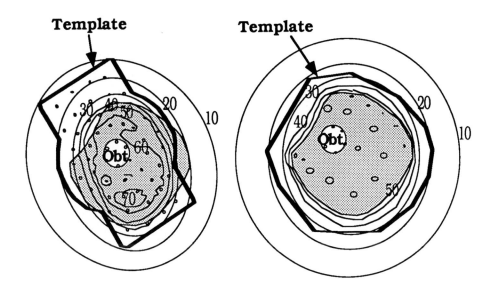

Fig. 9.29. With standard templates (left), the needle pattern is predetermined and can result in hot spots and lack of target coverage while customized templates (right) can be designed to provide optimal dose uniformity and target coverage.

Case presentation

A 76-year-old woman was referred for consideration of radiation therapy for a squamous-cell carcinoma of the uterine cervix, stage IIIA. On examination, she was found to have a friable tumor mass involving the cervix and extending onto the vaginal canal down to the introitus. There was bilateral, medial parametrial involvement. The patient had undergone a supracervical hysterectomy 36 years prior to the diagnosis of malignant disease. Metastatic work-up revealed no rectal or bladder involvement and no extension beyond the pelvis. The patient received 5040 cGy to the whole pelvis via external-beam irradiation. At the completion of the course of external-beam treatment, there was essentially complete regression of the tumor mass in the cervix and vaginal walls.

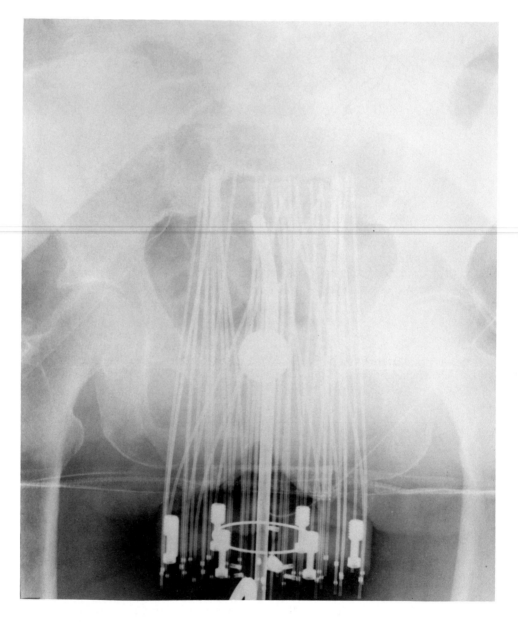

Fig. 9.30. Radiograph of perineal template using steel needles and a uterine tandem. As with all larger transperineal implants, the needles often change path as they encounter bone or a hard tumor mass and are thus deflected.

Approximately 3 weeks following the completion of external-beam irradiation, the patient was admitted for an interstitial template implant.*

Based on the configuration of the disease, it was elected to load only 27 of the 44 guide holes in the transperineal butterfly template. The guide holes in the most lateral aspects of the template were loaded with ten Ir-192 seeds each, but only in the deepest segment of the needles to provide coverage of the parametrial region. Difficulty was encountered in the insertion of some of these needles due to the intersecting bone which forced the needles to curve medially. The centrally located guide holes were loaded with ten Ir-192 seeds each, but only in the lower region surrounding the vagina. The central guide holes anterior and posterior to the vaginal obturator were not loaded, in an attempt to reduce the dose to the bladder and rectum. An intracavitary tandem, loaded with two cesium sources (14.4 and 10.5 mg Ra eq), was inserted into the remaining cervical canal (Fig. 9.30).

The sources remained in place 22 hours, delivering an estimated dose of 3080 cGy to point A, 1540 cGy to point B, and 1100 cGy at 0.5 cm depth in the vaginal mucosa. The maximum dose to the bladder was estimated to be 1500 cGy and to the rectum, approximately 1200 cGy.

The insertion of an interstitial template implant requires general anesthesia, while its removal can be made following administration of oral analgesics. The needles used in perineal templates must have a blind end to prevent the radioactive ribbons from projecting beyond the tip of the needle. If a loaded ribbon protrudes beyond the needle, it could be sheared off during the removal, causing sources to be left behind accidentally.

OTHER TEMPLATE IMPLANTS

Improved spacing and parallelism could be achieved in a breast implant if, for example, a template similar to that described for transperineal implants were used. Hollow tubes such as nasogastric tubes can also be used. The tubes are secured on the breast surface in the entrance and exit region. Holes are made at the desired spacing and the needles are pushed through the breast to the opposite side. Corresponding holes are made in the nasogastric tubes placed in the exit region and the exiting needles are pushed through these holes as well. The plastic tubing is inserted through the needle and the

---

*   In this text, the use of a standard transperineal template is described only because
    it is the standard method. Duke University Medical Center consistently uses
    customized rather than standardized templates.

needle is then withdrawn as previously described. The implant is then loaded in conventional fashion.

Small rectal lesions can be implanted using a similar technique. A nasogastric tube with needles pushed through the walls at equal spacing can be curved to form a semicircle (or alternatively, a circle) and placed overlying the lesion adjacent to the anal canal (Fig. 9.31). The nasogastric tube is secured by suturing it to the skin. The blind steel (or alternatively, plastic) needles are pushed in through the lesion (Fig. 9.32). A second plane of needles can be inserted in a similar fashion outside the first. Figure 9.32 illustrates such a two-plane rectal implant; it uses blind steel needles, but plastic needles would make the procedure more comfortable for the patient. The length of the needles is determined by the depth of the lesion. A similar technique can be used for implants of urethral or paravaginal lesions.

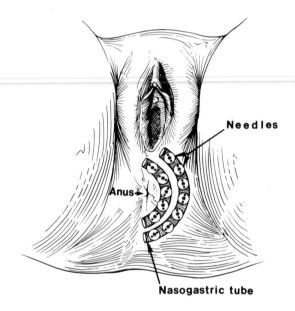

Fig. 9.31. An individualized template can be made of nasogastric tubing which is used to guide the spacing of the needles.

Case presentation

A 48-year-old female patient presented with a lesion 2 cm in diameter on the left lateral wall of the rectum 4 to 5 cm above the anal verge. A biopsy showed adenocarcinoma and the patient was diagnosed as having adenocarcinoma of the rectum, Stage A. She underwent a wide local excision followed by 4500 cGy to the whole pelvis via external-beam irradiation. This was followed approximately 2 weeks later by a two-plane, semicircular iridium implant. The inner semicircle contained four blind needles with eight Ir-192 seeds each, and the outer semicircle placed 1 cm farther out from the anus contained five needles with eight Ir-192 seeds each. The seeds were spaced 1 cm apart in the ribbon, and the needles were spaced 1 cm from each other. Figure 9.32 shows the anterior and lateral localization films obtained for dose-calculation purposes. The implant remained in place 21.5 hours delivering a minimum target-volume dose of 1500 cGy.

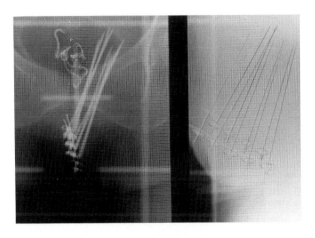

Fig. 9.32. Orthogonal radiographs of a rectal implant using two semicircles as shown in Fig. 9.31.

Case presentation

A 72-year-old female patient was referred for postoperative irradiation of a periurethral lesion. She underwent a radical hysterectomy 8 years prior to the referral for stage 1B carcinoma of the cervix. She did well until 2 years prior to her referral when she was found to have squamous-cell carcinoma of the vagina. This was thought to be a new primary tumor. The lesion was excised, but 1 year following the excision she was found to have a periurethral nodule just inside the introitus. This was also excised, leaving practically no vaginal canal, and she was referred for postoperative irradiation. Physical examination was unremarkable with the exception of the pelvic exam which revealed absence of the vagina and some induration in the right periurethral area. The patient was diagnosed as having squamous-cell carcinoma of the vagina, recurrent post local excision. She received 3000 cGy to the lesion via external-beam irradiation using two anterior oblique wedged fields. This was followed approximately 2 weeks later by an interstitial iridium implant.

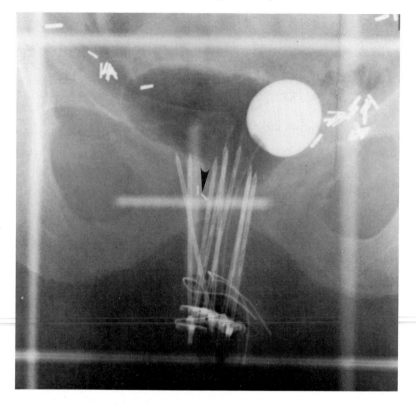

Fig. 9.33. A periurethral lesion implanted using a custom-designed template technique. Arrow indicates tumor-marking seeds.

The implant technique was similar to the one described for the rectal lesion. She had two planes forming two parallel semicircles from approximately five to one o'clock. There were four needles in the inner and five in the outer semicircle. Each needle was loaded with four Ir-192 seeds each, spaced 1 cm apart (Fig. 9.33). The implant remained in place 44 hours, delivering 3520 cGy to the volume encompassed by the 80 cGy/hr line.

These two cases were treated using the same technique although both the anatomy and the tumor distribution are very different. They are included to illustrate how one technique can easily be adapted to different situations.

A note of caution must be added regarding the removal of this kind of implant. Blind needles must be used to prevent the radioactive ribbons from exiting the deep end of an open needle and entering the tissue. During removal, the segment extending outside the needle can easily be sheared off and thus become lodged in the tissues as previously indicated (page 297). Surgical removal is the only option when available; this is difficult, embarrassing, and hazardous.

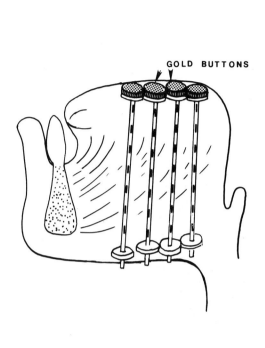

GOLD BUTTONS

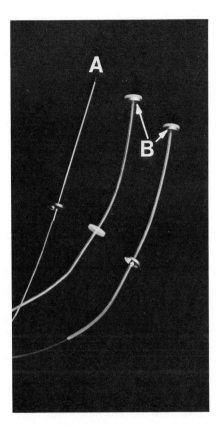

Fig. 9.34. Diagram of a gold-button implant in the tongue (left). A blind needle (right) (A) and two gold-button ribbons (B).

OTHER IMPLANT TECHNIQUES

GOLD-BUTTON TECHNIQUES

A gold-button technique is sometimes used for implants of head and neck lesions. Hollow steel needles are inserted into the neck through the tumor until they extend into the oral cavity. With one end of the needle projecting through the oral mucosa and the other end presenting on the skin surface, plastic tubes with a gold button attached to the already-sealed intraoral end and with a silk thread tied under the button, are threaded through the needles, starting at the intraoral end of the needle (Fig. 9.34). The steel needles are then removed, and the plastic tubes are left in place. Steel buttons are lightly crimped onto the tubes close to the skin surface. When all plastic tubes are fixed in place, all silk threads are brought through a Penrose drain which is taped to the patient's cheek. The loading of radioactive ribbons through the tubes is practically the same as described above for other techniques.

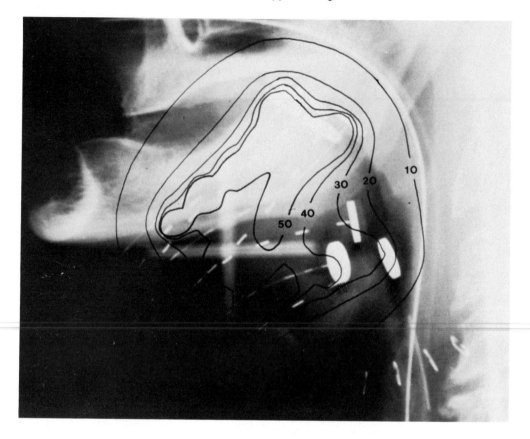

Fig. 9.35. Dose-rate distribution superimposed on a radiograph of an implant in the posterior one third of the tongue using a gold-button technique.

The gold-button technique serves a dual role: it spaces and retains the plastic tubes in place and protects overlying tissues against unnecessary irradiation and friction caused by the needles. This technique is most useful for interstitial therapy of oral and oropharyngeal tumors.

Case presentation

A 52-year-old female patient presented with squamous-cell carcinoma of the posterior tongue. She received 5000 cGy via external-beam irradiation followed by an interstitial implant using the gold-button technique previously described. Seven ribbons containing Ir-192 seeds each were inserted (Fig. 9.35). The first two seeds at the end nearest the gold button were spaced only 0.5 cm apart, and in the remainder of the ribbons the seeds were spaced 1 cm apart. The intention was to substitute higher loading near the end of the implant for the crossing needle.

LOOP TECHNIQUES

Alternatively, a loop technique can be used for implants in the oral cavity. This technique utilizes pairs of hollow steel needles which are inserted through the neck on either side of the mandible throughout the tumor volume. The needles protrude through the oral mucosa with the other end presenting on the skin surface. Open-ended plastic tubing, previously described, is threaded through each pair of needles so that the result is an inverted "U." The steel needles are removed, and the plastic tubes are left in place (Fig. 9.36). The fixation, localization, dose calculation, and loading procedures are essentially the same as previously described.

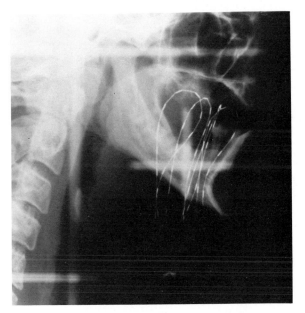 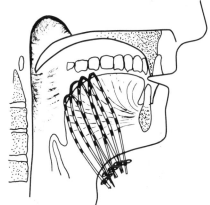

Fig. 9.36. Radiograph (left) and a diagram (right) of a loop implant in the anterior oral tongue. The implant consisted of four loops each holding eleven Ir-192 seeds.

REMOVAL OF INTERSTITIAL IMPLANTS

Removal of temporary interstitial implants requires care and skill, or seeds could accidentally be left in the patient. For the removal of implants using open-ended plastic tubing, such as shown for breast implants above, a special wire cutter, adjusted to clip only the outer plastic tube and to spare the seed ribbon, is used in the removal. The plastic tube should be cut between the skin surface and the button, revealing the radioactive ribbon which is then removed and the seeds counted before being placed in an appropriately shielded container. Following assurances that all seeds are removed, including a negative radiation survey of the patient, the plastic tube is cut near the skin on the opposite side, and the remaining portion is pulled out. Radioactive sources must always be removed before the plastic tube is pulled out so that in the rare event that a source (seed) is left behind, a pathway for its retrieval is still intact.

REMOVABLE INTERSTITIAL BRAIN IMPLANTS

Removable implants in the management of certain brain tumors are becoming an increasingly popular technique. Some solitary brain tumors can be cured by surgery and radiation therapy. Delivery of cancerocidal doses to large brain fields via external-beam irradiation is often prevented by the radiation toxicity in the surrounding normal brain tissue. External-beam irradiation can therefore be followed by a boost (higher dose to a smaller volume, page 179) via an interstitial implant using Ir-192 or other radionuclide. Interstitial implants, using low-energy, high-activity I-125 seeds, can be used to treat recurrent brain tumors in patients who have already received high-dose irradiation, and in whom it is therefore critical to tailor the dose distribution to the shape of the tumor. The relatively low energy of I-125 and rapid dose fall-off away from the seeds makes it more suitable for such tailoring than most other radionuclides.

Fig. 9.37. Three-dimensional representation of a brain tumor and the planned catheter placement. A point, through which the catheter must pass, is selected on each of two images (A and B). These points must be selected so that the catheter also pass through the tumor at the desired locations on all other images.

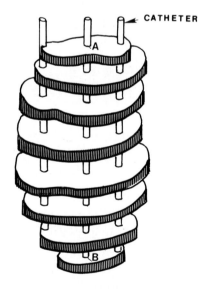

Although not practiced extensively, interstitial brachytherapy has been used to treat brain tumors since the early 1900s (Bernstein 1981). In the last several decades, stereotactic implantation of radioisotopes, primarily to treat low-grade gliomas, has been practiced particularly in Europe (Talairach 1955, Mundinger 1961, 1963, 1968, 1970, Szikla 1979). The integration of stereotactic systems with computerized tomography scanners, with which tumor targets can be visualized and precisely implanted, and the availability of possibly more effective isotopes are some factors which make the continued use and refinement of brachytherapy attractive in treatment of malignant brain tumors (Mundinger 1978, MacKay 1982).

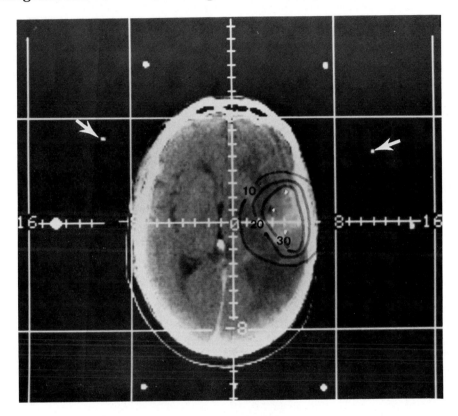

Fig. 9.38. A contrast-enhanced CT obtained with the stereotactic frame in place immediately prior to a brain implant. The bars of the frame (seen as light spots in the periphery of the skull) are used as reference points.

The procedure is very labor-intensive and requires special equipment and computerized treatment-planning systems. Very high-activity I-125 seeds (approximately 40 mCi/seed) are typically used, although other isotopes can also be used. This requires special ordering of seeds several days prior to the procedure. Efforts to minimize the number of seeds in order to limit the cost of the procedure are made by optimized planning of seed placement. Three-dimensional viewing of the target volume is possible with some treatment-planning computer software, but a manual 3-D reconstruction, although time consuming, can be made (Fig. 9.37).

Prior to the actual insertion of the catheters, a stereotactic frame is attached to the patient's cranium (Gutin 1981, 1982, 1984). A contrast-enhanced CT study is then obtained throughout the tumor volume (Fig. 9.38).

Placement of the catheters or tubes holding the radioactive seeds is chosen from at least two CT images. The points selected for a given catheter, with respect to reference points of the frame, are entered into the computer that drives the stereotactic device. The computer calculates the coordinates and angles necessary for precise placement of the catheters, and after setting these parameters on the stereotactic frame, each catheter is pushed through the tumor to the desired depth. A hole drilled through the cranium permits the introduction of the catheter into the brain. When the catheter is in place, it is sutured to the scalp to prevent motion. This procedure is carried out in the operating room under light sedation and local anesthesia.

Following recovery, the position of the catheters is verified radiographically. Dose distributions are calculated using dummy seeds inserted in afterloading tubes which fit inside the catheters. When the placement of the dummy seeds is acceptable, they are replaced by identical inserts carrying the active seeds, which remain in place for several days until the desired dose is delivered.

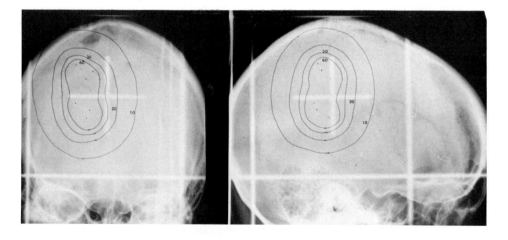

Fig. 9.39. Orthogonal localization films of an I-125 implant of a recurrent brain tumor with the dose-rate distribution superimposed. The dose in this patient was calculated to the 30 cGy/hr line as seen in the dose distribution.

<u>Case presentation</u>

A 32-year-old female patient was referred for consideration of stereotactic brain implant of a recurrent astrocytoma. Three years prior to the referral she underwent resection of a Grade I - II malignant astrocytoma. This was followed by 5900 cGy via external-beam irradiation. Approximately 2 years later she presented with a recurrence which was resected and showed Grade III - IV astrocytoma. She was subsequently given seven cycles of chemotherapy, but failed again.

Three stereotactically controlled catheters were inserted into the tumor in the operating room. She was then brought to the simulator room where orthogonal radiographs (Fig. 9.39), using dummy seeds, were obtained. Two high-intensity (40 mCi) I-125 seeds were inserted in each catheter. The implant was left in place 144 hours, delivering 8640 cGy at the 60 cGy/hr line, which enclosed the lesion and a 0.5 cm margin.

The choice of I-125 seeds in brain implants is primarily based on its relatively low energy which results in accentuated sparing of surrounding normal tissue. The cranium functions as a shield during the implant, and radiation which does have sufficient energy to penetrate the bone can effectively be stopped by a lead-shielded helmet. Personnel are easily protected by lead aprons, which are virtually useless for protection against commonly used isotopes other than I-125.

OPHTHALMIC PLAQUE TREATMENT

Treatment of ocular malignancies using Rn-222 seeds was described many years ago (Moore 1930). More recently, plaques using Co-60, Ru-106[*], Ir-192, or I-125 have been used for treatment of ocular melanomas (Stallard 1968, Bedford 1973, Lommatzsch 1974, Sealy 1976, Packer 1980, Brady 1984). Cobalt-60 plaques can be purchased in standard sizes and shapes while plaques with a seed-carrier insert can be individually made to fit the lesion (Fig. 9.40). The desired dose rate and dose pattern are calculated prior to the purchase of the seeds. The seeds are then loaded into the seed carrier in the planned pattern. The plaques have at least two suturing eyelets so that they can be anchored to the eye over the lesion. Figure 9.41 shows dose rates from a 16 mm diameter I-125 plaque, and a schematic representation of an ophthalmic implant. The thickness of the lesion is determined via ultrasound. The treatment is usually prescribed at the apex of the lesion and doses on the order of 8000 to 10,000 cGy are typically delivered over several days. The maximum dose is obviously at the base of the lesion which is

---

[*] Ruthenium-106

nearest the surface of the plaque. The dose to the sclera exceeds 40,000 cGy in some cases.

These plaques are inserted and removed in the operating room in a procedure which requires mild sedation and local anesthesia. The tumor margins, visualized when a light source is placed on the opposite side, are marked on the sclera. The dose to the operating surgeon is limited by the use of a transparent dummy plaque, with suture eyelets identical to that of the hot plaque. The dummy is sutured to the sclera over the tumor such that it can be removed while the sutures remain in the tissues. A second transillumination procedure, verifying that the tumor shadow lies within the boundaries of the transparent plaque, is made before the dummy plaque is removed. The dummy plaque is replaced by the hot plaque which is quickly anchored to the eye by threading the sutures through the matching eyelets. This type of plaque treatment has also been described for treatment of retinoblastoma (Stallard 1948, Ellsworth 1969).

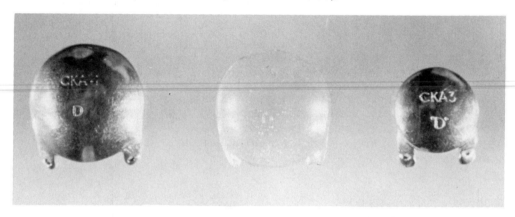

Fig. 9.40. Cobalt-60 eye plaques (10 and 15 mm in diameter) with a plastic dummy (above). I-125 eye plaque with the seed carrier loaded and in place inside the gold shield (right). Also see Fig. 8.4.

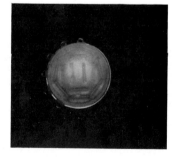

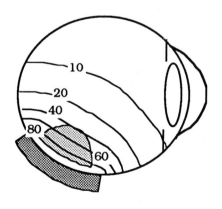

Fig. 9.41. Dose-rate distribution (cGy/hr) resulting from a I-125 loading with 13 seeds containing 1 mCi/seed.

A strontium-90 ophthalmic applicator, primarily used for treatment of pterygium, a benign condition of the conjunctiva, has been described in Chapter 8 (pages 225 and 229).

PERMANENT INTERSTITIAL IMPLANTS

The advantage of permanent implants is that the seeds can be placed in inaccessible tumors where removal would be impractical or impossible. An example of this would be a deep pelvic or abdominal tumor where the radioactive sources can be implanted during a surgical procedure. Removal would require another surgical procedure within a few days, which the patient's condition may not permit.

Radioisotopes with relatively short half-life are best suited for permanent implants because most of the dose is deposited early on before the seeds have a chance of becoming displaced. Iodine-125, which also has relatively low energy, is beneficial in implants of tumors near radiosensitive organs where a very rapid fall-off of dose is desired. Low-activity I-125 seeds implanted in the prostate (Fig. 9.42), where the proximity of the rectum prevents high doses from being delivered via external-beam treatment, are sometimes used (Whitmore 1972, Shipley 1981, Kumar 1986). Permanent implants of I-125 seeds in other pelvic, abdominal, or lung tumors can also be used (Shipley 1980).

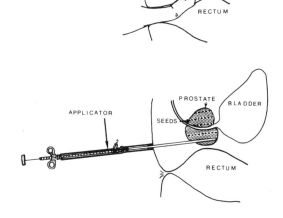

Fig. 9.42. Permanent implant of I-125 seeds in the prostate. Digital palpation is employed to prevent rectal-wall puncture and to guide the needles in the prostate (upper). A gun-type device is then used to deposit the seeds with uniform spacing as each needle is withdrawn (lower).

Since devices such as those used to insert and maintain seed spacing in the removable implants previously described cannot be used in permanent implants, other devices built to insert and guide the spacing of permanently implanted seeds have been developed (Scott 1977, 1981, Hawliczek 1991).

In one of these, a semi-automatic gun-type applicator is used in an attempt to obtain a uniform distribution of the seeds within the tumor. The I-125 seeds are preloaded into magazines, each of which carries up to fourteen seeds. The magazine fits into a slot in the applicator. Hollow stainless-steel needles are inserted through the tumor parallel to each other at the desired spacing. The gun is connected to a needle, and the depth of the needle into the tissue is read from a gauge on the gun. The stylet in the gun is advanced to force a seed from the magazine, through the needle and into the tissue. As the needle is withdrawn and the trigger of the gun is squeezed, another seed is deposited. The needle is removed when the desired length of each path has been implanted. When all needles have been loaded and the implant is completed, no needles remain. This technique is particularly useful for deep-seated tumors in the pelvis and in the abdomen.

PERMANENT IMPLANTS IN THE PELVIS

Case presentation

A 60-year-old female patient was referred for radiation therapy of a periurethral recurrence of a squamous-cell carcinoma of the cervix. She underwent a full course of radiation therapy to the whole pelvis via external-beam treatment and two intracavitary Cs-137 insertions 9 years prior to presentation. An earlier recurrence was treated by a radical hysterectomy.

Under general anesthesia, seventeen steel needles were placed in the tumor in a cylindrical fashion. These were afterloaded with I-125 seeds using the gun-type applicator previously described. A total of sixty-four seeds were inserted. The average activity was 0.62 mCi per seed (Fig. 9.43). This delivered 4000 cGy to the implanted volume. The patient was instructed to collect and submit all urine for survey to detect radioactive seeds which could possibly have been excreted in the urine.

Dose calculation for a large number of seeds is very complicated and the I-125 seeds are also very difficult to visualize on a radiograph, even under optimal conditions. A technique referred to as the dimension averaging technique has been developed and used for many years in permanent implants (Henschke 1968, Anderson 1976). In this technique, the total activity in mCi of I-125, is taken to be five times the average of three mutually perpendicular dimensions, in cm, of a treatment region encompassing the tumor. In a 4 x 5 x2 cm tumor, the average dimension is 3.66 cm, therefore, 18.3 (3.66 x 5) mCi I-125 is needed. The number of seeds required is given by dividing the total activity needed by the available seed strength. Seeds are usually between 0.4 and 0.6 mCi. Prescription for the spacing of the seeds can be obtained from an I-125 Spacing Nomograph (Anderson 1976).

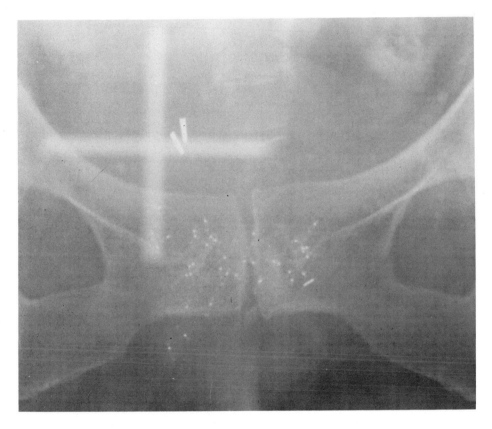

Fig. 9.43. Iodine-125 seeds permanently implanted in a recurrent periurethral lesion.

PERMANENT IMPLANT IN THE LUNG

Gold (Au-198) seeds, described on page 225, are also suitable for permanent implants due to the very short half-life (2.7 days from Table 8.1 on page 222). Although the use of I-125 seeds in implants of bronchial lesions appears more popular (Hilaris 1971, 1975, 1979, 1981, 1983, 1985, Scott 1975 A), gold seeds are also used. Serious difficulty is sometimes encountered in precise placement of the seeds in lung implants due to the long distance over which one must manipulate the instrument and the seeds. Optimized distribution rules for gold implants have been studied (Dale 1976).

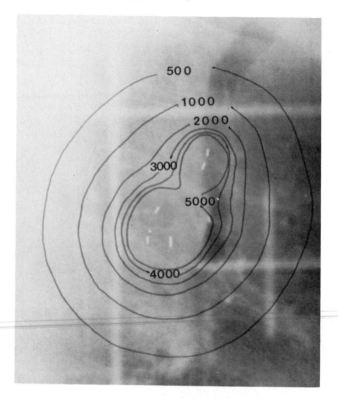

Fig. 9.44. Eight Au-198 seeds implanted in a recurrent lesion in the trachea just above the branching off of the right main stem bronchus. The numbers along the lines of the superimposed dose distribution on this lateral radiograph represent the total dose delivered, in cGy. A diagram (below) shows the tumor location.

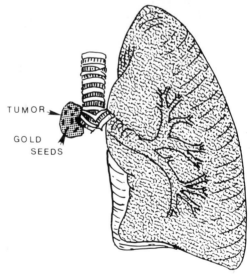

Case presentation

A 56-year-old male patient was referred for consideration of a bronchial implant of a recurrent squamous-cell carcinoma of the lung. The patient received 5500 cGy to the primary lesion in the right upper lobe via external-beam irradiation approximately 1 year prior to the consultation.

Bronchoscopy revealed a mass growing into the right side of the trachea approximately 1 cm above the branching off of the right main stem bronchus. Further external-beam irradiation was precluded because the normal-tissue tolerance in this region had been reached.

The patient was taken to the operating room where 8 Au-198 seeds were inserted via a bronchoscope. A long steel needle, especially designed for this type of implant, was used. Each seed contained 5.8 mCi at the time of the procedure. The implant delivered a minimum tumor dose of 3000 cGy (Fig. 9.44). This procedure was carried out in an attempt at palliating symptoms of bleeding and coughing.

PERMANENT IMPLANTS IN THE HEAD AND NECK

Gold seeds, permanently implanted, can be effective in the treatment of very small lesions in the oral cavity, particularly as an alternative to a more invasive procedure in patients who cannot undergo general anesthesia.

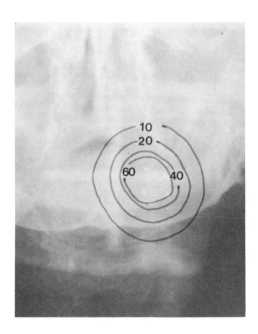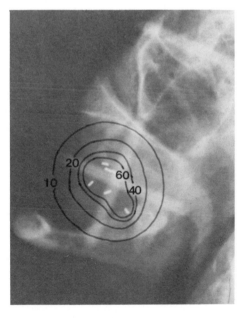

Fig. 9.45. Six Au-198 seeds permanently implanted in a recurrent lesion in the floor of the mouth of an 88-year-old female patient. The numbers along the lines in the superimposed dose distribution represent the total dose in Gy delivered to the tumor.

Case presentation

An 88-year-old female patient was referred for radiation therapy of a recurrent squamous-cell carcinoma of the floor of the mouth. She had received 6000 cGy via external-beam irradiation 8 years prior to this recurrence. The patient had a history of congestive heart failure, so an implant requiring general anesthesia was precluded. Examination of the oral cavity revealed a 2.5 x 3.5 cm lesion on the left oral tongue with extension into the buccal gingival sulcus. Under local anesthesia, six Au-198 seeds were inserted in the lesion (Fig. 9.45). Each seed had an activity of 2.8 mCi at the time of the insertion, and dose calculations showed that the minimum tumor dose from the implant was 4000 cGy. The patient tolerated the procedure very well despite her age and was able to return home the same day without requiring hospitalization.

PERMANENT IMPLANTS USING ABSORBABLE SUTURES

Another technique for permanent seed implantation has been described and consists of inserting absorbable sutures with I-125 seeds interspaced at 1 cm distances (Harter 1975, Scott 1975 B, Goode 1979, Palos 1980). This method is primarily used for relatively flat tumors of the bladder, chest wall, etc. A technique utilizing I-125 seeds impregnated in absorbable gel foam which is sewn in place with an absorbable vicryl mesh has also been described (Marchese 1984).

INTRALUMINAL IMPLANTS

Insertion of a plastic tube, holding radioactive sources, into the lumen of a tube-shaped organ such as the bronchus, the esophagus, or the biliary tract is referred to as an intraluminal implant (Ikeda 1979, Fletcher 1981, Herskovic 1981, Conroy 1982, Johnson 1985, Syed 1987).

Obstructing lesions in the bile duct require high radiation doses to a very limited volume. Insertion of Ir-192 seed ribbons into a percutaneously placed intracholangial catheter can be used in this treatment (Herskovic 1981, Conroy 1982, Johnson 1985) (Fig. 9.46). The radioactive ribbon is inserted under fluoroscopic guidance. Contrast is introduced to determine the dimensions of the bile duct for dose calculation purposes. The implant remains in place until approximately 5000 cGy is delivered at 5 mm from the center of the catheter. The rapid fall-off of dose allows high mucosal dose to be delivered without adverse effects.

Insertion of radioactive sources in the bronchus or trachea to treat obstructing bronchial tumors was first described by Yankauer using radium (Yankauer 1922) and more recently by Schray et al. using iridium (Schray 1985). An afterloading tube is inserted under fiberoptic bronchoscopy guidance. A lead marker in the leading end of the tube indicate the depth of insertion on radiographs. Following radiographic verification of location and determination of the length of the radioactive ribbon using dummy seeds, the Ir-192 seed ribbon is inserted (Fig. 9.47). The dose is usually calculated at 0.5 cm from the center of the seed ribbon and a dose of 3000 cGy is delivered in approximately 2 days.

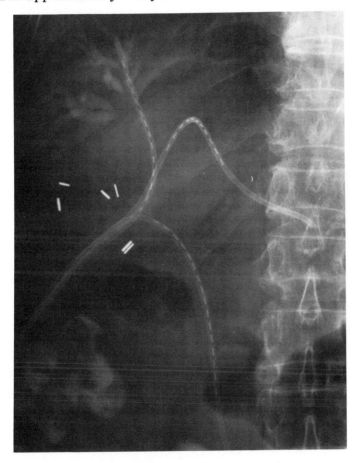

Fig. 9.46. Intraluminal Ir-192 treatment of obstructive biliary duct tumor. The radioactive ribbons are inserted via an intracholangial catheter.

Placement of radioactive sources in the esophagus to boost the dose in small esophageal lesions, or for palliation of symptoms in patients with recurrent tumors is sometimes used in desperate attempts to prolong survival in patients with this dismal prognosis (Fig. 9.48). Syed et al. reported 37 patients with primary esophageal carcinoma treated with external-beam irradiation to 45 to 50 Gy followed by intraluminal irradiation delivering 25 to 35 Gy in two applications, and 10 patients with recurrent esophageal carcinoma treated with only two intraluminal applications delivering 50 to 60 Gy. The dose was calculated at 0.5 cm from the outer surface of the applicator. Both groups also received 5-flourouracil infusion. Eighty-one percent (38/47) of these patients had excellent palliation of symptoms and were able to swallow until dying of metastatic disease (Syed 1987).

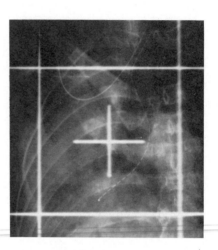

Fig. 9.47. A bronchial Ir-192 seed ribbon containing 23 seeds spaced 0.5 cm apart is placed inside an afterloading tube. Note the leading lead marker. This ribbon was left in place 48 hrs, delivering 3000 cGy at 0.5 cm from the center of the seed-ribbon.

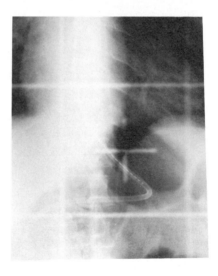

Fig. 9.48. Intraluminal implant to treat an esophageal tumor.

REMOTE-CONTROL AFTERLOADING DEVICES AND TECHNIQUES

All afterloading techniques described in the previous section require handling of radioactive sources during the preparation and actual loading of the sources into the previously inserted apparatus. Direct handling of the radioactivity is eliminated by using a remotely controlled afterloading technique. Such equipment, developed during the early 1960s, has gained increased popularity in recent years. These units were first designed for use in gynecologic brachytherapy (Henschke 1964, O'Connell 1965, 1967, Wakabayashi 1971, Liversage 1976, Howard 1979, Utley 1984) but more recent models can be used for other sites as well. Other remote-control afterloading units use high-activity linear sources which are similarly inserted but are programmed to oscillate within the applicator (Henschke 1966, Seay 1972) so that they remain longer at a segment requiring a higher dose than at segments requiring a lower dose.

Remote-control afterloading systems can be used with various types of applicators, not only those designed for gynecologic brachytherapy, but also for those used in interstitial brachytherapy. The applicators used in gynecologic brachytherapy are similar in design to the conventional tandem and ovoid system. Remote afterloading eliminates any contact with the radioactive material for the clinical staff. The ease with which the sources are loaded and unloaded makes it possible to return them to the shielded system while personnel work near the patient, thus minimizing staff exposure (Grigsby 1991).

Remote-control afterloading units consist of a lead-shielded storage for radioactive sources, several channels for source transport, a remote loading and unloading system, and a variety of applicators which are inserted in the patient in the usual fashion. Following radiographic verification of their position using dummy sources, the optimal source configuration and dose distribution are determined and the desired loading is programmed on a microcomputer. The sources, shaped as pellets or tubes, are automatically arranged as programmed within each channel, with inactive spacers between the active pellets to achieve the desired spacing. Each source-transport tube is coupled to each receptor of the apparatus in the patient, who remains in an adjoining room during the treatment. After all personnel have left the treatment room and the door is closed, the treatment is initiated from a remote-control switch. The sources and spacers are transported via a pneumatic transport system into the applicator within a few seconds. The unloading of the sources is also accomplished via remote control and requires only a few seconds. Sedation is seldom needed, and multiple treatments are given on an out-patient basis.

HANDLING AND CARE OF RADIOACTIVE SOURCES

The safe handling of radioactivity has been a matter of concern in hospitals for many years. The generally very small, innocent-looking sources can cause considerable harm to uninformed and unsuspecting persons, but they present little danger when strict regulations with respect to handling and storage are enforced and proper facilities are provided; it is particularly necessary to have a carefully planned source-handling room (often called a "radium room") in order to minimize exposure to personnel (Farmer 1964).

An adequate inventory of sources and source activities must always be maintained for gynecologic implants. The sources should be stored in a locked room in an inaccessible area. A shielded safe with several drawers, only one of which is opened at a time, will minimize exposure to personnel who must open the safe for loading and unloading. Each drawer should contain approximately the same amount of activity to minimize exposure while a certain drawer is opened for source removal or return. Color coding of the sources simplifies identification, thus reducing the exposure time and the chances for potential errors. Only the color-coded end should be visible when the drawer is opened and the remainder of the source should be behind sufficient lead to prevent unnecessary exposure. Long-handled instruments must also be used to maintain the greatest possible distance between the source and the operator.

A lead-shielded work space immediately adjacent to the safe is necessary so that the person loading the sources into the apparatus can stand behind the shield while handling the sources using long instruments. The shield should be high enough to shield the person up to the shoulders. A lead glass window above that allows visualization of the work area and also provides some shielding of the face and head. A lamp with a magnifying glass attached is very useful when serial numbers on the sources must be verified. A clamp to hold the tubes or apparatus when the sources are being loaded, is a practical way of reducing the number of persons needed for loading.

It is a good practice to limit the number of persons with access to the safe. An inventory log book is necessary to maintain strict control of where the sources are at any given time. Routine checks of the inventory must be made to verify that all sources are in the correct location.

Sources or seeds with short half-lifes that are purchased for a certain implant are handled somewhat differently. Iridium seeds, for example, are purchased in nylon ribbons, while I-125 and Au-198 seeds usually are shipped as individual seeds. Immediately upon arrival, all seeds should be counted to ensure that nothing has been lost during transport. Shipping documents will indicate activity per seed on a certain date, as measured by the supplier. However, it is recommended that the user also determine the activity of each source before use. The seeds must be kept in a shielded and locked cabinet until they are returned to the supplier or are otherwise disposed of except, of course, when they are in the patient.

The number of seeds, the activity, and the container identification must be part of the record keeping. When the seeds are inserted into the patient, the number of seeds used, the time of the insertion, and the patient's name are noted along with the physician's name. The same information is noted at the time of removal. In addition to counting the removed seeds, the patient must be surveyed by using a sensitive survey meter to verify that no radioactivity is left behind. This negative survey must be noted in the patient's chart.

As soon as possible following removal from the patient, the sources should be returned to the supplier or otherwise disposed of. Gold-198 and I-125 seeds, which are not usually returnable, should be removed from the active area and placed in a shielded and locked place to decay and to prevent mix-up with current seeds.

The time for preparation and loading of the sources into the patient must be kept to a minimum. Specially-designed loading mechanisms can be built to minimize the exposure. Mirrors can be used to allow source preparation to be carried out behind lead shields via indirect visualization. All radioactive sources and seeds must be handled very carefully to avoid scratching, bending, or breaking. Utmost care must be taken not to cut through a seed during these procedures. Some radioactive eye plaques, for example, must not be handled by any other part than by the suture eyelets to avoid scratching of the very thin platinum shell over the radioactive material. Wipe tests of such eye plaques, to verify that no leakage has occurred, are necessary before each implant. Any leakage would result in radioactive deposits on the eye. A wipe test consists of careful wiping of the source with a moist cotton ball and then testing for the presence of radioactivity on the cotton ball, using a sensitive counter. These tests should be performed by a radiation safety officer or a physicist, depending on the organization in the institution, and the results kept in a log.

REFERENCES

Ampuero, F., Doss, L.L., Khan, M., Skipper, B., Hilgers, R.D., The Syed-Neblett interstitial template in locally advanced gynecologic malignancies, Int. J. Radiat. Oncol. Biol. Phys. 9, 1897 (1983).

Anderson, L.L., Spacing nomograph for interstitial implants of I-125 seeds Medical Physics 3, 48 (1976).

Anderson L.L., Wagner, L.K., Schauber, T.H., Memorial Hospital methods of dose calculations for 192-Ir, in Modern Interstitial and Intracavitary Radiation Cancer Management, George, F.W., III, (ed.), Masson, New York, NY, 1981.

Anderson, L.L., Hilaris, B.S., Wagner, L.K., A nomograph for planar implant planning, Endocurietherapy/Hyperthermia Oncology 1, 9 (1985).

Béclère, A., La radiothérapie des fibromes utérins, Trans. Int. Cong. Med. Section 22 pt. 2, 199, London, UK, (1914).

Bedford, M.A., The use and abuse of cobalt plaques in the treatment of choroidal malignant melanomata, Trans. Ophthalmol. Soc. U.K. 93, 139 (1973).

Bentel, G.C., Nelson, C.E., Noell, K.T., Treatment Planning and Dose Calculation in Radiation Oncology, Pergamon Press, Inc. Elmsford, NY, 1989.

Bentel, G.C., Oleson, J.R., Clarke-Pearson, D., Soper, J.T., Montana, G.S., Transperineal templates for brachytherapy treatment of pelvic malignancies - a comparison of standard and customized templates, Int. J. Radiat. Oncol. Biol. Phys. 19,751 (1990).

Bernstein, M., Gutin, P.H., Interstitial irradiation of brain tumors: A review, Neurosurgery 9, 741 (1981).

Boyer, A.L., Wang, C.C., Gitterman, M., A Luer lock afterloading device for iridium-192 brachytherapy, Int. J. Radiat. Oncol. Biol. Phys. 6, 511 (1980).

Brady, L.W., Shields, J.A., Augsburger, J.J., Day, J.L., Saunders, W. M., Castro, J.R., Munzenrider, J.E., Grogoudas, E., Posterior uveal melanomas, Radiation Oncology Annual, Phillips, T.L., Pistenmaa, D.A. (Eds.), Raven Press, New York, NY, 1984.

Calle, R., Pilleron, J.P., Schlienger, P., Vilcoq, J.R., Conservative management of operable breast cancer: Ten years' experience at the Foundation Curie, Cancer 42, 2045 (1978).

Chassagne, D., Wilson, J.F., Brachytherapy of carcinomas of the nasal vestibule (Editorial), Int. J. Radiat. Oncol. Biol. Phys. 10, 761 (1984).

Conroy, R.M., Shahbazian, A.A., Edwards, K.C., Moran, E.M., Swingle, K.F., Lewis, G.J., Pribam, H.F.W., A new method for treating carcinomatous biliary obstruction with intracatheter radium, Cancer 49, 1321 (1982).

Cunningham, D.E., Stryker, J.A., Velkley, D.E., Chung, C.K., Routine clinical estimation of rectal, rectosigmoidal, and bladder doses from intracavitary brachytherapy in the treatment of carcinoma of the cervix, Int. J. Radiat. Oncol. Biol. Phys. 7, 653 (1981).

Dale, R.G., Calculation by computer of dose-distributions for superficial gold-198 implants and the derivation of optimized distribution rules, Brit. J. Radiol. 49, 533 (1976).

Ellsworth, R.M., The practical management of retinoblastoma, Trans. Am. Ophthalmol. Soc. 67, 462 (1969).

Farmer, F.T., Haggith, J.W., The design of a protective radium and radioisotope laboratory, Brit. J. Radiol. 37, 938 (1964).

Feder, B.H., Syed A.M.N., Neblett, D., Treatment of extensive carcinoma of the cervix with the 'transperineal parametrial butterfly': A preliminary report on the revival of Waterman's approach, Int. J. Radiat. Oncol. Biol. Phys. 4, 735 (1978).

Fisher, B., Montague, E., Redmond, C., other NSABP investigators, Comparison of radical mastectomy with alternative treatments of primary breast cancer: A first report of results from a prospective randomized clinical trial, Cancer 39, 2827 (1977).

Flemming, P., Syed, A.M.N., Neblett, D., Puthawala, A., George, F.W. III, Townsend, D., Description of an afterloading Ir-192 interstitial-intercavitary technique in the treatment of carcinoma of the vagina, Obstet. Gynecol. 55, 525 (1980).

Forssell, G., Radium behandling av maligna tumörer i kvinnliga genitalia, Hygien 74, 445 (1912).

Fletcher, G.H., Brown, T.C., Rutledge, F.N., Clinical significance of rectal and bladder dose measurements in radium therapy of cancer of the uterine cervix, Am. J. Roentgenol. 79, 421 (1958).

Fletcher, G.H., Textbook of Radiology, (3rd ed.), Lea & Febiger, Philadelphia, PA, 1980.

Fletcher, M.S., Dawson, J.L., Wheeler, P.G., Brinkley, D., Nunnerly, H., Williams, R., Treatment of high bile duct carcinoma by internal radiotherapy with Ir-192 wire, Lancet 2, 172 (1981).

Fu, K.K., Newman, H., Phillips, T.L., Treatment of locally recurrent carcinoma of the nasopharynx, Radiology 117, 425 (1975).

Gillin, M.T., Kline, R.W., Wilson, J.F., Cox, J.D., Single and double plane implants: A comparison of the Manchester system with the Paris system, Int. J. Radiat. Oncol. Biol. Phys. 10, 921 (1984).

Goode, R., Fee, W., Goffinet, D., Martinez, A., Radioactive suture in the treatment of head and neck cancer, The Laryngoscope 89, 349 (1979).

Gray, M.J., Kottmeier, H.L., Rectal and bladder injuries following therapy for carcinoma of the cervix at the Radiumhemmet, Am. J. Obstet. Gynecol. 74, 1294 (1957).

Grigsby, P.W., Perez, C.A., Eichling, J., Purdy, J., Slessinger, E., Reduction in radiation exposure to nursing personnel with the use of remote afterloading brachytherapy devices, Int. J. Radiat. Oncol. Biol. Phys. 20, 627 (1991).

Gutin, P.H., Phillips, T.L., Hosobuchi, Y., Wara, W.M., MacKay, A.R., Weaver, K.A., Lamb, S., Hurst, S., Permanent and removable implants for brachytherapy of brain tumors, Int. J. Radiat. Oncol. Biol. Phys. 7, 1371 (1981).

Gutin, P.H., Dormandy, R.H., Jr., A coaxial catheter system for afterloading radioactive sources for the interstitial irradiation of brain tumors, (Technical Note), J. Neurosurg. 56, 734 (1982).

Gutin, P.H., Phillips, T.L., Hosobuchi, Y., Local treatment of malignant brain tumors by removable stereotactically implanted radioactive isotopes, Progress in Radio-Oncology II, Karcher, K.H., Kogelnik, H.D., Reinartz, G., (Eds.), Raven Press, New York, NY, 1982.

Gutin, P.H., Phillips, T.L., Wara, W.M., Leibel, S.A., Hosobuchi, Y., Levin, V.A., Weaver, K., Lamb, S., Brachytherapy of recurrent malignant brain tumors with removable high activity iodine-125 sources, J. Neurosurg. 60, 61 (1984).

Hamberger, A.D., Unal, A., Gershenson, D.M., Fletcher, G.H., Analysis of the severe complications of irradiation of carcinoma of the cervix: Whole pelvis irradiation and intracavitary radium, Int. J. Radiat. Oncol. Biol. Phys. 9, 367 (1983).

Harris, J.R., Botnick, L., Bloomer, W.D., Chaffey, J.T., Hellman, S., Primary radiation therapy for early breast cancer: The experience of the Joint Center for Radiation Therapy, Int. J. Radiat. Oncol. Biol. Phys. 7, 1549 (1981).

Harter, D.J., Delclos, L., Sealed sources in synthetic absorbable suture, Radiology 116, 721 (1975).

Hawliczek, R., Neubauer, J., Schmidt, W.F.O., Grunert, P., Coia, L.R., A new device for interstitial ^{125}iodine seed implantation, Int. J. Radiat. Oncolo. Biol. Phys. 20, 621 (1991).

Henschke, U.K., Hilaris, B.S., Mahan, G.D., Afterloading in interstitial and intracavitary radiation therapy, Am. J. Roentgenol. 90, 386 (1963).

Henschke, U.K., Hilaris, B.S., Mahan, G.D., Remote afterloading with intracavitary applicators, Radiology 83, 344 (1964).

Henschke, U.K., Hilaris, B.S., Mahan, G.D., Intracavitary radiation therapy of cancer of the uterine cervix by remote afterloading with cycling sources, Am. J. Roentgenol. 96, 45 (1966).

Henschke, U.K., Cevc, P., Dimension averaging, a simple method for dosimetry of interstitial implants, Radiobiol. Radiother. 9, 287 (1968).

Herskovic, A., Heaston, D., Engler, M.J., Fishburn, R.I., Jones, R.S., Noell, K.T., Irradiation of biliary carcinoma, Radiology 139, 219 (1981).

Hilaris, B.S., Luomanen, R.K., Beattie, E.J., Integrated irradiation and surgery in the treatment of apical lung cancer, Cancer 27, 1369 (1971).

Hilaris, B.S., Martini, N., Batata, M.A., Beattie, E.J., Interstitial irradiation for unresectable carcinoma of the lung, Ann. Thorac. Surg. 20, 491 (1975).

Hilaris, B.S., Martini, N., Loumanen, R.K., Endobronchial interstitial implantation, Clinical Bulletin 9, 17 (1979).

Hilaris, B.S., Martini, N., Interstitial brachytherapy in cancer of the lung: A 20 year experience, Int. J. Radiat. Oncol. Biol. Phys. 5, 1951 (1979).

Hilaris, B.S., Martini, N., Nori, D., Beattie, E.J. Jr., The place for radiotherapy in the treatment of lung cancer, World J. Surg. 5, 675 (1981).

Hilaris, B.S., Nori, D., Beattie, E.J., Martini, N., Value of perioperative brachytherapy in the management of non-oat cell carcinoma of the lung, Int. J. Radiat. Oncol. Biol. Phys. 9, 1161 (1983).

Hilaris, B.S., Gomez, J., Nori, D., Anderson, L.L., Martini, N., Combined surgery, intraoperative brachytherapy, and postoperative external beam radiation in stage III non-small cell lung cancer, Cancer 55, 1226 (1985).

Howard, N., Cathetron: High intensity cobalt, Int. J. Radiat. Oncol. Biol. Phys. 5, 1885 (1979).

Ibrahim, E., Chassagne, D., Cachin, Y., Haie, C., Les epithélioma du seuil narinaire: A propos de 36 cas traités à l'Institute Gustave - Roussy de 1961 a 1975, Les Cahiers D'O.R.L. XVII, 109 (1982).

Ikeda, H., Kuroda, C., Uchida, H., Miyata, Y., Masaki, N., Shigematsu, Y., Monden, M., Okamura, J., Intraluminal irradiation with iridium-192 wires for extrahepatic bile duct carcinoma: A preliminary report, Nippon Igaku Hoshasen Gakkai Zasshi 39, 1356 (1979).

Johnson, D.W., Safai, C., Goffinet, D.R., Malignant obstructive jaundice: Treatment with external beam and intracavitary radiotherapy, Int. J. Radiat. Oncol. Biol. Phys. 11, 411 (1985).

Karolis, C., Reay-Young, P.S., Walsh, W., Velautham, G., Silicone Plesiotherapy molds, Int. J. Radiat. Oncol. Biol. Phys. 9, 569 (1983).

Kumar, P.P., Good, R.R., Rainbolt, C., Epstein, B.E., Chu, W.K., Jones, E.O., Cascione, C.J., Hussain, M.B., Low morbidity following transperineal percutaneous template technique for permanent iodine-125 endocurie therapy of prostate cancer, Endocurietherapy/Hyperthermia Oncology 2, 119 (1986).

Kwan, D.K., Kagan, A.R., Olch, A.J., Chan, P.Y.M., Hintz, B.L., Wollin, M., Single and double plane iridium-192 interstitial implants: Implantation guidelines and dosimetry, Medical Physics 10, 456 (1983).

Lee, K.H., Kagan, A.R., Nussbaum, H., Wollin, M., Winkley, J.H., Norman, A., Analysis of dose, dose-rate and treatment time in the production of injuries by radium treatment for cancer of the uterine cervix, Brit. J. Radiol. 49, 430 (1976).

Levene, M.B., Interstitial therapy of breast cancer, Int. J. Radiat. Oncol. Biol. Phys. 2, 1157 (1977).

Lichter, A.S., Dillon, M.B., Rosenshein, N.B., Order, S.E., The use of custom molds for intracavitary treatment of carcinoma of the cervix, Int. J. Radiat. Oncol. Biol. Phys. 4, 874 (1978).

Liversage, W.E., Martin-Smith, P., Ramsey, N.W., The treatment of uterine carcinoma using the cathetron, Brit. J. Radiol. 40, 887 (1976).

Lommatzsch, P., Treatment of choroidal melanomas with Ru-106, Rh-106 beta ray applicators, Surg. Ophthalmol. 19, 85 (1974).

MacKay, A.R., Gutin, P.H., Hosobuchi, Y., Norman, D., Computed tomography-directed stereotaxy for biopsy and interstitial irradiation of brain tumors (Technical Note), Neurosurg. 11, 38 (1982).

Marchese, M.J., Nori, D., Anderson, L.L., Hilaris, B.S., A versatile permanent planar implant technique utilizing iodine-125 seeds imbedded in Gel-foam, Int. J. Radiat. Oncol. Biol. Phys. 10, 747 (1984).

Marinello, G., Valero, M., Leung, S., Pierquin, B., Comparative dosimetry between iridium wires and seed ribbons, Int. J. Radiat. Oncol. Biol. Phys. 11, 1733 (1985).

Martinez, A., Cox, R.S., Edmundson, G.K., A multiple-site perineal applicator (MUPIT) for treatment of prostatic, anorectal, and gynecologic malignancies, Int. J. Radiat. Oncol. Biol. Phys. 10, 297 (1984).

Martinez, A., Edmundson, G.K., Cox, R.S., Gunderson, L.L., Howes, A.F., Combination of external beam irradiation and the multiple-site perineal applicator (MUPIT) for treatment of locally advanced or recurrent prostatic, anorectal and gynecologic malignancies, Int. J. Radiat. Oncol. Biol. Phys. 11, 391 (1985).

Million, R.R., Mauderli, W., Bruno, F.P., Modification of technique for bladder and rectal measurements in carcinoma of the cervix, Radiology 60, 921 (1966).

Montana, G.S., Fowler, W.C., Varia, M.A., Walton, L.A., Kirsch, M., Halle, S.J., McCafferty, B., Carcinoma of the cervix stage IB: Results of treatment with radiation therapy, Int. J. Radiat. Oncol. Biol. Phys. 9, 45 (1983).

Montana, G.S., Fowler, W.C., Varia, M.A., Walton, L.A., Mack, Y., Analysis of results of radiation therapy for stage II carcinoma of the cervix, Cancer 5, 956 (1985).

Montana, G.S., Fowler, W.C., Varia, M.A., Walton, L.A., Mack, Y., Shemansky, L., Carcinoma of the cervix stage III: Results of radiation therapy, Cancer 1, 148 (1986).

Moore, R.F., Choroidal sarcoma treated by the intraocular insertion of radon seeds, Brit. J. Ophthalmol. 14, 145 (1930).

Mundinger, F., Langzeitergebnisse der stereotaktischen Radio-Isotopenbestrahlung von Hypophysentumoren. Strahlentherapie 116, 523 (1961).

Mundinger, F., Die interstitielle Radioisotopen-Bestrahlung von Hirntumoren mit vergleichenden Langzeitergebnissen zur Röntgentiefentherapie, Acta. Neurochir. 11, 89 (1963).

Mundinger, F., Ergebnisse der primär und kombiniert operativ-stereotaktischen Radioisotopenbestrahlung von Hypophysenadenomen. Vortrag I; Jahrestagung d. Ges f. Nuklearmedizin, Freiburg , Germany (1963).

Mundinger, F., Die stereotaktischoperative Behandlung des Parkinson-Syndroms, Pathophysiologie, Ergebnisse und Indikationsstellung, Med. Klin. 29, 1181 (1963).

Mundinger, F., Diskussionsbemerkung zu den Resultaten der Hypophysektomie mit statistischen Auswertungen, Tag Ges f. Nuklearmedizin, Freiburg, Germany 17, 19, 10 (1963).

Mundinger, F., Dynamics of technetium 99m in normal and pathological CSF-spaces with digital autofluoroscope (Gammacamera), Meeting Brit. German Neurological Societies, London, UK, 1968.

Mundinger, F., The Treatment of Brain Tumors with Interstitially Applied Radioactive Isotopes, Radionuclide applications in Neurology and Neurosurgery, Wange, Y., Paoletti, P., (Eds.), Charles C. Thomas, Inc., Springfield, IL, 1970.

Mundinger, F., Birg, W., Ostertag, C.B., Treatment of small cerebral gliomas with CT aided stereotaxic curie therapy, Neuroradiology 16, 564 (1978).

O'Connell, D., Howard, N., Joslin, C.A.F., Ramsey, N.W., Liversage, W.E., A new remotely controlled unit for the treatment of uterine carcinoma, Lancet 2, 570 (1965).

O'Connell, D., Howard, N., Joslin, C.A.F., Ramsey, N.W., Liversage, W.E., The treatment of uterine carcinoma using the cathetron, Brit. J. Radiol. 40, 882 (1967).

Orton, C.G., Wolf-Rosenblum, S., Dose dependence of complication rates in cervix cancer radiotherapy, Int. J. Radiat. Oncol. Biol. Phys. 12, 37 (1986).

Packer, S., Rotman, M., Radiotherapy of choroidal melanoma with iodine-125, Ophthalmology 87, 582 (1980).

Packer, S., Rotman, M., Fairchild, R.G., Albert, D.M., Atkins, H.L., Chan, B., Irradiation of choroidal melanoma with iodine-125 ophthalmic plaque, Arch. Ophthalmol. 98, 1453 (1980).

Palos, B.B., Pooler, B.A., Goffinet, D.R., Martinez, A., A method for inserting I-125 seeds into absorbable sutures for permanent implantation in tissue, Int. J. Radiat. Oncol. Biol. Phys. 6, 381 (1980).

Perez, C.A., Breaux, S., Bedwinek, J.M., Madoc-Jones, H., Camel, H.M., Purdy, J.A., Walz, B.J., Radiation therapy alone in the treatment of carcinoma of the uterine cervix II: Analysis of complications, Cancer 54, 235 (1984).

Pierquin, B., Dutreix, A., Paine, C.H., Chassagne, D., Marinello, G., Ash, D., The Paris system in interstitial radiation therapy, Acta. Radiol. Oncol. 17, 33 (1978).

Pierquin, B., Chassagne, D.J., Chahbazian, C.M., Wilson, J.F., Brachytherapy, Warren H. Green, Inc., St. Louis, MO, 1979.

Pierquin, B., Owen, R., Maylin, C., Otmezquine, Y., Raynal, M., Muller, N., Hannoun, S., Radical radiation therapy of breast cancer, Int. J. Radiat. Oncol. Biol. Phys. 6, 17 (1980).

Pitts, H.C., Waterman, G.W., Report of results of radium treatment of carcinoma of cervix, Am. J. Obstet. Gynecol. 29, 607 (1930).

Pourquier, H., Dubois, J.B., Delard, R., Cancer of the uterine cervix: Dosimetric guidelines for prevention of late rectal and rectosigmoid complications as a result of radiotherapeutic treatment, Int. J. Radiat. Oncol. Biol. Phys. 8, 1887 (1982).

Prosnitz, L.R., Goldenburg, I.S., Packard, R.A., Levene, M.B., Harris, J., Hellman, S., Wallner, P.E., Brady, L.W., Mansfield, C.M., Kramer, S., Radiation therapy as initial treatment for early stage cancer of the breast without mastectomy, Cancer 39, 917 (1977).

Roswit, B., Malsky, S.J., Reid, C.B., Amato, C.G., Gobels, R., In vivo radiation dosimetry: Review of a 12 year experience, Radiology 97, 413 (1970).

Schray, M.F., McDougall, J.C., Martinez, A. , Edmundson, G.K., Cortese, D.A., Management of malignant airway obstruction: clinical and dosimetric considerations using an iridium-192 afterloading technique in conjunction with the neodymium laser, Int. J. Radiat. Oncol. Biol. Phys. 11, 403 (1985).

Scott, W.P., Cervicovaginal irradiator - a triple applicator, Am. J. Roentgenol. 96, 52 (1966).

Scott, W.P., Simplified interstitial therapy technique (Vicryl I-125) for unresectable lung cancer, Radiology 117, 734 (1975 A).

Scott, W.P., Interstitial therapy, using non-absorbable (iridium-192 nylon ribbon) and absorbable (I-125 'Vicryl') suturing techniques, Am. J. Roentg. Radiat. Ther. Nucl. Med. 124, No. 4, (1975 B).

Scott, W.P., A spacer/injector needle for I-125 and other radioactive sources in permanent seed implant, Radiology 122, 832 (1977).

Scott, W.P., Implanter for radioactive sources, Int. J. Radiat. Oncol. Biol. Phys. 7, 263 (1981).

Sealy, R., le Roux, P.L.M., Rapley, F., Hering, E., Shackleton, D., Sevel, D., The treatment of ophthalmic tumours with low energy sources, Brit. J. Radiol. 49, 551 (1976).

Seay, D.G., Hilbert, J.W., Moeller, J., Alderman, S.J., von Essen, C.F., Therapy using a new remote-controlled high-intensity afterloading device, Radiology 105, 709 (1972).

Shipley, W.U., Nardi, G.L., Cohen, A.M., Ling, C.C., Iodine-125 implant as boost therapy in patient irradiated for localized pancreatic carcinoma: A comparative study to surgical resection, Cancer 45, 709 (1980).

Shipley, W.U., Kopelson, G., Novack, D.J., Ling, C.C., Dretler, S.P., Prout, G.R., Jr., Preoperative irradiation, lymphadenectomy, and I-125 implant for selected patients with localized prostatic carcinoma: A correlation of implant dosimetry with clinical results, J. Urol. 24, 639 (1981).

Smith, H.S., Lapinski, M.V., Barr, C.E., A simplified method for intracavitary radiation for recurrent nasopharyngeal carcinoma, Radiology 131, 534 (1979).

Stallard, H.B., Radiotherapy of malignant intraocular neoplasms, Brit. J. Ophthalmol. 32, 618 (1948).

Stallard, H.B., Malignant melanoblastoma of the choroid, Mod. Prob. Ophthalmol. 7, 18 (1968).

Strockbine, M.F., Hancock, J.E., Fletcher, G.H., Complications in 831 patients with squamous cell carcinoma of the intact uterine cervix treated with 3000 rad or more whole pelvis radiation, Am. J. Roentgenol. 58, 293 (1970).

Suit, H.D., Moore, E.B., Fletcher, G.H., Worsnop, B., Modification of Fletcher ovoid system for afterloading using standard size radium tubes (milligram and microgram), Radiology 81, 126 (1963).

Syed, A.M.N., Feder, B.H., Technique of afterloading interstitial implants, Radiologica Clinica 46, 458 (1977).

Syed, A.M.N., Puthawala, A., Neblett, D., George, F.W.III, Myint, U.S., Lipsett, J.A., Jackson, B.R., Flemming, P.A., Primary treatment of carcinoma of the lower rectum and anal canal by combination of external irradiation and interstitial implant, Radiology 128, 199 (1978).

Syed, A.M.N., Feder, B.H., George, F.W., Neblett, D., Iridium-192 afterloaded implant in the retreatment of head and neck cancers, Brit. J. Radiol. 51, 814 (1978).

Syed, A.M.N., Puthawala, A., Tansey, L.A., Shanberg, A.M., Neblett, D., McNamara, C., Temporary iridium-192 implantation in the management of carcinoma of the prostate, Brachytherapy Oncology, Hilaris, B., Batata, M. (Eds.) New York Memorial Sloan-Kettering Cancer Center, New York, NY, 1983.

Syed, A.M.N., Puthawala, A.A., Severance, S.R., Zamost, B.J., Intraluminal irradiation in the treatment of esophageal cancer, <u>Endocurietherapy/ Hyperthermia Oncology</u> 3, 105 (1987).

Szikla, G. (Ed.) <u>Stereotactic Cerebral Irradiation</u>, Elsevier/North Holland, Amsterdam, Netherlands, 1979.

Talairach, J., Ruggiero, G., Aboulker, J., David, M., A new method of treatment of inoperable brain tumours by stereotaxic implantation of radioactive gold - a preliminary report, <u>Brit. J. Radiol.</u> 28, 62 (1955).

Utley, J.F., von Essen, C.F., Horn, R.A., Moeller, J.H., High dose rate afterloading brachytherapy in carcinoma of the uterine cervix, <u>Int. J. Radiat. Oncol. Biol. Phys.</u> 10, 2259 (1984).

Villasanta, U., Complications of radiotherapy for carcinoma of the uterine cervix, <u>Am. J. Obstet. Gynecol.</u> 114, No. 66, 717 (1972).

Vora, N., Forell, B., Desai, K., Bradley, W., Technique to maintain separation of mandibular loops in interstitial implantation of head and neck tumors, <u>Int. J. Radiat. Oncol. Biol. Phys.</u> 9, 261 (1983).

Wakabayashi, M., High dose rate intracavitary radiotherapy using the Ralstron, <u>Hokkaido Univ. Med. Lib. Series</u>, Vol 4., Hokkaido Univ. School of Medicine, Sapporo, Japan, 1971.

Wang, C.C., Schulz, M.D., Management of locally recurrent carcinoma of the nasopharynx, <u>Radiology</u> 86, 900 (1966).

Wang, C.C., Busse, J., Gitterman, M., A simple afterloading applicator for intracavitary irradiation for carcinoma of the nasopharynx, <u>Radiology</u> 115, 737 (1975).

Whitmore, W.F., Hilaris, B.S., Grabstald, H., Retropubic implantation of I-125 in the treatment of prostatic cancer, <u>J. Urol.</u> 108, 918 (1972).

Zwicker, R.D., Schmidt-Ullrich, R., Schiller, B., Planning of Ir-192 seed implants for boost irradiation of the breast, <u>Int. J. Radiat. Oncol. Biol. Phys.</u> 11, 2163 (1985).

Yankauer, S., Two cases of lung tumor treated bronchoscopically, <u>New York Medical Journal and Medical Record</u> 115, 741 (1922).

PROBLEMS

1. Afterloading techniques were developed primarily to reduce

    a) the possibilities of errors in loading
    b) the time required for the implant
    c) exposure to personnel

2. Radioactive sources frequently used in tandems and ovoids are in the shape of

    a) tubes
    b) seeds
    c) needles

3. Radioactive isotopes used in tandems and ovoids are usually

    a) iridium-192
    b) cobalt-60
    c) cesium-137
    d) strontium-90

4. Point "A" is defined in gynecologic implants to be a point located

    a) 2 cm cephalad of the external cervical os and 5 cm lateral to the patient's midline

    b) 2 cm cephalad of the external cervical os and 2 cm lateral to the patient's midline

    c) 2 cm cephalad of the external cervical os and 5 cm lateral to the uterine tandem

    d) 2 cm cephalad of the external cervical os and 2 cm lateral to the uterine tandem

5. In which of the following situations is the use of a tandem and ovoid *least* useful

    a) in a patient with a large exophytic lesion in the cervix, extending into the vaginal apex

    b) in a patient who has undergone a radical hysterectomy for squamous cell carcinoma of the cervix and now has a recurrence in the vaginal apex

c) in a patient who has undergone a supracervical hysterectomy and now has a recurrence in the cervical stump

6. Open-ended plastic tubing can be inserted and loaded

   a) in implants where the tube can exit the tissue on the opposite side
   b) in transperineal implants where there is no exit on the opposite side
   c) in a brain implant where there is no exit on the opposite side

7. Ophthalmic plaques can be constructed for use with

   a) cobalt-60
   b) iodine-125
   c) ruthenium-106
   d) iridium-192
   e) all of the above

8. High-activity iodine-125 seeds (40 mCi/seed) are frequently used in

   a) ophthalmic plaques
   b) brain implants
   c) lung implants
   d) esophageal implants

9. Isotopes used in permanent implants are most frequently

   a) iodine-125 and gold-198
   b) iridium-192 and gold-198
   c) cesium-137 and iridium-192
   d) radium-226 and iodine-125

10. Isotopes used in permanent implants are selected primarily because of their

    a) specific activity
    b) half-value thickness
    c) half-life
    d) durability

11. Customized transperineal templates are superior to standard templates because

    a) they are easier to load
    b) they are more comfortable for the patient

c) they can be designed to cover the target and loaded to deliver better dose uniformity
d) they can be designed to better cover the target and spare more normal tissue

12. Surface molds can be used to treat all of the following tumors *except*

   a) a deep-seated tumor in the pelvic side wall
   b) a lesion on the hard palate
   c) a lesion in an exenterated orbit
   d) a 1 cm deep lesion in the preauricular region

13. Remote afterloading apparatus was first designed for

   a) high-dose rate treatment in any site
   b) gynecologic implants
   c) intraoperative use
   d) low-dose rate treatment in any implant

14. To produce approximately the same dose rate on the surface of an ovoid the source activity must

   a) be decreased as the ovoid diameter increases
   b) be increased as the ovoid diameter decreases
   c) be increased as the ovoid diameter increases
   d) not be changed

15. In ophthalmic plaque treatment of ocular melanoma the scleral dose may exceed

   a)   80,000 cGy
   b)   60,000 cGy
   c)   40,000 cGy
   d) 100,000 cGy

16. When handling radioactive sources, long-handled instruments must be used to

   a) reduce the time spent loading
   b) reduce the exposure to the hands of the loader
   c) increase the distance to the patient and thus reduce exposure to the patient
   d) increase the speed of loading

17. Which of the following statements *best* describes the proper removal of an implant

    a) the radioactive sources and the apparatus holding the sources are all removed simultaneously
    b) the radioactive sources are removed first and then the apparatus holding the sources
    c) the apparatus holding the radioactive sources is not removed until all radioactive sources are accounted for and a negative survey has been obtained
    d) the order in which the implant sources and apparatus is removed is not important as long as the patient does not experience any pain

18. The use of intraluminal implants has been described for various sites *except* for the

    a) esophagus
    b) duodenum
    c) biliary duct
    d) bronchus

19. The isotope most frequently used in nasopharyngeal implants is

    a) cesium-137
    b) gold-198
    c) iodine-125
    d) strontium-90

20. The use of radium is rapidly being abandoned because

    a) it is difficult to buy
    b) it is especially hazardous
    c) the half-life is too long
    d) it is too expensive

SOLUTIONS

1. c
2. a
3. c
4. d
5. b
6. a
7. e

8. b
9. a
10. c
11. c
12. a
13. b
14. c

15. c
16. b
17. c
18. b
19. a
20. b

APPENDIX

TABLE A.1

PERCENTAGE DEPTH DOSE DATA FOR
COBALT-60, SSD 80 cm

| Depth (cm) | Field size (side of square field, cm) | | | | | | |
	5.0	**8.0**	**10.0**	**12.0**	**15.0**	**18.0**	**20.0**
0.5	100.0	100.0	100.0	100.0	100.0	100.0	100.0
1.0	97.0	97.8	98.1	98.3	98.4	98.4	98.4
2.0	91.3	92.7	93.2	93.6	93.8	93.9	94.0
3.0	85.6	87.6	88.3	88.7	89.2	89.5	89.6
4.0	80.2	82.5	83.3	83.9	84.6	85.0	85.2
5.0	74.8	77.4	78.4	79.2	80.0	80.5	80.9
6.0	69.5	72.3	73.5	74.3	75.3	76.0	76.5
7.0	64.4	67.5	68.7	69.7	70.7	71.6	72.2
8.0	59.4	62.7	64.0	65.1	66.4	67.4	68.1
9.0	55.0	58.2	59.6	60.7	62.1	63.3	64.2
10.0	50.7	54.0	55.5	56.8	58.3	59.5	60.4
11.0	46.9	50.1	51.7	53.0	54.6	55.9	56.9
12.0	43.2	46.4	48.0	49.4	51.0	52.5	53.5
13.0	40.0	43.2	44.8	46.2	47.8	49.3	50.3
14.0	36.8	40.1	41.7	43.1	44.8	46.3	47.3
15.0	34.1	37.2	38.9	40.2	41.9	43.5	44.5
16.0	31.5	34.5	36.1	37.5	39.2	40.8	41.9
17.0	29.3	32.2	33.8	35.1	36.8	38.4	39.5
18.0	27.1	29.9	31.5	32.8	34.5	36.2	37.3
19.0	25.1	27.8	29.3	30.6	32.3	34.0	35.2
20.0	23.1	25.7	27.2	28.5	30.2	32.0	33.1
25.0	16.3	18.4	19.7	20.9	22.4	23.9	25.0
30.0	10.6	12.3	13.4	14.4	15.7	17.1	18.0

TABLE A.2

PERCENTAGE DEPTH DOSE FOR
4 MV PHOTONS, SSD 80 CM

Depth (cm)	Field size (side of square field, cm)						
	5.0	**8.0**	**10.0**	**12.0**	**15.0**	**18.0**	**20.0**
1.0	100.0	100.0	100.0	100.0	100.0	100.0	100.0
2.0	96.4	97.0	97.2	97.3	97.5	97.6	97.7
3.0	91.2	92.2	92.5	92.7	93.0	93.3	93.5
4.0	95.5	86.9	87.4	87.8	88.4	88.9	89.2
5.0	80.0	81.8	82.4	82.8	83.2	83.8	84.1
6.0	74.4	76.8	77.7	78.2	78.7	79.3	79.6
7.0	69.3	72.0	73.0	73.7	74.4	74.9	75.3
8.0	64.7	67.6	68.6	69.3	70.0	70.8	71.3
9.0	60.2	63.3	64.3	65.1	66.0	66.9	67.6
10.0	56.4	59.3	60.5	61.4	62.4	63.3	63.9
11.0	52.5	55.5	56.7	57.6	58.7	59.7	60.3
12.0	48.7	51.8	53.1	54.1	55.2	56.2	56.9
13.0	45.4	48.4	49.8	50.8	51.9	53.0	53.7
14.0	42.3	45.3	46.7	47.7	48.8	49.9	50.6
15.0	39.5	42.3	43.7	44.7	45.9	47.0	47.7
16.0	36.8	39.5	40.8	41.8	43.0	44.2	45.0
17.0	34.4	37.0	38.3	39.3	40.6	41.8	42.6
18.0	32.1	34.6	35.9	37.0	38.2	39.4	40.2
19.0	29.8	32.4	33.7	34.7	36.0	37.1	37.9
20.0	27.7	30.1	31.5	32.5	33.8	35.0	35.8
25.0	19.8	21.8	22.9	23.9	25.0	26.0	26.7
30.0	13.9	15.6	16.5	17.3	18.4	19.4	20.1

TABLE A.3

TISSUE-AIR RATIOS FOR COBALT-60

Field size (side of square field, cm)

Depth (cm)	0.0	5.0	8.0	10.0	12.0	15.0	18.0	20.0	30.0	35.0
0.5	1.000	1.012	1.022	1.030	1.039	1.049	1.056	1.060	1.080	1.090
1.0	0.966	0.994	1.012	1.023	1.033	1.044	1.052	1.056	1.076	1.086
2.0	0.904	0.957	0.982	0.995	1.007	1.020	1.028	1.033	1.056	1.067
3.0	0.845	0.919	0.949	0.964	0.977	0.993	1.002	1.008	1.035	1.049
4.0	0.792	0.880	0.914	0.931	0.946	0.963	0.974	0.981	1.013	1.029
5.0	0.741	0.839	0.877	0.895	0.912	0.931	0.944	0.951	0.988	1.007
6.0	0.694	0.797	0.838	0.857	0.875	0.895	0.910	0.919	0.963	0.985
7.0	0.649	0.753	0.798	0.818	0.837	0.859	0.875	0.885	0.935	0.960
8.0	0.608	0.710	0.757	0.778	0.798	0.822	0.841	0.852	0.907	0.935
9.0	0.570	0.670	0.716	0.739	0.759	0.785	0.805	0.818	0.880	0.911
10.0	0.534	0.631	0.678	0.701	0.723	0.750	0.771	0.784	0.849	0.881
11.0	0.501	0.595	0.642	0.665	0.687	0.716	0.738	0.752	0.820	0.854
12.0	0.469	0.559	0.606	0.629	0.652	0.681	0.705	0.719	0.791	0.827
13.0	0.440	0.527	0.574	0.598	0.620	0.650	0.674	0.689	0.762	0.798
14.0	0.412	0.495	0.541	0.566	0.589	0.619	0.643	0.658	0.733	0.770
15.0	0.387	0.467	0.512	0.536	0.559	0.589	0.614	0.629	0.705	0.743
20.0	0.278	0.345	0.383	0.405	0.427	0.457	0.483	0.500	0.584	0.626
25.0	0.211	0.265	0.296	0.316	0.335	0.362	0.386	0.402	0.479	0.517
30.0	0.144	0.185	0.209	0.226	0.244	0.268	0.290	0.304	0.374	0.409

TABLE A.4

TISSUE-AIR RATIOS FOR 4 MV PHOTONS

Depth (cm)	Field size (side of square field, cm)								
	0.0	5.0	8.0	10.0	11.0	12.0	15.0	17.0	20.0
1.0	0.999	1.017	1.029	1.036	1.039	1.042	1.051	1.055	1.061
2.0	0.973	1.004	1.022	1.031	1.035	1.039	1.049	1.055	1.061
3.0	0.928	0.972	0.994	1.004	1.009	1.014	1.025	1.031	1.040
4.0	0.881	0.933	0.959	0.971	0.977	0.982	0.996	1.004	1.015
5.0	0.835	0.892	0.923	0.936	0.942	0.947	0.960	0.967	0.978
6.0	0.780	0.848	0.885	0.902	0.909	0.915	0.928	0.936	0.947
7.0	0.734	0.807	0.847	0.866	0.874	0.880	0.896	0.905	0.915
8.0	0.690	0.769	0.812	0.831	0.839	0.846	0.862	0.871	0.884
9.0	0.655	0.731	0.775	0.795	0.803	0.810	0.828	0.839	0.854
10.0	0.612	0.697	0.743	0.763	0.771	0.779	0.799	0.810	0.825
11.0	0.582	0.663	0.707	0.729	0.738	0.747	0.767	0.779	0.794
12.0	0.552	0.628	0.672	0.695	0.705	0.714	0.736	0.747	0.763
13.0	0.521	0.597	0.641	0.664	0.675	0.684	0.706	0.717	0.733
14.0	0.490	0.566	0.610	0.634	0.644	0.653	0.676	0.688	0.704
15.0	0.462	0.538	0.581	0.604	0.615	0.623	0.646	0.659	0.676
16.0	0.435	0.510	0.553	0.575	0.585	0.593	0.617	0.630	0.643
17.0	0.413	0.486	0.527	0.549	0.559	0.568	0.592	0.605	0.623
18.0	0.392	0.462	0.501	0.524	0.534	0.543	0.567	0.580	0.598
19.0	0.370	0.437	0.476	0.498	0.509	0.518	0.542	0.555	0.573
20.0	0.348	0.413	0.450	0.473	0.483	0.492	0.517	0.530	0.548
21.0	0.332	0.394	0.430	0.452	0.462	0.471	0.495	0.509	0.526
22.0	0.315	0.375	0.410	0.431	0.441	0.450	0.474	0.487	0.504
23.0	0.299	0.356	0.389	0.410	0.420	0.428	0.453	0.466	0.483
24.0	0.282	0.337	0.369	0.389	0.398	0.407	0.431	0.444	0.461
25.0	0.269	0.322	0.353	0.372	0.381	0.390	0.413	0.426	0.443
26.0	0.255	0.306	0.336	0.355	0.364	0.372	0.395	0.408	0.424
27.0	0.242	0.291	0.320	0.338	0.347	0.355	0.377	0.390	0.406
28.0	0.228	0.275	0.304	0.322	0.330	0.338	0.359	0.372	0.388
29.0	0.214	0.260	0.287	0.305	0.313	0.320	0.341	0.354	0.370
30.0	0.201	0.244	0.271	0.288	0.296	0.303	0.323	0.336	0.352

TABLE A.5

TISSUE-MAXIMUM RATIOS FOR 10 MV PHOTONS

Depth (cm)	Field size (side of square field, cm)										
	0.0	5.0	6.0	8.0	10.0	12.0	15.0	17.0	20.0	25.0	30.0
1.0	0.835	0.859	0.864	0.874	0.884	0.888	0.893	0.896	0.903	0.913	0.922
2.0	0.956	0.968	0.970	0.971	0.972	0.975	0.980	0.981	0.982	0.985	0.985
2.5	1.000	1.000	1.000	1.000	1.000	1.000	1.000	1.000	1.000	1.000	1.000
3.0	0.983	1.000	1.000	1.000	1.000	1.000	1.000	1.000	1.000	1.000	1.000
4.0	0.955	0.992	0.992	0.993	0.993	0.993	0.993	0.993	0.993	0.994	0.994
5.0	0.914	0.962	0.963	0.965	0.966	0.967	0.968	0.970	0.971	0.972	0.973
6.0	0.885	0.929	0.933	0.935	0.938	0.940	0.944	0.947	0.949	0.950	0.951
7.0	0.856	0.899	0.905	0.910	0.913	0.916	0.920	0.921	0.924	0.928	0.931
8.0	0.826	0.868	0.878	0.884	0.888	0.891	0.895	0.900	0.906	0.908	0.910
9.0	0.800	0.840	0.850	0.858	0.862	0.865	0.872	0.876	0.883	0.885	0.889
10.0	0.772	0.812	0.823	0.830	0.836	0.842	0.850	0.856	0.864	0.862	0.869
11.0	0.746	0.785	0.798	0.807	0.814	0.818	0.825	0.828	0.843	0.845	0.849
12.0	0.722	0.760	0.771	0.781	0.791	0.797	0.803	0.813	0.821	0.823	0.829
13.0	0.696	0.735	0.749	0.759	0.768	0.772	0.783	0.788	0.801	0.803	0.809
14.0	0.674	0.708	0.725	0.736	0.745	0.752	0.762	0.767	0.774	0.783	0.790
15.0	0.651	0.685	0.700	0.712	0.720	0.730	0.740	0.746	0.755	0.765	0.771
16.0	0.630	0.665	0.676	0.690	0.701	0.710	0.720	0.727	0.734	0.744	0.751
17.0	0.608	0.640	0.656	0.669	0.680	0.689	0.700	0.708	0.714	0.726	0.735
18.0	0.586	0.616	0.634	0.648	0.659	0.669	0.680	0.690	0.695	0.707	0.717
19.0	0.568	0.595	0.613	0.628	0.639	0.649	0.661	0.670	0.676	0.689	0.699
20.0	0.550	0.574	0.593	0.609	0.620	0.632	0.642	0.651	0.658	0.670	0.680
21.0	0.531	0.552	0.573	0.580	0.601	0.611	0.622	0.626	0.640	0.653	0.662
22.0	0.512	0.531	0.552	0.570	0.581	0.591	0.603	0.606	0.621	0.637	0.645
23.0	0.494	0.514	0.535	0.550	0.565	0.574	0.587	0.595	0.608	0.619	0.632
24.0	0.477	0.494	0.515	0.532	0.545	0.555	0.570	0.578	0.589	0.601	0.615
25.0	0.456	0.477	0.498	0.516	0.530	0.539	0.553	0.560	0.570	0.583	0.598
30.0	0.390	0.395	0.416	0.434	0.448	0.558	0.474	0.482	0.494	0.510	0.522

TABLE A.6

EQUIVALENT SQUARES OF RECTANGULAR FIELDS

Short axis (cm)

Long axis (cm)	1	2	3	4	5	6	7	8	9	10	11	12	13	14	15	16	17	18	19	20	22	24	26	28	30
1	1.0																								
2	1.4	2.0																							
3	1.6	2.4	3.0																						
4	1.7	2.7	3.4	4.0																					
5	1.8	3.0	3.8	4.5	5.0																				
6	1.9	3.1	4.1	4.8	5.5	6.0																			
7	2.0	3.3	4.3	5.1	5.8	6.5	7.0																		
8	2.1	3.4	4.5	5.4	6.2	6.9	7.5	8.0																	
9	2.1	3.5	4.6	5.6	6.5	7.2	7.9	8.5	9.0																
10	2.2	3.6	4.8	5.8	6.7	7.5	8.2	8.9	9.5	10.0															
11	2.2	3.7	4.9	5.9	6.9	7.8	8.6	9.3	9.9	10.5	11.0														
12	2.2	3.7	5.0	6.1	7.1	8.0	8.8	9.6	10.3	10.9	11.5	12.0													
13	2.2	3.8	5.1	6.2	7.2	8.2	9.1	9.9	10.6	11.3	11.9	12.5	13.0												
14	2.3	3.8	5.1	6.3	7.4	8.4	9.3	10.1	10.9	11.6	12.3	12.9	13.5	14.0											
15	2.3	3.9	5.2	6.4	7.5	8.5	9.5	10.3	11.2	11.9	12.6	13.3	13.9	14.5	15.0										
16	2.3	3.9	5.2	6.5	7.6	8.6	9.6	10.5	11.4	12.2	13.0	13.7	14.3	14.9	15.5	16.0									
17	2.3	3.9	5.3	6.5	7.7	8.8	9.8	10.7	11.6	12.4	13.2	14.0	14.7	15.3	15.9	16.5	17.0								
18	2.3	4.0	5.3	6.6	7.8	8.9	9.9	10.8	11.8	12.7	13.5	14.3	15.0	15.7	16.3	16.9	17.5	18.0							
19	2.3	4.0	5.4	6.6	7.8	8.9	10.0	11.0	11.9	12.8	13.7	14.5	15.3	16.0	16.7	17.3	17.9	18.5	19.0						
20	2.3	4.0	5.4	6.7	7.9	9.0	10.1	11.1	12.1	13.0	13.9	14.7	15.5	16.3	17.0	17.7	18.3	18.9	19.5	20.0					
22	2.3	4.0	5.5	6.8	8.0	9.1	10.3	11.3	12.3	13.3	14.2	15.1	16.0	16.8	17.6	18.3	19.0	19.7	20.3	20.9	22.0				
24	2.4	4.1	5.5	6.8	8.1	9.2	10.4	11.5	12.5	13.5	14.5	15.4	16.3	17.2	18.0	18.8	19.6	20.3	21.0	21.7	22.9	24.0			
26	2.4	4.1	5.5	6.9	8.1	9.3	10.5	11.6	12.6	13.7	14.7	15.7	16.6	17.5	18.4	19.2	20.1	20.9	21.6	22.4	23.7	24.9	26.0		
28	2.4	4.1	5.6	6.9	8.2	9.4	10.5	11.7	12.8	13.8	14.8	15.9	16.8	17.8	18.7	19.6	20.5	21.3	22.1	22.9	24.4	25.7	27.0	28.0	
30	2.4	4.1	5.6	6.9	8.2	9.4	10.6	11.7	12.8	13.9	15.0	16.0	17.0	18.0	18.9	19.9	20.8	21.7	22.5	23.3	24.9	26.4	27.7	29.0	30.0

TABLE A.7

SCATTER-AIR RATIOS (SAR): CO-60

----

r, Field radius in cm at depth (cm)

Depth (cm)	1.0	2.0	3.0	4.0	5.0	6.0	7.0	8.0	9.0	10.0	11.0	12.0
0.5	0.007	0.014	0.019	0.026	0.032	0.037	0.043	0.048	0.054	0.058	0.063	0.067
1.0	0.013	0.025	0.037	0.048	0.058	0.066	0.073	0.078	0.084	0.089	0.094	0.098
2.0	0.023	0.045	0.064	0.080	0.091	0.102	0.110	0.116	0.122	0.127	0.133	0.139
3.0	0.032	0.061	0.084	0.103	0.118	0.130	0.139	0.147	0.154	0.161	0.166	0.172
4.0	0.038	0.071	0.099	0.121	0.137	0.151	0.162	0.170	0.179	0.186	0.191	0.197
5.0	0.041	0.076	0.107	0.134	0.152	0.166	0.178	0.189	0.198	0.206	0.212	0.218
6.0	0.042	0.080	0.114	0.141	0.160	0.176	0.190	0.201	0.211	0.219	0.226	0.234
7.0	0.042	0.081	0.115	0.143	0.164	0.181	0.196	0.209	0.220	0.229	0.239	0.246
8.0	0.041	0.080	0.114	0.142	0.165	0.185	0.199	0.214	0.225	0.236	0.246	0.254
9.0	0.040	0.078	0.112	0.140	0.164	0.183	0.200	0.216	0.228	0.240	0.251	0.260
10.0	0.038	0.075	0.109	0.136	0.161	0.181	0.199	0.215	0.229	0.242	0.252	0.262
11.0	0.036	0.071	0.104	0.132	0.157	0.178	0.197	0.213	0.227	0.241	0.252	0.262
12.0	0.035	0.069	0.099	0.128	0.153	0.174	0.194	0.210	0.225	0.239	0.251	0.261
13.0	0.034	0.066	0.095	0.124	0.149	0.170	0.190	0.207	0.223	0.237	0.249	0.260
14.0	0.032	0.063	0.063	0.092	0.120	0.168	0.186	0.204	0.220	0.235	0.247	0.258
15.0	0.031	0.060	0.089	0.116	0.140	0.162	0.182	0.200	0.216	0.231	0.244	0.255

Continued

r, Field radius in cm at depth (cm)

Depth (cm)	13.0	14.0	15.0	16.0	17.0	18.0	19.0	20.0	21.0	22.0	23.0	24.0
0.5	0.070	0.073	0.076	0.078	0.080	0.082	0.084	0.085	0.086	0.087	0.088	0.088
1.0	0.101	0.104	0.107	0.109	0.112	0.114	0.116	0.118	0.119	0.120	0.121	0.122
2.0	0.142	0.146	0.149	0.152	0.154	0.156	0.158	0.160	0.161	0.162	0.164	0.166
3.0	0.176	0.180	0.184	0.187	0.190	0.193	0.195	0.198	0.200	0.202	0.203	0.204
4.0	0.201	0.205	0.210	0.215	0.218	0.222	0.225	0.228	0.231	0.233	0.235	0.237
5.0	0.224	0.229	0.235	0.240	0.245	0.248	0.252	0.255	0.258	0.261	0.263	0.264
6.0	0.241	0.246	0.252	0.257	0.262	0.265	0.269	0.272	0.275	0.278	0.280	0.282
7.0	0.254	0.260	0.267	0.273	0.278	0.282	0.287	0.290	0.294	0.296	0.299	0.302
8.0	0.263	0.271	0.278	0.285	0.289	0.294	0.298	0.301	0.305	0.309	0.311	0.313
9.0	0.269	0.277	0.284	0.292	0.298	0.303	0.308	0.312	0.316	0.319	0.322	0.324
10.0	0.271	0.279	0.288	0.295	0.302	0.308	0.314	0.318	0.324	0.327	0.331	0.333
11.0	0.272	0.280	0.289	0.296	0.304	0.311	0.316	0.322	0.328	0.331	0.334	0.337
12.0	0.272	0.281	0.290	0.297	0.305	0.312	0.318	0.324	0.330	0.333	0.337	0.340
13.0	0.270	0.280	0.290	0.298	0.306	0.313	0.319	0.325	0.332	0.335	0.340	0.342
14.0	0.268	0.279	0.288	0.297	0.305	0.313	0.320	0.326	0.333	0.337	0.341	0.344
15.0	0.266	0.277	0.286	0.295	0.303	0.311	0.318	0.325	0.331	0.336	0.340	0.344

TABLE A.8

SCATTER-AIR RATIOS (SAR): VARIAN CLINAC 4 MV X-RAYS (LEAD FLATNESS FILTER)

Depth (cm)	r, Field radius at depth (cm)								
	1.0	**2.0**	**3.0**	**4.0**	**5.0**	**6.0**	**7.0**	**8.0**	**9.0**
1.2	0.007	0.013	0.020	0.026	0.033	0.039	0.046	0.052	0.058
2.0	0.020	0.035	0.047	0.055	0.064	0.073	0.080	0.088	0.093
3.0	0.027	0.048	0.067	0.081	0.093	0.102	0.111	0.118	0.125
4.0	0.032	0.058	0.079	0.097	0.112	0.125	0.136	0.145	0.152
5.0	0.034	0.063	0.089	0.110	0.127	0.141	0.154	0.165	0.173
6.0	0.035	0.067	0.095	0.119	0.137	0.155	0.170	0.181	0.190
7.0	0.035	0.068	0.098	0.125	0.146	0.163	0.180	0.193	0.203
8.0	0.035	0.069	0.101	0.128	0.152	0.170	0.187	0.201	0.213
9.0	0.035	0.069	0.102	0.131	0.156	0.174	0.192	0.207	0.220
10.0	0.034	0.068	0.102	0.132	0.158	0.177	0.195	0.210	0.224
11.0	0.034	0.067	0.101	0.131	0.158	0.178	0.196	0.213	0.227
12.0	0.034	0.066	0.100	0.130	0.157	0.178	0.197	0.215	0.229
13.0	0.033	0.065	0.098	0.128	0.155	0.177	0.196	0.214	0.230
14.0	0.033	0.063	0.095	0.125	0.152	0.175	0.195	0.212	0.229
15.0	0.032	0.062	0.093	0.122	0.148	0.171	0.192	0.210	0.226
16.0	0.031	0.060	0.090	0.118	0.144	0.168	0.188	0.206	0.223
17.0	0.030	0.059	0.087	0.114	0.140	0.163	0.184	0.202	0.220
18.0	0.030	0.057	0.084	0.110	0.135	0.159	0.179	0.197	0.215
19.0	0.029	0.056	0.081	0.107	0.132	0.154	0.175	0.193	0.211
20.0	0.028	0.054	0.079	0.104	0.128	0.150	0.170	0.188	0.206

Continued

Depth (cm)	r, Field radius at depth (cm)								
	10.0	**11.0**	**12.0**	**13.0**	**14.0**	**15.0**	**16.0**	**20.0**	**25.0**
1.2	0.062	0.066	0.068	0.070	0.072	0.073	0.075	0.077	0.079
2.0	0.098	0.103	0.105	0.107	0.108	0.110	0.112	0.115	0.118
3.0	0.130	0.134	0.137	0.140	0.141	0.143	0.146	0.150	0.154
4.0	0.157	0.161	0.164	0.168	0.171	0.174	0.180	0.188	0.195
5.0	0.179	0.185	0.189	0.193	0.197	0.200	0.206	0.214	0.222
6.0	0.196	0.202	0.207	0.212	0.216	0.220	0.228	0.237	0.246
7.0	0.211	0.217	0.223	0.228	0.233	0.237	0.246	0.257	0.268
8.0	0.222	0.230	0.236	0.242	0.247	0.252	0.261	0.272	0.283
9.0	0.230	0.239	0.246	0.252	0.258	0.263	0.273	0.283	0.296
10.0	0.236	0.246	0.253	0.259	0.265	0.271	0.282	0.291	0.303
11.0	0.240	0.252	0.258	0.266	0.272	0.278	0.289	0.300	0.315
12.0	0.242	0.255	0.263	0.271	0.277	0.283	0.295	0.308	0.318
13.0	0.243	0.256	0.266	0.274	0.281	0.288	0.299	0.314	0.325
14.0	0.243	0.256	0.267	0.275	0.283	0.289	0.302	0.316	0.330
15.0	0.241	0.255	0.266	0.275	0.283	0.290	0.302	0.316	0.330
16.0	0.239	0.252	0.264	0.273	0.282	0.289	0.302	0.316	0.325
17.0	0.235	0.249	0.261	0.270	0.279	0.287	0.301	0.314	0.323
18.0	0.230	0.245	0.257	0.267	0.276	0.284	0.300	0.312	0.320
19.0	0.226	0.240	0.252	0.262	0.272	0.281	0.297	0.310	0.318
20.0	0.221	0.235	0.247	0.257	0.267	0.276	0.293	0.306	0.314

Reproduced with permission from Saylor and Ames: *Dosage Calculation in Radiation Therapy,* Courtesy Williams & Wilkins Co., Baltimore, MD, 1978.

SUBJECT INDEX